Advances in Glucuronide Conjugation

FALK SYMPOSIUM 40

Advances in Glucuronide Conjugation

EDITED BY

S. Matern
Department of Internal Medicine III
University of Aachen
West Germany

K. W. Bock
Department of Pharmacology and Toxicology
University of Göttingen
West Germany

W. Gerok
University Medical Clinic
University of Freiburg
West Germany

Proceedings of the 40th Falk Symposium held at Titisee, West Germany, May 31st to June 2nd, 1984

MTP PRESS LIMITED
a member of the KLUWER ACADEMIC PUBLISHERS GROUP
LANCASTER / BOSTON / THE HAGUE / DORDRECHT

Published in the UK and Europe by
MTP Press Limited
Falcon House
Lancaster, England

British Library Cataloguing in Publication Data

Falk Symposium *(40th: 1984: Titisee)*
Advances in glucuronide conjugation : proceedings of the 40th Falk Symposium held at Titisee, West Germany, May 31st to June 2nd, 1984.
1. Glucuronides
I. Title II. Matern S. III. Bock, K. W.
IV. Gerok, W.
612′.015 QP702.G57

ISBN 0–85200–901–1

Published in the USA by
MTP Press
A division of Kluwer Boston Inc
190 Old Derby Street
Hingham, MA 02043, USA

Library of Congress Cataloging in Publication Data

Falk Symposium (40th: 1984: Titisee, Germany)
Advances in glucuronide conjugation.

Includes bibliographies and indexes.
1. Glucuronides—Synthesis—Congresses.
2. Metabolic conjugation—Congresses. I. Matern, S.
II. Bock, K. W. (Karl Walter), 1935– . III. Gerok,
W. (Wolfgang), 1926– . IV. Title. [DNLM:
1. Glucuronates—metabolism—congresses. W3 FA17 40th
1984a/QU84 F191 1984a]
QP702.G572F35 1984 599′.0149 84–26145

ISBN 0–85200–901–1

Phototypesetting by Titus Wilson, Kendal, Cumbria
Printed in Great Britain by Butler & Tanner Limited, Frome and London

Contents

Preface

This book comprises the lectures and poster abstracts of the Falk Symposium No. 40, held May 31st–June 2nd, 1984, at Kurhaus Titisee, Black Forest, West Germany.

Glucuronide conjugation of drugs and endogenous compounds is the most versatile and quantitatively the most important of the conjugation reactions, leading in general to biologically inactive, water-soluble products which are readily eliminated from the organism. It was the aim of the conference to bring together specialists involved in various aspects of glucuronide conjugation. These aspects included studies on multiple iso-enzymes of UDP-glucuronosyltransferase, factors determining glucuronide formation in the intact cell and the whole organism, studies in man on the identification and fate of glucuronides of drugs and endogenous compounds such as bilirubin, bile acids and bile alcohols. In this way it was possible to present a comprehensive up-to-date survey of glucuronide conjugation, ranging from enzyme studies to pathophysiological aspects of glucuronide disposition in patients.

Our sincere thanks go to Dr Herbert Falk and his Foundation whose generous sponsorship made the symposium possible. Fourteen years after the first Falk Symposium on 'Icterus' this symposium again dealt with the conjugation of bilirubin, one of Dr Falk's special interests. We also greatly acknowledge the skilled organization of the meeting by Dr Falk who provided excellent facilities for scientific communication and generous hospitality in the pleasant atmosphere of the Black Forest.

S. Matern
K. W. Bock
W. Gerok

List of Contributors

M. S. ADACHI
Department of Biopharmacy
Meiji College of Pharmacy
Nozawa-Setagaya-Ku
Tokyo 154
Japan

P. ADRIAENSEN
Department of Medical Research – KU Leuven
Laboratory of Hepatology
Campus Gasthuisberg
Herestraat 49,
B-3000 Leuven
Belgium

B. ANTOINE
Laboratoire de Biochimie Pharmacologie–
Unité Associée au CNRS No 597
Centre du Medicament
30 Rue Lionnois
F-54000 Nancy
France

I. M. ARIAS
Department of Physiology
Tufts University School of Medicine
136 Harrison Avenue
Boston MA 02111
USA

M. AXELSON
Department of Clinical Chemistry
Karolinska Hospital
Stockholm

P. BACK
Medizinische Universitätsklinik
Hugstetter Str. 55
7800 Freiburg i. Br.
West Germany

G. C. BARR
Department of Biochemistry
University of Dundee
Dundee DD1 4HN
UK

P. D. BERK
Department of Haematology
Mount Sinai School of Medicine
1 Gustave L. Levy Place
New York, NY 10029
USA

M. D. BERMAN
Brockton Veterans Administration Hospital
940 Belmont Street
Brockton, MA 02401
USA

N. BLANCKAERT
Department of Laboratory Medicine/ Medicine–L518A
UCSF Medical Center
San Francisco, CA 94143
USA

K. W. BOCK
Zentrum Pharmakologie und Toxikologie
Universität Göttingen
Kreuzbergring 57
3400 Göttingen
West Germany

B. S. BOCK-HENNIG
Zentrum Pharmakologie und Toxikologie
Universität Göttingen
Kreuzbergring 57
3400 Göttingen
West Germany

J. BÖTTCHER
Kreiskrankenhaus
6640 Merzig
West Germany

R. A. BRANCH
Division of Clinical Pharmacology
Vanderbilt University School of Medicine
Nashville, TN 37232
USA

S. BROUWER
Department of Pharmacology
State University of Groningen
Bloemsingel 1
9713 BZ Groningen
The Netherlands

G. BRUNNER
Medizinische Hochschule Hannover
Abt. Gastroenterologie im Oststadtkrankenhaus
Podbielskistr. 380
3000 Hannover 51
West Germany

B. BURCHELL
Department of Biochemistry
Medical Sciences Institute
University of Dundee
Dundee, DD1 4HN
Scotland

J. CALDWELL
Department of Pharmacology
St. Mary's Hospital Medical School
Norfolk Place
London, W2 1PG
UK

M. C. CAREY
Gastroenterology Division RBO13
Brigham and Women's Hospital
Harvard Medical School
75 Francis Street
Boston, MA 02115
USA

G. CARRERA
INSERM U. 87
2 Rue F. Magendie
31400 Toulouse
France

S. CECCHETTI
Department of Medicine
University of California, San Diego
225 Dickinson Street
San Diego, CA 92103
USA

G. M. COHEN
Toxicology Unit
Department of Pharmacology
School of Pharmacy
University of London
29/39 Brunswick Square
London, WC1N 1AX
UK

C. COLIZZI
Department of Surgical Pathology
University of Pisa
56100 Pisa
Italy

J. L. CONVERSE
Department of Medicine
University of California, San Diego
225 Dickinson Street
San Diego, CA 92103
USA

J. CUMMINGS
Department of Clinical Oncology
University of Glasgow
Horselethill Road
Glasgow
UK

J. CUYPERS
Department of Medical Research
Laboratory of Hepatology – KU Leuven
Campus Gasthuisberg
Herestraat 49
B-3000 Leuven
Belgium

M. D'ARCY DOHERTY
Toxicology Unit, School of Pharmacy
University of London
29/39 Brunswick Square
London, WC1N 1AX
UK

P. V. DESMOND
Department of Medicine and Gastroenterology
St. Vincents Hospital
Fitzroy, Victoria 3065
Australia

G. DEVIS
Academic Hospital
Laarbeeklaan 101
1090 Bruxelles
Belgium

H.-J. DIETRICH
Ziegelstr. 41
7320 Göppingen
West Germany

R. L. DILLS
Department of Pharmacology, Toxicology and Therapeutics
University of Kansas Medical Center
Kansas City, KS 66103
USA

S. DRAGACCI
Université de Nancy 1
Faculté des Sciences Pharmaceutiques et Biologiques
7 Rue Albert-Lebrun
54001 Nancy Cedex
France

G. J. DUTTON
Department of Biochemistry
Medical Sciences Institute
The University
Dundee, DD1 4HN
Scotland

B. EGESTAD
Department of Physiological Chemistry
Karolinska Institutet
Box 60 400, S-104 01 Stockholm
Sweden

J. ELIS
Institute of Pharmacology
Czechoslovak Academy of Sciences
Albertov 4
Prague 2
CSSR

K. ELISOVA
Department of Pharmacology
Medical Faculty
Charles University
Albertov 4
Prague 2
CSSR

W. ELLRICHMANN
Abt. f. Innere Medizin
Krankenhaus Bethanien
4600 Dortmund 30
West Germany

L. ERIKSSON
Department of Pathology
Karolinkska Institutet
Huddinge University Hospital
191 86 Huddinge
Sweden

C. N. FALANY
Department of Pharmacology
The University of Iowa
Bowen Science Building
Iowa City, IA 52242
USA

B. FAYE
Université de Nancy 1
Faculté des Sciences Pharmaceutiques et Biologiques
7 Rue Albert-Lebrun
54001 Nancy Cedex
France

U. FEMFERT
Ruhr-Universität Bochum
Medizinische Universitätsklinik 'Bergmaunsheil Bochum'
Abteilung Gastroenterologie und Hepatologie
4630 Bochum 1
Hunscheidstrasse 1
West Germany

J. FEVERY
Laboratory of Hepatology
Department of Medical Research
University of Leuven
B-3900 Leuven
Belgium

G. FISCHER
Zentrum Pathologie der Universität
Robert-Koche-Strasse 40
3400 Göttingen
West Germany

R. FLEISCHMANN
Medizinische Universitätsklinik
Otfried-Müller-Str. 10
7400 Tübingen
West Germany

A. FOLIOT
INSERM U 24
Hôpital Beaujon
100 Bd Gl Leclerc
92118 Clichy Cedex
France

C. FORSTHOVE
Biochemisches Institut
Universität Freiburg
Hermann-Herderstrasse 7
D-7800 Freiburg im Breisgau
West Germany

S. FOURNEL
Laboratoire de Biochimie
Pharmacologique associé au CRNS
Centre du Médicament
30 Rue Lionnois
54000 Nancy
France

B. GAWRONSKA-SKLARZ
Department of Pharmacology
Pomeranian Medical Academy
70-111 Szczecin
Poland

W. GEROK
Medizinische Universitätsklinik
Hugstetter Str. 55
7800 Freiburg i. Br.
West Germany

L. GIULIANI
Department of Surgical Pathology
University of Pisa
56100 Pisa
Italy

J. L. GOLLAN
Gastroenterology Division
Harvard Medical School and Brigham
and Women's Hospital
75 Francis Street
Boston, MA 02115
USA

M. GOOSENS
Department of Medical Research – KU
Leuven
Laboratory of Hepatology
Campus Gasthuisberg
Herestraat 49
B-3000 Leuven
Belgium

E. R. GORDON
Liver Study Unit
Yale Medical School
333 Cedar Avenue
New Haven, CT 06510
USA

A. B. GRAHAM
Department of Pharmaceutical
Chemistry
University of Strathclyde
Glasgow, G1 1XW
UK

Z. GREGUS
Department of Pharmacology,
Toxicology and Therapeutics
University of Kansas Medical Center
Kansas City, KS 66103
USA

D. GURANTZ
Department of Medicine
University of California, San Diego
225 Dickinson Street
San Diego, CA 92103
USA

G. H. HAGE
Prins Hendrikplein 2
7316 AM – Apeldoorn
The Netherlands

L. R. HAGEY
Department of Medicine
University of California, San Diego
225 Dickinson Street
San Diego, California 92103
USA

W. HAGMANN
Biochemisches Institut der Universität
Hermann-Herder-Str. 7
7800 Freiburg i. Br.
West Germany

T. HALLINAN
Department of Biochemistry
RFHSM
University of London
Rowland Hill Street
London NW3 2PF
UK

O. HÄNNINEN
Department of Physiology
University of Kuopio
70211 Kuopio 21
Finland

S. C. HAUSER
Gastroenterology Division
Harvard Medical School and Brigham
and Women's Hospital
75 Francis Street
Boston, MA 02115
USA

G. A. HAZELTON
Department of Pharmacology, Toxicology and Therapeutics
University of Kansas Medical Center
Kansas City, KS 66103
USA

G. HEDENBORG
Department of Clinical Chemistry
Karolinska Sjukhuset
S-104 01 Stockholm
Sweden

M. HEGER
Universitätsklinikum der Gesamthochschule Essen
Hufelandstr. 55
4300 Essen 1
West Germany

K. P. M. HEIRWEGH
Laboratory of Hepatology
Katholieke Universiteit of Leuven
Campus Gasthuisberg
Teaching and Research Building
Herestraat 49
B-3000 Leuven
Belgium

R. HENDERIX
Department of Medical Research – KU Leuven
Laboratory of Hepatology
Campus Gasthuisberg
Herestraat 49
B-3000 Leuven
Belgium

J. J. HJELLE
Department of Pharmacology, Toxicology and Therapeutics
University of Kansas Medical Center
Kansas City, KS 66103
USA

A. F. HOFMANN
Division of Gastroenterology
Department of Medicine
UCSD Medical Center (H-811D)
225 Dickinson Street
San Diego, CA 92103
USA

J. B. HOUSTON
Department of Pharmacy
University of Manchester
Manchester, M13 9PL
UK

S. HUIJGHEBAERT
Department of Medicine
University of California, San Diego
225 Dickinson Street
San Diego, CA 92103
USA

M. R. JACKSON
Department of Biochemistry
Medical Sciences Institute
The University of Dundee
Dundee, DD1 4HN
Scotland

P. L. M. JANSEN
Division of Gastroenterology and Liver Diseases
St. Radboud Hospital
University of Nijmegen
6500 HB Nijmegen
The Netherlands

M. J. T. JONES
Department of Hematology
Mount Sinai School of Medicine
1 Gustave L. Levy Place
New York, NY 10029
USA

R. JAUCH
F. Hoffmann-La Roche and Co.
4002 Basel
Switzerland

K. KAMISAKA
III Internal Medicine
Tokyo Medical and Dental University
Tokyo
Japan

G. KARLAGANIS
Institut für Klinische Pharmakologie Inselspital
Murtenstr. 35
3010 Bern
Switzerland

D. KEPPLER
Biochemisches Institut der Universität Freiburg
Hermann-Herder-Str. 7
7800 Freiburg i. Br.
West Germany

C.-L. KIANG
Department of Hematology
Mount Sinai School of Medicine
1 Gustave L. Levy Place
New York, NY 10029
USA

R. B. KIRKPATRICK
Division of Gastroenterology-Hepatology
Department of Internal Medicine
Veterans Administration Medical Center
Iowa City, IA 52240
USA

C. D. KLAASSEN
Department of Pharmacology, Toxicology and Therapeutics
University of Kansas Medical Center
Kansas City, KS 66103
USA

U. KOIVUSAARI
Department of Physiology
University of Kuopio
PO Box 6
SF-70211 Kuopio 21
Finland

A. SJ. KOSTER
Rijksuniversiteit Utrecht
Department of Pharmacology and Pharmacotherapy
Faculty of Pharmacy
State University of Utrecht
Catharijnesingel 60
3511 GH Utrecht
The Netherlands

H. D. KUNTZ
Ruhr-Universität Bochum
Medizinische Universitätsklinik 'Bergmannsheil Bochum'
Abteilung Gastroenterologie und Hepatologie
4630 Bochum 1
Hunscheidtstrasse 1
West Germany

V. LAPOSTOLLE
Université de Bordeaux II
Laboratoire des Interactions Cellulaires Physiopathologie–Pharmakologie
Université de Bordeaux II,
146 Rue Leo Saignant
33076 Bordeaux-Cedex
France

J. LEAKEY
Department of Biochemistry
Medical Sciences Institute
University of Dundee
Dundee, DD1 4HN
Scotland

W. LILIENBLUM
Department of Pharmacology and Toxicology
University of Göttingen
Kreuzbergring 57
D-3400 Göttingen
West Germany

P. LINDSTRÖM-SEPPÄ
Department of Physiology
University of Kuopio
PO Box 6
SF-70211 Kuopio 21
Finland

L. McCARTHY
Department of Biochemistry
University of Dundee
Dundee, DD1 4HN
UK

A. LUEDTKE
Arzt f. Chirurgie
Städt. Krankenhaus Lüneburg
Bögelstr. 1
2120 Lüneburg
West Germany

P. I. MACKENZIE
Laboratory of Developmental Pharmacology
NICHD
National Institutes of Health
Building 10, Room 6C-101
Bethesda, MA 20205
USA

J. MAGDALOU
Laboratoire de Biochemie Pharmacologie associée au CNRS
Centre du Médicament
30 Rue Lionnois
54000 Nancy
France

G. MANINI
Boehringer Biochemia
Robin S.p.A.
Direzione Medica
Via S. Uguzzone, 5
20126 Milano
Italy

H. MATERN
Medizinische Universitätsklinik
Hugstetter Str. 55
7800 Freiburg i. Br.
West Germany

S. MATERN
Medizinische Universitätsklinik
Hugstetter Str. 55
7800 Freiburg i. Br.
West Germany

G. MAU
Riehenstr. 40
7850 Lörrach
West Germany

J. A. T. P. MEUWISSEN
Department of Medical Research – KU Leuven
Laboratory of Hepatology
Campus Gasthuisberg
Herestraat 49
B-3000 Leuven
Belgium

P. J. MEIER-ABT
Abt. Klin. Pharmakologie
Medizinische Klinik
Universitätsspital
8091 Zürich
Switzerland

V. MESA
Academisch Ziekenhuis
St. Rafael
Capucijnenvoer 35
3000 Leuven
Belgium

L. VON MEYERINCK
Pharmakologisches Institut der Universität Hamburg
Martinistr. 52
2000 Hamburg 20
West Germany

E. MICHELOTTI
Department of Medicine
University of California, San Diego
225 Dickinson Street
San Diego CA 92103
USA

M. MISTRY
Department of Pharmacy
University of Manchester
Manchester, M13 9PL
UK

M. MITCHELL
Department of Medicine
Johns Hopkins University
Baltimore
Maryland
USA

S. MITJAVILA
Laboratoire de Physiologie I
Univ. Paul Sabatier
INSERM U 87
2 Rue François Magendie
31400 Toulouse
France

K. MOHRI
Department of Biopharmacy
Meiji College of Pharmacy
Nozawara, Setagaya-Ku
Tokyo 154
Japan

H. MORATH
Schlüsselbad Klinik
Renchtalstr. 2
7605 Bad Peterstal
West Germany

G. J. MULDER
Department of Toxicology
University of Leiden
Sylvius Laboratories
PO Box 9503
2300 RA Leiden
The Netherlands

M. MURACA
Istituto di Medicina Interna
Policlinico Universitario
35100 Padova
Italy

A. MYARA
Laboratoire de Biochimie
Hôpital Saint Joseph
7 Rue P. Larousse
75674 Paris Cedex 14
France

H. NAUTA
Laboratory of Biophysics
State University of Utrecht
PO Box 80.000
3508 TA Utrecht
The Netherlands

A. NORMAN
Karolinska Institute
Department of Clinical Chemistry
Karolinska Sjukhuset
10401 Stockholm
Sweden

P. M. NOVIKOFF
Department of Pathology
Albert Einstein College of Medicine
1300 Morris Park Avenue
Bronx, NY 10461
USA

A. B. NOVIKOFF
Department of Pathology
Albert Einstein College of Medicine
1300 Morris Park Avenue
Bronx, NY 10461
USA

H. OKUDA
Department of Hematology
Mount Sinai School of Medicine
1 Gustave L. Levy Place
New York, NY 10029
USA

P. OPOLON
Unité de Recherches d'Hépatologie
INSERM U 9
Hôpital St. Antoine
184 Rue du Fbg. St. Antoine
75571 Paris Cedex 12
France

I. S. OWENS
Department of Health and Human Services
National Institutes of Health
Building 10, Room 6C–101
Bethesda, MD 20205
USA

G. M. PACIFICI
Instituto di Patologia Generale
Universita di Pisa
Via Roma 55
56100 Pisa
Italy

K. R. PALMER
Department of Gastroenterology
Central Middlesex Hospital
Acton Lane, Park Royal
London
UK

M. PARQUET
INSERM U 9
Hôpital St. Antoine
184 Rue de Fbg. St. Antoine
75571 Paris Cedex 12
France

J. PAUSCH
Medizinische Universitätsklinik
Hugstetter Str. 55
7800 Freiburg i. Br.
West Germany

W. H. M. PETERS
Division of Gastroenterology
St. Radboud Hospital
6500 HB Nijmegen
The Netherlands

P. PETTERSSON
Department of Physiological Chemistry
Karolinska Institutet
Box 60 400
S-104 01 Stockholm
Sweden

B. PFRIEME
Langgasse 68
6330 Wetzlar
West Germany

H. POPPER
Gustave L. Levy Distinguished Service Professor
Mount Sinai School of Medicine
1 Gustave L. Levy Place
New York, NY 10029
USA

R. PREISIG
Institut für Klinische Pharmakologie der Universität Bern
Murtenstr. 35
3010 Bern
Switzerland

L. F. PRESCOTT
University Department of Therapeutics and Clinical Pharmacology
The Royal Infirmary
Edinburgh, EH3 9YW
Scotland

A. RANE
Department of Clinical Pharmacology
Huddinge Hospital
Karolinska Institute
14186 Huddinge
Sweden

H. REMMER
Institut für Toxikologie
Universität Tübingen
Wilhelmstrasse 56
7400 Tübingen
West Germany

J. ROY CHOWDHURY
Department of Medicine
Albert Einstein College of Medicine
1300 Morris Park Avenue
Bronx, NY 10461
USA

N. ROY CHOWDHURY
Department of Medicine
Albert Einstein College of Medicine
1300 Morris Park Avenue
Bronx, NY 10461
USA

G. L. RICCI
Gastroenterologia
Clinica Medica 2
Policlinico Umberto I
Università di Roma
00161 Roma
Italy

G. ROßNAGEL
Deutsches Krebsforschungszentrum
Institut für Toxikologie und Chemotherapie
Im Neuenheimer Feld 280
6900 Heidelberg
West Germany

W. ROTH
Abt. Biochemie
G. Pharmacokinetik and Metabolismus
Dr. Karl Thomae GmbH
Postfach 1755
7950 Biberach/Riss
West Germany

P. SALVÁ
Laboratorios Dimefar, SA
C/. Pujol, 22
Barcelona 22
Spain

E. SCHENK
Triererstr. 7
6619 Weiskirchen
West Germany

G. SCHIRMER
Institut für Pharmakologie und Toxikologie der Universität
Kreuzbergring 57
3400 Göttingen
West Germany

A. SCHMOLDT
Institut für Rechtsmedizin der Universität Hamburg
Martinistrasse 52
2000 Hamburg 54
West Germany

R. SCHÜPPEL
Institut für Pharmakologie und Toxikologie
Technische Universität
Mendelssohnstr. 1
3300 Braunschweig
West Germany

C. SCHIESSEL
Biochemisches Institut
Universität Freiburg
Hermann-Herderstrasse 7
D-7800 Freiburg im Breisgau
West Germany

E. SCHOLTENS
Department of Pharmacology
State University of Groningen
Bloemsingel 1
9713 BZ Groningen
The Netherlands

M. SCHWENK
Institut für Toxikologie
Universität Tübingen
Wilhelmstrasse 56
7400 Tübingen
West Germany

G. SCOTT
Drug Metabolism Research Unit
Department of Pharmacy (Pharmaceutical Chemistry)
University of Strathclyde
Glasgow, G1 1XW
UK

I. SCRAGG
Department of Biochemistry
Medical Sciences Institute
The University of Dundee
Dundee, DD1 4HN
UK

K.-J. SEROKA
Bahnhofstr. 5
2308 Preetz
West Germany

K. D. R. SETCHELL
Section of Mass Spectrometry
MRC Clinical Research Centre
Harrow, Middlesex, HA1 3UJ
UK

D. SHEMIN
Northwestern University
Department of Biochemistry and Molecular Biology
Evanston, IL 60201
USA

A. SIEG
Medizinische Universitätsklinik
Bergheimer Str. 58
6900 Heidelberg 1
West Germany

H. C.-P. SIEGERS
Institut für Toxikologie der Medizinische Hochschule Lübeck
Ratzeburger Allee 160
2400 Lübeck 1
West Germany

G. SIEST
Centre du Médicament Unité de Recherche Associée au CNRS n. 597
Université de Nancy 1
30 Rue Lionnois
54000 Nancy
France

J. SJÖVALL
Department of Physiological Chemistry
Karolinksa Institutet
Box 60 400
104 01 Stockholm
Sweden

S. SKREDE
Institute of Clinical Biochemistry
Rikshspitalet
University of Oslo
Norway

W. SOMMER
Marktgasse 19
3000 Bern
Switzerland

U. STÄRZ
Medizinische Universitätsklinik
Otfield-Müller-Strasse 10
D-7400 Tübingen
West Germany

J. O. SVENSSON
Department of Clinical Pharmacology
Huddinge University Hospital
S-141 86 Huddinge
Sweden

A. TANGERMANN
Department of Medicine
Division of Gastroenterology and Liver Diseases
Katholieke Universiteit
Sint Radboudziekenhuis
6500 HB Nijmegen
Netherlands

N. TAVOLONI
Department of Hematology
Mount Sinai School of Medicine
1 Gustave L. Levy Place
New York, NY 10029
USA

F. TEGTMEIER
Department of Gastroenterology and Hepatology
Medizinische Hochschule Hannover
Krankenhaus Oststadt
Podbielskistrasse 380
D-3000 Hannover 51
West Germany

T. R. TEPHLY
The Toxicology Center
Department of Pharmacology
The University of Iowa
Bowen Science Building
Iowa City, IA 52242
USA

J. THOMASSIN
Laboratoire de Biochimie Pharmacologique Associé au CNRS
Centre du Médicament
30 Rue Lionnois
54000 Nancy
France

F. TRIVIN
Laboratoire de Biochimie
Hôpital Saint Joseph
7 Rue de P. Larousse
75674 Paris Cedex 14
France

H. UEHLEKE
Leit. Direktor Abt. Toxikologie
Bundesgesundheitsamt
Thielallee 88
1000 Berlin 33
West Germany

T. UESUGI
Department of Biopharmacy
Meiji College of Pharmacy
Nozawa, Setagaya-Ku
Tokyo 154
Japan

D. ULLRICH
Zentrum für Pharmakologie und Toxikologie der Universität
Kreuzbergring 57
3400 Göttingen
West Germany

F. VANSTAPEL
Department of Laboratory Medicine L-518
UCSF Medical Center
San Francisco, CA 94143
USA

D. VELASQUEZ
Department of Gastroenterology
Medizinische Hochschule Hannover
Krankenhaus Oststadt
Podbielskistrasse 380
D-3000 Hannover 51
West Germany

J. B. WATKINS III
Medical Sciences Program
Pharmacology Section
Myers Hall 306
Indiana University School of Medicine
Bloomington, IN 47405
USA

J. G. WEITERING
Department of Pharmacology
State University of Groningen
Bloemsingel 1, 9713 BZ Groningen
The Netherlands

J. WIDÉN
Department of Clinical Pharmacology
Huddinge University Hospital
S-141 86 Huddinge
Sweden

G. WECKBECKER
Biochemisches Institut
Hermann-Herder-Str. 7
7800 Freiburg i. Br.
West Germany

M. WIESSLER
Institut für Toxikologie und Chemotherapie
Deutsches Krebsforschungszentrum
Im Neuenheimer Feld 280
6900 Heidelberg
West Germany

G. C. WOOD
Drug Metabolism Research Unit
Department of Pharmacy
University of Strathclyde
Glasgow, G1 1XW
Scotland

Y. B. YOON
Department of Medicine
University of California, San Diego
225 Dickinson Street
San Diego, CA 92103
USA

M. YOUNES
Institut für Toxikologie
Medizinische Hochschule Lübeck
Ratzeburger Allee 160
2400 Lübeck 1
West Germany

P. Y. ZAUGG
Department of Clinical Pharmacology
University of Berne
Murtenstrasse 35
CH-3010 Berne
Switzerland

1
Introduction

G. J. DUTTON

It is a great pleasure to contribute an Introduction to this volume of papers presented at the Falk Symposium on Advances in Glucuronide Conjugation. I do not intend to summarize the papers, nor to give personal impressions of them; Hans Popper does that at the end of the volume, where he combines an unrivalled knowledge of the liver with the candidly perceptive eye of a non-specialist. Nor do I wish to add yet one more general review to those already existing on the subject. I intend only to indicate briefly why I consider the study of glucuronidation important today. Support by the Falk Foundation of basic research on liver function is both generous and discriminating, and it is fitting, when acknowledging the generosity, to suggest why this particular subject should have been chosen.

Pharmacologically and toxicologically, of course, glucuronidation is of great interest. The range of compounds glucuronidated is enormous, and the capacity of the body to glucuronidate them very large. This aspect is summarized by Caldwell's paper (Chapter 2). Anyone studying the metabolism of drugs, pesticides, food additives, pollutants or carcinogens must acquaint themselves with the elements of glucuronidation as a bodily process, and with its assay.

As Caldwell points out, endogenous compounds also are glucuronidated. Indeed, at the time I began work on the subject, the glucuronidation of steroids as a means of biologically inactivating them, of transporting their glucuronides to 'target tissues' for hydrolysis, and of excreting them was considered much more clinically important than glucuronidation as a 'detoxicatory' mechanism for use with foreign compounds. Despite the ceaseless torrent of xenobiotic aglycones pouring out today from the industrial organic chemistry laboratory, the endogenous examples still hold their own, as the equal spate of papers on, say, bilirubin glucuronidation emphasizes. (It is interesting to note that, 39 meetings ago, the 1st Falk Symposium was concerned with the subject of Jaundice). The clinical chemist, then, must also know of the recent advances in glucuronide conjugation.

The above appeals largely to those involved in animal physiology. Plants indulge in glucuronidation, extensively in building up their secondary tissues, and occasionally in conjugating, for some as yet unclear reason, certain of their own metabolic products. The molecule of glucuronic acid, free and combined, is, therefore, not strange to plant biologists or to the paper industry; though the present volume is not directly relevant to that aspect.

Glucuronic acid and its derivatives are of considerable interest to the organic chemist. Karl Meyer, many years ago, pointed out the curious physicochemical properties of the free acid, and pleaded for greater attention to be paid to those of its conjugates; particularly to the possible enzymically controlled change of the glucuronide's ionized form to and from any lactonized form in passage through membranes. The recent discovery of aglycone migration from C-1 to other positions should stimulate work in this strangely neglected area. Glucuronide conjugates can be rewarding models for the physical organic chemist.

The biochemist, of course, has been especially interested in the biosynthesis of glucuronides since the discovery of the major formative reaction:

$$\text{UDP-glucuronic acid} + \text{aglycone} \rightleftharpoons \text{aglycone glucuronide} + \text{UDP}$$

Those aspects of intermediary metabolism concerning the formation of pentoses, ascorbic acid and the hexuronic acid-containing polysaccharides require knowledge of the synthesis and various fates of UDP-glucuronic acid, including the one denoted above.

However, the major biochemical interest for workers on glucuronide conjugation is the enzyme catalysing the reaction, UDP-glucuronosyltransferase. The interest is broadly divided into two fields; that of the enzyme mechanism and its regulation, and that of the 'multiplicity' of the enzyme protein(s).

Both these approaches offer more than a specialist's appeal. They throw light on two outstanding problems in biochemistry today, and so contribute to the current widespread interest in the process of glucuronidation.

The enzyme is bound to, and probably in, the endoplasmic reticulum membrane and, like some other enzymes similarly situated, exhibits 'latency' in the fresh microsomal preparation; on perturbation of the microsomes, activity assayed *in vitro* can rise several-fold, before subsiding to zero on continued perturbation. One great question confronting modern biochemistry, of how far *in vitro* studies can be related to, or grossed up into, the *in vivo* situation, is well exemplified by asking what is the 'real' activity of UDP-glucuronosyltransferase *in vivo*? Many studies are attempting to answer this. They compare overall glucuronidation in intact cells or organs with that in microsomal preparations treated with, hopefully, '*in vivo*' concentrations of, hopefully, endogenous substrates and activators. They may also construct model systems, employing the purified enzyme reconstituted with phospholipid and seeing how far along the road to life it may be coaxed. Remarkable success has been claimed, and sometimes attained, in these model studies, and their stimulus to thought has been welcome. A dichotomy has declared itself between the concept of an enzyme constrained by its conformation in a membrane of variably-controlled fluidity; and that of an enzyme whose activity is constrained by the regulated access of one or both substrates, with an accompanying retinue of porters. The distinction seems rather of theoretical, or dialectical, convenience, and is now perhaps counter-productive. Certainly an enzyme in a membrane is susceptible to subtleties of control not available to its simpler cytosolic brethren, and several forms of regulatory constraint have probably evolved. However, a new Michaelis–Menten treatment of kinetics for such insoluble enzymes may be needed for full understanding. More biophysical studies will be required, but already UDP-glucuronosyltransferase is a popular model for enzymologists.

The question of the 'multiplicity' of UDP-glucuronosyltransferase is also one of specialized appeal for the biochemist and protein chemist, besides its obvious interest to the pharmacologist and clinician seeking to extrapolate data from substrate to substrate, tissue to tissue, or species to species.

I believe that this family of enzymes, with its wide distribution in the tissues, and its span of substrates from endogenous molecules to the most bizarre of xenobiotics, will provide a key to the mapping of that new development, 'enzyme ecology'.

One must presume that an enzyme system found in any given metabolic niche in the body is the one that will do its job there the most effectively; e.g. that the selection of lactate dehydrogenase forms found in muscle is better suited to the character and concentration of impinging ions and metabolic associates there, than would be the forms found, say, in liver; and vice versa. This would suppose what is increasingly becoming likely, i.e. that enzymes, and proteins generally, may exist not as a single 'ideal' chemical compound, but as a number, large or small, of forms around that ideal, analogous to the spectrum of strains and subspecies in the members of a plant community exposed to an environmental gradient. The profile of enzyme forms encountered in any metabolic situation (e.g. age or tissue) is that best adapted for efficient functioning there.

Obviously, in the critical pathways of intermediary metabolism this profile cannot change markedly without the likelihood of a deleterious effect upon the organism; the whole pathway has evolved together. These enzymes respond only to the internal environment, which varies within strict limits. A slight change in this internal environment, through dietary, seasonal or hormonal influence, will lower some forms and raise others in the profile. In this way, the metabolic pattern may change somewhat with time; in the case of ontogeny, for example, as a programmed sequence. I have termed these the 'core' enzymes; mutability in their profile through non-specific inducers, or in their structure, at the gene or post-translationally, is to be discouraged.

Where the organism is exposed to the greatly-varying external environment, however, such mutability is beneficial. Enzymes dealing with incoming xenobiotic molecules from the diet, the air and so on, may be expected to possess a wide spectrum of forms, a selection of which can safely be induced in response to any particular environmental challenge. I have termed this the 'peripheral' metabolic area. Such an arrangement benefits the organism by an inner homeostasis and an outer flexibility.

The great interest in the UDP-glucuronosyltransferase family is that it may be regarded as a core enzyme when we consider those activities dealing with such biologically potent and highly-evolved endogenous molecules as the various steroids and bilirubin; and also as a peripheral enzyme when we consider, say, those activities dealing with drugs. From this point of view, the 'endogenous' activities of the enzyme should be the most easy to identify as specific (as for the different steroid C-positions) and the 'xenobiotic' activities should be the most difficult to characterize. These latter may be numerous, and possess some overlapping specificity; and a swarm of unsuspected forms may indeed be induced, either from zero or from very low levels, by xenobiotics arriving at the periphery.

Evidence so far obtained from the isolation of specific UDP-glucuronosyltransferases is consistent with the idea of core and peripheral forms; as is the parallel work on those cytochrome P-450 activities associated with steroids or porphyrins and those dealing with xenobiotics.

Allied to the above concept is that of 'priority', whereby in stress the less essential metabolic functions would be shed to conserve the more vital; analogous to the priority in blood supply to various tissues during exposure to cold, when the core organs take precedence over the peripheral ones. Clearly, glucuronidation of core substrates such as bilirubin would be expected to possess priority over that of xenobiotics. This is indeed seen in liver disease, and has been known for many years.

Evolutionary selection in a gradually-changing external environment may be presumed to have brought about the core and peripheral enzyme populations and the order of priorities. Today's external molecular environment has changed very suddenly, and we are bombarded by the quite novel creations of the organic chemist. The biological value of their metabolic change is unpredictable; and they may well, by stimulating mutation or induction untested by evolution, penetrate these defence mechanisms. We must expect trouble for the organism if, because of unlucky mutation or induction by xenobiotics, a new form or profile of forms of core enzyme appears and tries to engage in core metabolism. Especially in the fetus, which from its situation indulges wholly in core metabolism, such an attempt is likely to result in death or teratogenic change.

Therefore, the study of glucuronide conjugation (or, more strictly, glucuronic acid conjugation) invites a wide range of work and promises insight into many fields of great current interest. It is no surprise that the 40th Falk Symposium has been dedicated to examining recent advances in so absorbing a subject. The excellent papers which follow should be read against the wider background so cursorily sketched out here.

Section 1 Glucuronide Conjugation in Biotransformation

Chairman: G. J. Dutton

2
Glucuronic acid conjugation in the context of the metabolic conjugation of xenobiotics

J. CALDWELL

INTRODUCTION

The chemical environment in which living organisms exist contains two types of compounds, *nutrients* and *anutrients*, or *xenobiotics*. It is the purpose of this paper to consider the biological fates of such anutrient chemicals, and particularly to consider the significance of the metabolic conjugation reactions in this context.

Xenobiotics which enter the living organism may undergo one or more of four distinct fates:

(1) Enzymic metabolism
(2) Elimination unchanged
(3) Spontaneous chemical transformation
(4) Accumulation unchanged

Although the third and fourth possibilities are very important when they occur, the great majority of xenobiotics undergo enzymic metabolism and/or are eliminated unchanged, the relative proportions of these two options being variable.

Characteristically, the enzymic metabolism of xenobiotics is a biphasic process, involving a plethora of reactions which may be divided into two distinct types[1]. The compound undergoes initially a Phase I, or functionalization, reaction of oxidation, reduction or hydrolysis, the product of which is then subjected to a Phase II, or conjugation, reaction (Figure 2.1) These latter are biosynthetic reactions, in which the xenobiotic is linked with an endogenous moiety to give a characteristic product, known as a conjugate. In certain cases, the products of Phase I metabolism may be eliminated without conjugation, while yet other xenobiotics possess within their structures a group suitable for

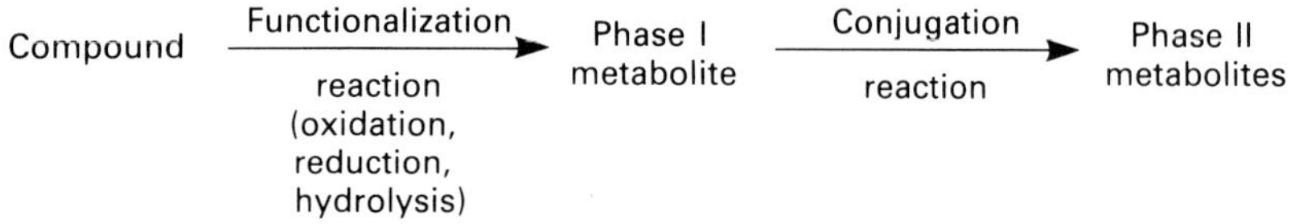

Figure 2.1 The biphasic sequence of xenobiotic metabolism

Phase II metabolism directly, and thus undergo only conjugation reactions. The elimination products of xenobiotics may thus comprise the unchanged compound, Phase I metabolites, Phase II metabolites, and the products of both Phase I and Phase II reactions. In the majority of cases, xenobiotics are characteristically eliminated in the form of conjugates[2].

It is now generally accepted that, in mammals, there are seven major conjugation reactions which xenobiotics may undergo, whose substrate and co-substrate requirements and phylogenetic distribution are reasonably well-known[2,3]. Each of these reactions is also of significance in the disposition of endogenous compounds and biosynthesis. In addition, there are a number of so-called 'novel' conjugation reactions, which are presently viewed as being restricted in their occurrence to particular combinations of substrate(s) and species[3–6]. It is to be stressed that in the future, as further knowledge is acquired, some at least of the 'novel' reactions may attain the status of the major reactions. The major reactions are listed in Table 2.1, which also

Table 2.1 The major conjugation reactions of xenobiotic metabolism

Reaction	*Endogenous role*
Glucuronidation	Biosynthesis, detoxication, e.g. bilirubin
Sulphation	Biosynthesis, steroid metabolism, detoxication, e.g. indoxyl
Methylation	Biosynthesis, detoxication, e.g. catecholamines
Acetylation	Biosynthesis, intermediary metabolism
Cyanide detoxication	Vitamin B_{12} metabolism
Glutathione conjugation	Leukotriene synthesis, maintenance of redox potential
Amino acid conjugations	Detoxication of endogenous acids, especially in amino acidurias

indicates their significance in intermediary biochemistry. Table 2.2 presents some examples of novel conjugations.

The major conjugation reactions all involve the participation of a transferase enzyme, specific for the endogenous conjugating agent in question; the required energy is supplied either by the conjugating agent being present in a high-energy form (generally a nucleotide), or by the prior metabolic activation of the xenobiotic substrate[3]. Of the major conjugations, only the glutathione conjugation and the various amino acid conjugations fall into the latter category. The xenobiotic substrate for conjugation must possess within its structure an appropriate functional group for linkage to the conjugating agent, which may either be chemically stable, e.g. hydroxyl (alcoholic, phenolic or carboxylic),

Table 2.2 Some novel metabolic conjugation reactions

Conjugation with:
Carbohydrates, e.g. xylose, ribose, galactose
Acyl groups, e.g. formyl, succinyl, stearoyl
Amino acids, e.g. histidine, alanine, glutamic acid, valine, serine
Formation of:
Methylthio conjugates
Hybrid fatty acids
Hybrid triglycerides

amino or thiol, or chemically reactive, e.g. oxirane (epoxide or arene oxide) or carbonium ion.

THE GLUCURONIC ACID CONJUGATION

Of the major conjugation reactions, it is reasonable to view the glucuronic acid mechanism as the most versatile, in terms of (1) the range of xenobiotics which it may accept, (2) its wide phylogenetic distribution, (3) its distribution through the tissues of the body and (4) its capacity in pharmacokinetic terms.

Biochemistry

The glucuronic acid incorporated into the conjugate derives from the endogenous nucleotide uridine diphosphate glucuronic acid[7] (UDPGA), in which the glucuronic acid moiety is in the pyranose form and has the protons on C-1 and C-2 *cis* to each other, i.e. it is in the α-form. During the process of conjugation, the configuration of the glucuronic acid is inverted to the β-form, with the C-1 and C-2 protons *trans* to each other, and the xenobiotic residue is attached to C-1, giving rise to a 1-*O*-substituted β-D-glucopyranosiduronate[8]. Glucuronic acid conjugation is effected by the enzyme UDP-glucuronosyltransferase (UDPGT) which is found bound to membranes, notably the endoplasmic reticulum, in the liver and a variety of other tissues[9]. This reaction is shown in Figure 2.2.

UDPGT activity is largely recovered in the microsomal fraction of tissue homogenates, and is at least partially latent. Its activity may be enhanced by lipolytic agents and detergents, which disrupt membrane structure, and the degree of latency depends upon the tissue, mode of preparation, substrate and the activating agent used[9]. It appears that the latency of the enzyme *in vivo* is controlled by UDP-*N*-acetylglucosamine[10]. Evidence for the functional heterogeneity of UDPGT has accumulated over many years, from studies of species and strain variations, substrate specificity, ontogenesis, tissue distribution, induction, inhibition and activation[11]. Although progress with this problem was hindered by the membrane-bound nature of the enzyme, at least three forms have now been purified to apparent homogeneity, these being differentially inducible and have different, but partially overlapping, substrate specificities. Other evidence from studies of differential induction[12] and substrate specificity[13] indicates the existence of yet further forms. Rapid progress

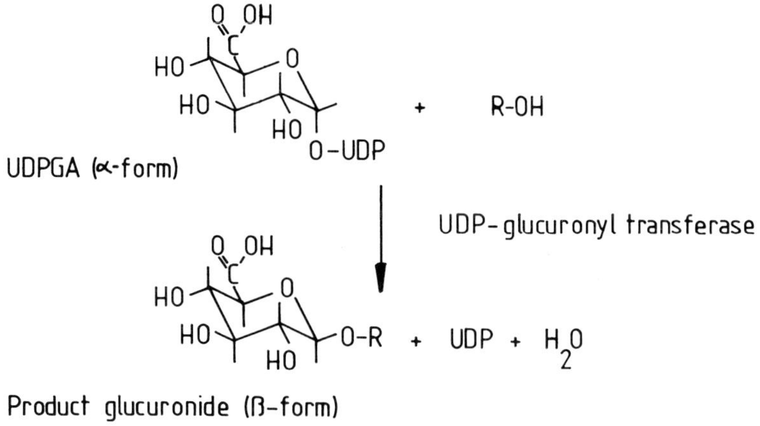

Figure 2.2 The reaction sequence of glucuronic acid conjugation

is currently being made in the immunochemistry and molecular biology of these multiple forms of UDPGT, and accounts are to be found in the proceedings of a recent symposium in Dundee, Scotland[14] and the present conference.

The existence of multiple UDPGTs with (partially) overlapping substrate specificities renders assays of microsomal glucuronidation activity towards particular substrates confusing as measures of specific UDPGT forms. Recommendations for the use of standardized assay conditions to reduce such confusion have recently been made[15].

Xenobiotic substrates for glucuronidation

The various UDPGTs have the capacity to transfer glucuronic acid from UDPGA to a tremendous variety of compounds, sharing in common the possession of a potentially ionizable proton which is replaced by glucuronic acid. Examples of these, classified in terms of the functional group in which the replaceable proton is found, are listed in Table 2.3. Many of these examples refer to classes of glucuronides known for many years, e.g. trichloroethanol, the first glucuronide to be discovered[16], phenols and carboxylic acids, but it is to be noted that new classes of glucuronides are still being discovered. Thus, the quaternary *N*-glucuronide of the tertiary amine drug, cyproheptadine[17] and the *C–C*–glucuronides of the pyrazlone drugs phenylbutazone, feprazone and sulphinpyrazone[18,19] (Kubo and Hasegawa, personal communication) represent newly discovered classes of glucuronide, resistant to classical analytical methods and characterized by physicochemical methods.

Chemistry and analytical methodology of glucuronides

Glucuronides are generally thought of as chemically stable entities which are readily excreted from the body. Their identification depends in the most part upon colour reactions, notably with naphthoresorcinol (Tollen's reagent) and their lability to the hydrolytic enzyme β-glucuronidase, which is widely avail-

Table 2.3 Types of compounds giving rise to glucuronic acid conjugates

Functional group	*Example*
Hydroxyl	
Primary alcohol	trichloroethanol
Secondary alcohol	propranolol
Tertiary alcohol	*tert*-butanol
Alicyclic alcohol	cyclohexanol
Terpenoid alcohol	menthol
Phenol	phenol
Terpenoid phenol	eugenol
Enol	4-hydroxycoumarin
Aliphatic hydroxylamine	*N*-hydroxychlorphentermine
Aromatic hydroxylamine	2-napthylhydroxylamine
Hydroxamic acid	*N*-hydroxy-2-acetamidofluorene
Carboxylic acid	
Alkyl	2-ethylhexanoic acid
Aromatic	benzoic acid
Heterocyclic	nicotinic acid
Arylacetic	Indole-3-acetic acid
Arylpropionic	hydratropic acid
Aryloxybutyric	clofibric acid
Carbamic acid	tocainide carbamate
Amino functions	
Aromatic	aniline
Azaheterocyclic	sulphisoxazole
Carbamate	meprobamate
Sulphonamide	sulphadimethoxine
Hydroxylamine *N*-	*N*-hydroxy-2-acetamidofluorene
Tertiary aliphatic	cyproheptadine
Urea	dulcin
Sulphur functions	
Thiol	2-mercaptobenzothiazole
Dithioic acid	*N.N*-diethyldithiocarbamic acid
Carbon centres	
Pyrazolone ring	phenylbutazone

able commercially from mammalian, molluscan and bacterial sources. However, it is important to appreciate that this enzyme does not cleave all glucuronides: the C–*C*-glucuronides are totally resistant, while certain of the *N*-glucuronides listed in Table 2.3 are of variable lability. In the case of the ester (acyl) glucuronides, their ability to serve as substrates for β-glucuronidase is variable due to their isomerization.

As has been stated earlier, UDPGT catalyses the synthesis of 1-*O*-substituted β-D-glucopyranosiduronates, and it is these which are substrates for β-glucuronidase. Ester glucuronides exhibit an interesting isomerization, in which the acyl moiety originally attached to C-1 migrates under mild alkaline (pH 7–9) conditions successively from C-1 to C-2, C-2 to C-3 and C-3 to C-4[20,21]. The products of this unidirectional reaction, the C-2, C-3 and C-4 isomers, are no longer substrates for β-glucuronidase, although they are, like the parent C-1 forms, hydrolysed by mild alkali (pH 10 and above for at least 30 minutes)[20,21]. Recognition of this intramolecular rearrangement is important to guide the design and execution of studies of compounds likely to give rise to ester glucuronides. Interestingly, the rearrangement may also occur *in vivo*, in the bladder when the urine pH is above 7 (notably in herbivorous species)[22], in the bile[20] or in the blood, notably in cases of renal insufficiency[23]. Some possible consequences of this intramolecular rearrangement of ester glucuronides will be commented upon later. A number of ester glucuronides have been shown to undergo this reaction, and is suspected to occur for a considerable number more, since discrepancies between the extent of hydrolysis of a glucuronide by β-glucuronidase and by mild alkali are common. Examples are presented in

Table 2.4 Ester glucuronides known or suspected to undergo intramolecular rearrangement to β-glucuronidase resistant isomers

Established for:	
Bilirubin	Isoxepac
Clofibric acid	WY-18251
Probenecid	Fenclofenac
Zomepirac	Valproic acid
Suspected for:	
Benzoic acid	Diphenylacetic acid
Hydratropic acid	Fenoprofen
Indomethacin	Indol-3-ylacetic acid
1- and 2-napthylacetic acids	

Table 2.4. The rate of rearrangement is dependent upon the acyl group in question, but the features determining its extent are unknown[24]. The intramolecular rearrangement must be considered as a general feature of the chemistry of ester glucuronides.

Phylogenetic distribution of glucuronic acid conjugation

The glucuronic acid conjugation mechanism exhibits a wide distribution through living organisms, and has been found to be involved in the metabolism of xenobiotics in mammals, birds, amphibians, reptiles and fish[2], but does not occur in insects or molluscs, where it is replaced by the analogous reaction of glucoside formation[25]. Additionally, the reaction has been reported to occur in plants[8]. The greatest amount of information is available for the order *Mammalia*, and although in general all mammals have the capacity to form glucuronides, there exist a number of species, and of genetically stable mutants within certain species, which exhibit an at least partial inability to conjugate xenobiotics with glucuronic acid, and examples are listed in Table 2.5. It is noteworthy that at least three unusual glucuronidation reactions involving *N* and *C* centres, are restricted in their occurrence to man and primate species. The N^1-glucuronidation of sulphadimethoxine and certain other sulphonamides occur only in man, monkey species (both Old and New World) and certain prosimians[26], while the quaternary *N*-glucuronide of cyproheptadine and the C–*C*-glucuronides of pyrazolones[18,19] (Kubo and Hasegawa, personal communication) are formed only by man and the chimpanzee.

Perhaps the best known instance of a so-called 'species defect' in glucuronidation is that in the cat. Although it was originally thought that this species was

Table 2.5 Inter- and intra-species differences in glucuronidation

Apparently restricted to man and primate species:
- Quaternary *N*-glucuronidation, e.g. cyproheptadine (man and apes)
- Sulphonamido *N*-glucuronidation, e.g. sulphadimethoxine (all primates)
- Pyrazolone *C*-glucuronidation, e.g. phenylbutazone (man and apes)

Defects in glucuronidation exist in:
- Wistar rat (androsterone)
- Gunn mutant of Wistar rat (many substrates)
- Cat and related feline species (substrate-specific)
- Man (1) Crigler–Najjar syndrome
  (2) Gilbert's syndrome

unable to form glucuronic acid conjugates of xenobiotics (the paper of Robinson and Williams[27] is entitled 'Do cats form glucuronides?'), it has been known for many years that cats form bilirubin glucuronides[28]. It is now clear that the defect of glucuronidation in the cat is only partial, and depends upon the substrate in question. This is illustrated for both ether and ester glucuronides in Table 2.6, which shows the ability of the cat to form the glucuronides of

Table 2.6 Dependence of the 'glucuronidation defect' in the cat upon the structure of the xenobiotic substrate

	% Dose glucuronidated by	
	Cat	*Rat*
Phenols		
Phenol	1	44
1-Naphthol	1	47
Phenolphthalein	60	98
Carboxylic acids		
1-Napththylacetic acid	0	79
Clofibric acid	2	82
Diphenylacetic acid	76	95

larger, more complex aglycones to approximately the same extent as the rat, and that the defect is restricted to smaller xenobiotic substrates.

The inability of the domestic cat (*Felis cattus*) to glucuronidate certain foreign compounds extends to a range of related species, and appears to be a biochemical characteristic of the cat-like carnivores, the super-family *Feloidea*. We have shown that this defect also occurs in the lion, lynx, civet and genet, but not in the hyena[29]. The ability of this latter carnivore to form the ester glucuronide of 1-napthylacetic acid is a finding of some taxonomic interest. The hyena is generally classified as a cat-like carnivore, but biochemically it lacks the feline defect in the glucuronic acid conjugation mechanism. Additionally, it shares with the dog an inability to acetylate aromatic amines, and thus in terms of pharmacotaxonomy[30], the hyena should be considered as a dog-like carnivore, in the super-family *Canoidea*.

In addition to the important inter-species differences in glucuronidation, it is noteworthy that Table 2.5 lists a number of intra-species (strain) differences in the occurrence of the glucuronic acid conjugation mechanism. These range in degree from the virtually complete defect observed in the human Crigler–Najjar syndrome to the defect in androsterone glucuronidation observed in certain outbred Wistar rats[31]. It is important to note that this latter defect is different from that seen in the Gunn mutant of the Wistar rat. A variety of explanations have been proferred for these various defects, the most popular of which involve either differences in the membrane environment of UDPGT or genetic polymorphisms of one or more forms of UDPGT. Although the contribution of variations in the membranes in which UDPGT is found must not be overlooked, in general the strain differences in UDPGT activities are supportive of the existence of multiple, independently regulated forms of this enzyme, the relative proportions of which may be highly variable between individual members of the same species.

THE BIOLOGICAL SIGNIFICANCE OF GLUCURONIC ACID CONJUGATION

Having established the significance of the glucuronic acid conjugation mechanism in terms of its phylogenetic distribution and wide range of xenobiotic substrates, and dealt briefly with its biochemistry, it is now appropriate to consider its biological significance. The significance of the major conjugation reactions of drug metabolism may be dealt with under three main headings[3] (1) a detoxication function, which may, however, fail under certain circumstances, (2) in some cases, the formation of biologically active conjugates and (3) their pharmacokinetic consequences. These various matters will now be considered in terms of the glucuronic acid mechanism, and are summarized in Table 2.7.

Table 2.7 The biological significance of the conjugation reactions

Metabolic conjugation leads to:		
(1) Readily excreted end-products of metabolism		
(2) Detoxication, which may be	(a) defective	
	(b) saturable	
(3) Metabolic activation, in a few cases		
(4) Pharmacokinetic implications, including		(a) saturation
		(b) enterohepatic circulation
		(c) presystemic elimination
		(d) drug–drug interactions

Detoxication

The biological properties of xenobiotics arise as a consequence of their interaction with important functional macromolecules of the body, e.g. hormone and neurotransmitter receptors, enzymes or excitable membranes. The nature, extent and consequences of such interactions are a function of the chemical structure of the xenobiotic in question. Thus, any process serving to change the structure of the xenobiotic molecules present in the organism may be expected to have an impact upon the biological activity of the parent foreign compound, and it is now well established that the fate of a xenobiotic is intimately related to its biological activity. The Phase I reactions of drug metabolism frequently do not cause great changes in the structure of xenobiotics, and thus it is not surprising that, in many cases, Phase I metabolites contribute towards the overall activity of the parent compound. However, the Phase II reactions of conjugation generally bring about substantial increases in both the polarity and water solubility of the substrate, and thereby lead to a loss of biological activity. This arises both from a reduction in affinity for biological target systems and/or from the facilitation of excretion in the urine or bile. This detoxication function of conjugation is well exemplified by the glucuronic acid mechanism, and is illustrated in Table 2.8, which compares

Table 2.8 The detoxication function of glucuronidation

	LD_{50}(mg/kg)	
	Cat	*Rabbit*
Phenol	80	250
Paracetamol	250	1200
1-Naphthol	100	9000
2-Naphthol	100	3000

the toxicity of selected aglycones in the rabbit, which glucuronidates them extensively, and the cat, which does not (*see* above). In each case, the compound is markedly more toxic to the cat than the rabbit, since the cat cannot compensate for the absence of the glucuronic acid conjugation by the use of alternative metabolic pathways[3].

In view of the fact that the glucuronic acid conjugation of the majority of substrates leads to their detoxication, in situations where the activity of this pathway is reduced, it is to be expected that changes in toxicity will ensue. The importance of species differences have already been illustrated with reference to the cat, and it is perhaps important to note that the human genetic variations in glucuronidation could influence the activity of drugs and other chemicals which undergo this conjugation. Although the Crigler–Najjar syndrome is a serious disorder, in which such 'failure of detoxication' of xenobiotics would probably have little significance in comparison with that of chronic unconjugated hyperbilirubinaemia, the situation could be different in the case of Gilbert's syndrome, since the majority of cases remain undiagnosed. It is possible that subjects with this defect of glucuronidation could be more at risk from adverse reactions to agents which undergo glucuronidation than are those in whom this pathway has normal activity. In addition, the abnormally low capacity for glucuronidation of xenobiotics could be of diagnostic value, especially for the purpose of detecting heterozygous 'carriers' of such defects[32]. It is beyond the scope of this brief review to deal with the ontogenesis of UDPGT and the glucuronic acid conjugation mechanism, but it is also interesting to note the toxicity of the antibiotic chloramphenicol to human neonates, especially premature infants, the so-called 'grey baby syndrome', which arises from their inability to effect the glucuronidation, and hence detoxication, of this drug[3].

It is now known that the polycyclic hydrocarbons undergo successive oxidations by the microsomal mono-oxygenases to produce carcinogenic metabolites.

In the case of benzo(a)pyrene, the ultimate carcinogen is most likely its 7,8-dihydrodiol-9,10-oxide, formed from the 7,8-dihydrodiol. This intermediate then undergoes either oxidation to the diol-epoxide or conjugation with glucuronic acid or sulphate. The conjugation options will thus prevent the formation of the ultimate carcinogenic metabolite, and it is possible that inter- and intra-species differences in the carcinogenicity of benzo(a)pyrene may arise from differences in the conjugation of the dihydrodiol[3].

Metabolic activation as a consequence of glucuronidation

As has been outlined above, in the majority of cases conjugation leads to the detoxication and inactivation of xenobiotics. However, there are exceptions to this general situation in which conjugation leads instead to the metabolic activation of the substrate in question. In one of three distinct ways (1) the conjugate is chemically stable, and retains the ability to undergo biologically important reversible interactions with the tissues, (2) conjugation contributes to the chemical reactivity of the substrate, leading to the formation of reactive species able to bind irreversibly to tissue components, or (3) the conjugate undergoes further metabolism leading to new types of biological activity. These possibilities have been discussed at length elsewhere[3-5], and examples of all three possibilities which involve the glucuronic acid conjugation mechanism will be discussed here.

As might be expected, examples of glucuronic acid conjugates which have biological activity *per se* are very unusual, and reports of such activity must be treated with caution in view of the high β-glucuronidase activity present in most tissues. However, it appears that the minor morphine metabolite, morphine-6-glucuronide does possess agonist activity against opiate receptors[33].

A number of chemical carcinogens, including arylamines, arylacetamides and allylbenzenes, require a biphasic metabolic activation to exert their activity. This involves an oxidation reaction, at the *N*-centre or at C-1 of the allyl side chain, followed by conjugation of the hydroxylated metabolite with either sulphate or glucuronic acid. The *O*-sulphate and *O*-glucuronide moieties are better leaving groups than is the hydroxyl group itself, so that the formation of the ultimate electrophilic carcinogenic metabolites is facilitated by conjugation[34]. It is to be noted that the contribution of glucuronidation to such metabolic activation is far less than that of the sulphation mechanism.

Glucuronides may also contribute to the activity of certain xenobiotics following further metabolism. This may simply arise from the release of the aglycone following hydrolysis, as occurs in the gastrointestinal tract during the enterohepatic circulation (see below), but may also result in the conjugate acting as a transport form of the compound, resulting in the expression of activity at sites not able to metabolize the xenobiotic. As well as undergoing glucuronic acid conjugation at the *N*-hydroxyl group, certain *N*-hydroxyarylamines undergo glucuronidation at the nitrogen atom to produce inactive conjugates which are excreted in the urine. However, these may be broken down in the urinary bladder by β-glucuronidase and, at the acid pH frequently encountered in the human bladder, may initiate tumour formation at a site different from that at which the metabolic activation occurred[35].

Pharmacokinetic implications of glucuronic acid conjugation

It is clear from the above discussion that the major conjugation reactions have a number of important consequences for the disposition and elimination of xenobiotics, which may be considered as pharmacokinetic implications, and these will be discussed with reference to the glucuronic acid conjugation.

Glucuronides are more polar and more water soluble than their aglycones, and thus their formation contributes to the elimination of the xenobiotic from the body. This may involve elimination in the urine, and certain glucuronides undergo active secretion by the kidney tubule[3]. In other cases, glucuronides may be excreted into the intestine via the bile. Compounds excreted by this route are characteristically amphipathic and of a certain minimum molecular weight, this latter varying with species[36]. Since most drugs are relatively small and lipid-soluble, the addition of a polar anionic group and the increase in molecular weight occurring as a consequence of glucuronic acid conjugation are of great significance for this route of excretion. Biliary excretion has a number of consequences in the disposition of xenobiotics. It leads in certain cases to the elimination of the compound and its metabolites in the faeces, but also may expose them to the many and varied metabolic activities of the gastrointestinal flora. The microflora have the ability to effect metabolic reactions not normally occurring within the tissues of the body, such as reductive dealkylation, dehydroxylation and heterocyclic ring fission[37]. Compounds excreted in the bile may also exert local actions within the gut, and examples whose biliary excretion depends upon their glucuronidation include the cathartic drug phenolphthalein, and indomethacin, an anti-inflammatory drug which causes intestinal ulceration[3].

The majority of glucuronides excreted in the bile undergo hydrolysis by bacterial β-glucuronidases, with the result that the aglycones can be reabsorbed, the so-called enterohepatic circulation. This can result in the appearance of secondary peaks in plasma level–time curves, in some cases associated with 'rebound effects' of drugs, retention of the compound in the body and delayed elimination[36].

The limited capacity of many of the major conjugation reactions, arising principally from limitations upon the supply of the endogenous conjugating agent in the appropriate form, results in their ready saturability. It is to be noted that the glucuronic acid mechanism appears to have the highest capacity of all the major conjugation reactions, and thus examples of the pharmacokinetic consequences of its saturation are hard to find. The toxicological sequelae of the failure of glucuronidation have been described above.

Although the liver is the major site of glucuronic acid conjugation, numerous other organs also have the ability to make a significant contribution to the overall glucuronidation capacity of the organism[38]. In particular, glucuronidation by the gastrointestinal mucosa may be responsible for route-of-administration related differences in metabolism[39].

CONCLUDING REMARKS

This short review has served to introduce the conjugation reactions, and the glucuronic acid mechanism in particular, in terms of their significance in the metabolic disposition of xenobiotics in the organism, and has indicated the significance which these reactions have for the biological properties of xenobiotics. The glucuronic acid conjugation is the most versatile of the xenobiotic conjugation reactions in terms of its distribution through living organisms and the range of xenobiotic substrates it is able to accept. It is a critical reaction for the detoxication, pharmacokinetic behaviour and elimination of many foreign compounds, and may on occasion be involved in their activation. The existence of a number of inter- and intra-species differences in glucuronidation capacity is of significance in highlighting the importance of this metabolic pathway, and also has an important bearing upon the biological activities in such species or strains of compounds normally undergoing glucuronidation.

Finally, it must not be overlooked that the major conjugation reactions all have important and well-defined roles in intermediary biochemistry, and they should, therefore, be viewed as interfaces between the biochemistry of endobiotic and xenobiotic compounds, which may be relevant to idiopathic disease. The metabolic conjugation reactions are virtually unexplored from the standpoint of their impact upon intermediary metabolism, although they all make use of essential biochemicals. In the case of the glucuronic acid mechanism, the possible interference by the conjugation of xenobiotics with the normal utilization of UDPGA has not been examined. It is to be expected that a fresh look at the conjugation reactions in this light may provide advances in biochemistry, pharmacology and pathology.

ACKNOWLEDGEMENTS

I am grateful to my colleagues Andrew Hutt, Philip Smith and Keith Sinclair for helpful discussion and literature references. The continuing advice and encouragement of Professor Robert Smith is acknowledged with pleasure. I thank SERC, FEMA (Washington, DC), Cilag-Chemie Stiftung and the Sir Halley Stewart Trust for financial support of our work in this area.

References

1. Williams, R. T. (1959). *Detoxication Mechanisms*, 2nd. edn. (London: Chapman & Hall)
2. Williams, R. T. (1967). The biogenesis of conjugation and detoxication products. In Bernfeld, P. (ed.). *Biogenesis of Natural Compounds*, 2nd. edn., pp. 590–639. (Oxford: Pergamon)
3. Caldwell, J. (1980). Conjugation reactions. In Jenner, P. and Testa, B. (eds.). *Concepts in Drug Metabolism*, Part A, pp. 211–50. (New York: Marcel Dekker)
4. Caldwell, J. (1982). Conjugation reactions in the metabolism of xenobiotics. In Arias, I., Popper, H., Schachter, D. and Shafritz, D. A. (eds.). *The Liver: Biology and Pathobiology*. pp. 281–95. (New York: Raven Press)
5. Caldwell, J. (1982). The conjugation reactions in foreign compound metabolism: definition, consequences and species variations. *Drug Metab. Rev.*, **13,** 745–78

6. Eadsforth, C. V. and Hutson, D. H. (1984). Formation of carbohydrate, sulfate and other conjugates. In Caldwell, J. and Paulson, G. D. (eds.). *Foreign Compound Metabolism*, pp. 173–86. (London: Taylor and Francis)
7. Storey, I. D. E. and Dutton, G. J. (1955). Uridine compounds in glucuronic acid metabolism. 2. The isolation and structure of 'uridine-diphosphate-glucuronic acid'. *Biochem. J.*, **59,** 279–88
8. Dutton, G. J. (1966). The biosynthesis of glucuronides. In Dutton, G. J. (ed.). *Glucuronic Acid Free and Combined*, pp. 186–299. (New York: Academic Press)
9. Dutton, G. J. (1980). *Glucuronidation of Drugs and Other Compounds*. (Boca Raton, FL: CRC Press)
10. Berry, C. S. (1978). Critical evaluation of UDP-*N*-acetyl-glucosamine and product glucuronides as allosteric effectors of UDP-glucuronyltransferase. In Aitio, A. (ed.). *Conjugation Reactions in Drug Biotransformation*, pp. 233–46. (Amsterdam: Elsevier)
11. Dutton, G. J., Wishart, G. J., Leakey, J. E. A. and Goheer, M. A. (1977). Conjugation with glucuronic acid and other sugars. In Parke, D. V. and Smith, R. L. (eds.). *Drug Metabolism from Microbe to Man*, pp. 71–90. (London: Taylor and Francis)
12. Bock, K. W., Lilienblum, W., Ullrich, D. and Fischer, G. (1984). Differential induction of UDP-glucuronosyltransferases and their 'permanent induction' in preneoplastic rat liver. *Biochem. Soc. Trans.*, **12,** 55–8
13. Boutin, J. A. (1983). Heterogeneite des UDP-glucuronosyl-transferase(s) chez l'animal et chez l'homme. *Doctoral Thesis*, University of Nancy, France
14. *Biochemical Society Transactions*, (1984), **12,** 1–106
15. Bock, K. W., Burchell, B., Dutton, G. J., Hanninen, O., Mulder, G. J., Owens, I. S., Siest, G. and Tephly, T. R. (1983). UDP-Glucuronosyltransferase activities. Guidelines for consistent interim terminology and assay conditions. *Biochem. Pharmacol.*, **32,** 953–6
16. Mering, E. V. and Musculus, A. (1875). Ueber einen neuen Körperim chloralharn. *Ber. Deut. Chem. Ges.*, **8,** 662–6
17. Fischer, L. J., Thies, R. L., Charkowski, D. and Donham, K. J. (1980). Formation and urinary excretion of cyproheptadine glucuronide in monkeys, chimpanzees and humans. *Drug Metab. Disp.*, **8,** 422–4
18. Richter, W. J., Alt, K. O., Dieterle, W., Faigle, J. W., Kriemler, H. P., Mory, H. and Winkler, T. (1975). *C*-glucuronides, a novel type of drug metabolites. *Helv. Chim. Acta*, **58,** 2512-17
19. Faigle, J. W. and Dieterle, W. (1977). The biotransformation of phenylbutazone (butazolidin). *J. Int. Med. Res.*, **5** (Suppl. 2), 2–14
20. Compernolle, F., van Hees, G. P., Blanckaert, N. and Heirwegh, K. P. M. (1978). Glucuronic acid conjugates of bilirubin IX-α in normal bile compared with post-obstructive bile. *Biochem. J.*, **171,** 185–201
21. Caldwell, J. and Sinclair, K. A. (1982). The formation of β-glucuronidase resistant glucuronides by the intramolecular rearrangement of glucuronic acid conjugates at mild alkaline pH. *Biochem. Pharmacol.*, **31,** 953–7
22. Caldwell, J., Hutt, A. J., Marsh, M. V. and Sinclair, K. A. (1983). Methodology for the isolation and characterization of amino acid and sugar conjugates of xenobiotic carboxylic acids. In Reid, E. and Leppard, J. P. (eds.). *Drug Metabolite Isolation and Determination*, pp. 161–79. (New York: Plenum Press)
23. Faed, E. M. and McQueen, E. G. (1978). Measurement of clofibric acid (CPIB) metabolites in the plasma of patients on clofibrate therapy. *Clin. Exp. Pharmacol. Physiol.*, **6,** 267–73
24. Janssen, F. W., Kirkman, S. K., Fenselau, C., Stogniew, M., Hofmann, B. R., Young, E. M. and Ruelius, H. W. (1982). Metabolic formation of *N*- and *O*-glucuronides of 3-(*p*-chlorophenyl)thiazolo-[3,2-a]benzimidazole-2-acetic acid. *Drug Metab. Disp.*, **10,** 599–604
25. Smith, J. N. (1977). Comparative detoxication of invertebrates. In Parke, D. V. and Smith, R. L. (eds.). *Drug Metabolism from Microbe to Man*, pp. 219–32. (London: Taylor and Francis)
26. Adamson, R. H., Bridges, J. W., Kibby, M. R., Walker, S. R. and Williams, R. T. (1970). The fate of sulphadimethoxine in primates compared with other species. *Biochem. J.*, **118,** 41–5
27. Robinson, D. and Williams, R. T. (1956). Do cats form glucuronides? *Biochem. J.*, **68,** 23P

28. Heirwegh, K. P. M. (1978). Formation, metabolism and significance of bilirubin IX-glycosides. In Aitio, A. (ed.). *Conjugation Reactions in Drug Biotransformation*, pp. 67–76. (Amsterdam: Elsevier)
29. Caldwell, J., Williams, R. T., Bassir, O. and French, M. R. (1978). Drug metabolism in exotic animals. *Eur. J. Drug Metab. Pharmacokin.*, **3,** 61–6
30. Caldwell, J. (1980). Comparative aspects of detoxication in mammals. In Jakoby, W. B. (ed.). *Enzymatic Basis of Detoxication*, Vol. 1, pp. 85–114. (New York: Academic Press)
31. Matsui, M. (1982). Variability in androsterone metabolism in Wistar rats, with special reference to the sulfated and glucuronidated metabolites. In Mulder, G. J., Caldwell, J., van Kempen, G. M. J. and Vonk, R. J. (eds.). *Sulfate Metabolism and Sulfate Conjugation*, pp. 181–8. (London: Taylor and Francis)
32. Schmid, R. and McDonagh, A. F. (1978). Hyperbilirubinaemia. In Wyngaarden, J. B. and Fredrickson, D. S. (eds.). *Metabolic Basis of Inherited Disease*, pp. 1221–57. (New York: McGraw-Hill)
33. Mori, M., Oguri, R., Yosimura, H., Shimomura, K., Kamata, O. and Ueki, S. (1972). Chemical synthesis and analgesic activity of morphine ethereal sulfates. *Life Sci.*, **11**(1), 525–33
34. Miller, J. A. and Miller, E. C. (1977). The concept of reactive electrophilic metabolites in chemical carcinogenesis. In Jollow, D. J., Kocsis, J. J., Snyder, R. and Vainio, H. (eds.). *Biological Reactive Intermediates*, pp. 6–24. (New York: Plenum)
35. Kadlubar, F. F., Miller, J. A. and Miller, E. C. (1977). Hepatic microsomal *N*-glucuronidation and nucleic acid binding of *N*-hydroxyarylamines in relation to urinary bladder carcinogenesis. *Cancer Res.*, **37,** 805–14
36. Smith, R. L. (1973). *The Excretory Function of Bile.* (London: Chapman and Hall)
37. Scheline, R. R. (1973). Metabolism of foreign compounds by gastrointestinal microorganisms. *Pharmacol. Rev.*, **25,** 451–523
38. Aitio, A. and Marniemi, J. (1980). Extrahepatic glucuronide conjugation. In Gram, T. E. (ed.). *Extrahepatic Metabolism of Drugs and Other Foreign Compounds*, pp. 365–87. (New York: SP Medical and Scientific Books)
39. Caldwell, J. and Marsh, M. V. (1982). Metabolism of drugs by the gastrointestinal tract. In George, C. F., Shand, D. G. and Renwick, A. G. (eds.). *Presystemic Drug Elimination*, pp. 29–42. (London: Butterworth Scientific)

3
Pharmacokinetics of glucuronidation in the rat *in vivo* and in intact perfused organs. Glucuronidation of 4-methylumbelliferome and harmol

G. J. MULDER, J. G. WEITERING, S. BROUWER AND
E. SCHOLTENS

INTRODUCTION

The study of pharmacokinetics of glucuronidation in whole, intact animals or in isolated perfused organs encompasses rather complicated systems in which various steps may become rate-limiting in the overall conjugation process. Figure 3.1 shows several of these steps in a model based on the hepatocyte; in the intact animal the pharmacokinetic behaviour can be determined through the elimination of the conjugate in bile and urine and the (steady-state) blood or plasma levels of the substrate. Briefly, the following potentially rate-limiting steps can be identified:

(1) *Blood flow* to the organ in which conjugation takes place; some drugs may change blood flow to certain organs selectively, or may reduce cardiac output as a whole. This will affect the conjugation of 'high extraction' drugs only[1,2].

(2) The *substrate concentration* in blood which is available for uptake by the cells. Protein binding may affect this availability[1].

(3) The *uptake* of the acceptor substrate by the cell, which may be simple diffusion (requiring sufficient lipid-solubility of the substrate), or carrier-mediated; also, back-transport from the interior of the cell back to blood may occur[3].

(4) Synthesis of the UDPGA precursor *UDP-glucose* from UTP and glucose-1-phosphate[4]. This step can be inhibited by D-galactosamine. Furthermore, fasting may limit the availability of glucose-1-phosphate in isolated hepatocytes or in the liver perfusion[5,6]; *in vivo* such an effect could not be found[7].

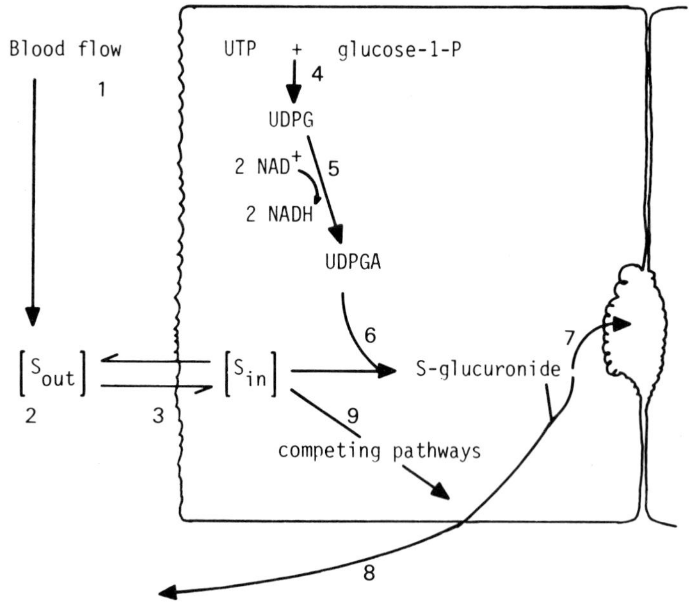

Figure 3.1 Potentially rate-limiting steps in glucuronidation in the intact cell. (1) Blood flow; (2) substrate concentration in blood; (3) uptake of substrate by cell; (4) synthesis of UDP glucose; (5) availability of UDP-glucuronic acid; (6) UDP-glucuronosyltransferase activity; (7) biliary excretion of glucuronide; (8) elimination of glucuronide in effluent blood

(5) Oxidation of UDP-glucose to UDP-glucuronic acid by UDPG-dehydrogenase, and *availability of UDPGA*. The dehydrogenase requires NAD^+, and, therefore, this step can be inhibited by ethanol, albeit only in the perfusion or the isolated hepatocyte preparation, since *in vivo* the balance between NAD^+ and NADH is not so easily disturbed. For some reason diethyl ether decreases the UDPGA concentration rapidly to approximately 10% of control, as do some other anaesthetics[8,9].

(6) The *UDP-glucuronosyltransferase* activity, which is dependent on the intracellular acceptor substrate concentration (not necessarily the same as the extracellular concentration; *see* reference 10), and the UDPGA concentration.

(7) Rate of elimination of the glucuronide conjugate in *bile*.

(8) Rate of elimination of the glucuronide conjugate in the *effluent blood*, and subsequently in *urine* (or bile after re-uptake by the liver).

(9) *Competition* with other reactions by which the substrate may be converted, in particular sulphation[11]; this may severely limit the availability of the acceptor substrate for glucuronidation.

(10) *Non-heterogeneous distribution* of glucuronidation activity in the organs, for instance a gradient of activity within the liver lobule. One has to keep in mind that a distribution of the transferase protein (determined, e.g. by immunochemical methods), is not the same as that of the overall glucuronidation activity, which includes UDPGA and acceptor substrate availability[12,13].

(11) A different substrate concentration-dependence of glucuronidation in *several organs* contributing to the overall conjugation of the substrate *in vivo*.

When the pharmacokinetics of glucuronidation is studied in an intact cell preparation or *in vivo*, one has to be aware of this complexity; for different substrates, different steps may be rate-limiting. This makes it rather hazardous to correlate *in vitro* determined K_m and V_{max} values for glucuronidation of a substrate, with the *in vivo* pharmacokinetics, even when steady-state experiments are being performed. In this chapter we will illustrate some of the problems with the substrates 4-methylumbelliferone (4-MU) and harmol (Figure 3.2), which have been studied in various *in vivo* and *in vitro* systems. 4-MU is a substrate which is mainly glucuronidated in the rat, while harmol is predominantly sulphated, unless very high doses are used.

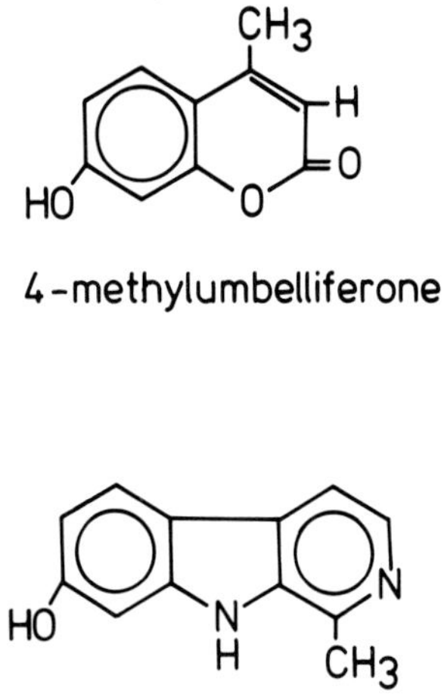

Figure 3.2 Structures of 4-methylumbelliferone (4-MU) and harmol

4-METHYLUMBELLIFERONE CONJUGATION *IN VIVO*; EFFECT OF INHIBITION OF SULPHATION, AND ß-NAPHTHOFLAVONE INDUCTION

4-Methylumbelliferone (Hymecromone; 7-hydroxy-4-methylcoumarin) is a drug used in man for its choleretic action. It is mainly glucuronidated in the rat *in vivo*[14–16], but some 20% is excreted as the sulphate conjugate at low doses (Table 3.1). However, at higher doses much less sulphation is observed; thus, only 6% sulphation was found when an infusion of 23 μmol min^{-1} kg^{-1} was given. Also in the rabbit the glucuronide is the main metabolite[14]. In some preliminary experiments we have studied conjugation of 4-MU under various conditions.

As is the case with other substrates of both glucuronidation and sulphation, the selective sulphation inhibitors 2,6-dichloro-4-nitrophenol (DCNP) and pentachlorophenol (PCP)[17,18] effectively reduce the sulphation of 4-MU; a higher degree of glucuronidation compensates for the loss of sulphation (Table 3.1). Ahotupa *et al.*[19] have suggested, based on *in vitro* work with UDP-glucuronosyltransferase, that PCP also inhibits UDP-glucuronosyltransferase activity very strongly. Now it has been shown in the past that many lipid soluble compounds may ('non-specifically') inhibit UDP-glucuronosyltransferase activity *in vitro*[4,20]. PCP and DCNP might cause a similar 'non-specific' inhibition. Therefore, we have investigated the effect of PCP and DCNP on the time-course of excretion of 4-MU metabolites in urine and bile: if glucuronidation were also affected by doses of PCP which caused pronounced inhibition of sulphation (Table 3.1), we would expect a slower excretion of the glucuronide

Table 3.1 Effect of DCNP and PCP on glucuronidation and sulphation of 4-methylumbelliferone (4-MU) in the rat *in vivo*

Pretreatment	*4-MU-sulphate (% of dose)*			*4-MU-glucuronide (% of dose)*		
	Bile	*Urine*	*Total*	*Bile*	*Urine*	*Total*
None	1.4±0.1	16.5±1.0	17.9	39±2	43±1	82
DCNP	0.3±0.1	3.8±0.3	4.1	51±1	45±1	96
PCP	0.5±0.1	3.9±0.1	4.4	55±2	40±2	95

Urine and bile were collected for 90 minutes after i.v. injection of 160 μmol/kg 4-methylumbelliferone in the jugular vein in pentobarbital-anaesthetized rats. The dose of both DCNP and PCP was 26 μmol/kg i.v. 5 min before the 4-MU injection into the tail vein. n = 4 in each group

conjugate in time. However, the results (Figure 3.3) clearly show that DCNP and PCP pretreatment cause the glucuronide conjugate to be excreted even faster (in bile) than in the controls: the additional glucuronide synthesized to compensate for the loss of sulphation appears in bile within a few minutes. Therefore, we feel that the inhibition (determined in microsomal preparations from rats pretreated with PCP) observed *in vitro* by Ahotupa *et al.*[19] does not result in relevant inhibition of glucuronidation *in vivo*, at least in our rats.

The glucuronidation of 4-MU (as measured *in vitro*) can be induced by β-naphthoflavone and similar inducers[21,22]. We have used this drug for induction of glucuronidation, and have pretreated rats with 100 mg/kg β-naphthoflavone (i.p.), 3 days before the experiment. The glucuronidation rate under those conditions was measured during steady-state infusion of 4-MU in 300 g rats (23 μmol $min^{-1} kg^{-1}$ i.v., after a priming dose of 165 μmol/kg). The results were somewhat unexpected: much less of the dose was recovered as the glucuronide than in the control rats. This suggested that alternative reactions were induced more by β-naphthoflavone than glucuronidation. Presumbly a non-fluorescent metabolite was formed since we did not detect anything besides the sulphate or glucuronide conjugate on our thin layer chromatography plates. This result seems to confirm the finding of Suolinna and Mäntylä[23], who reported that after pretreatment of rats with polychlorinated biphenyls a new 4-MU metabolite appeared.

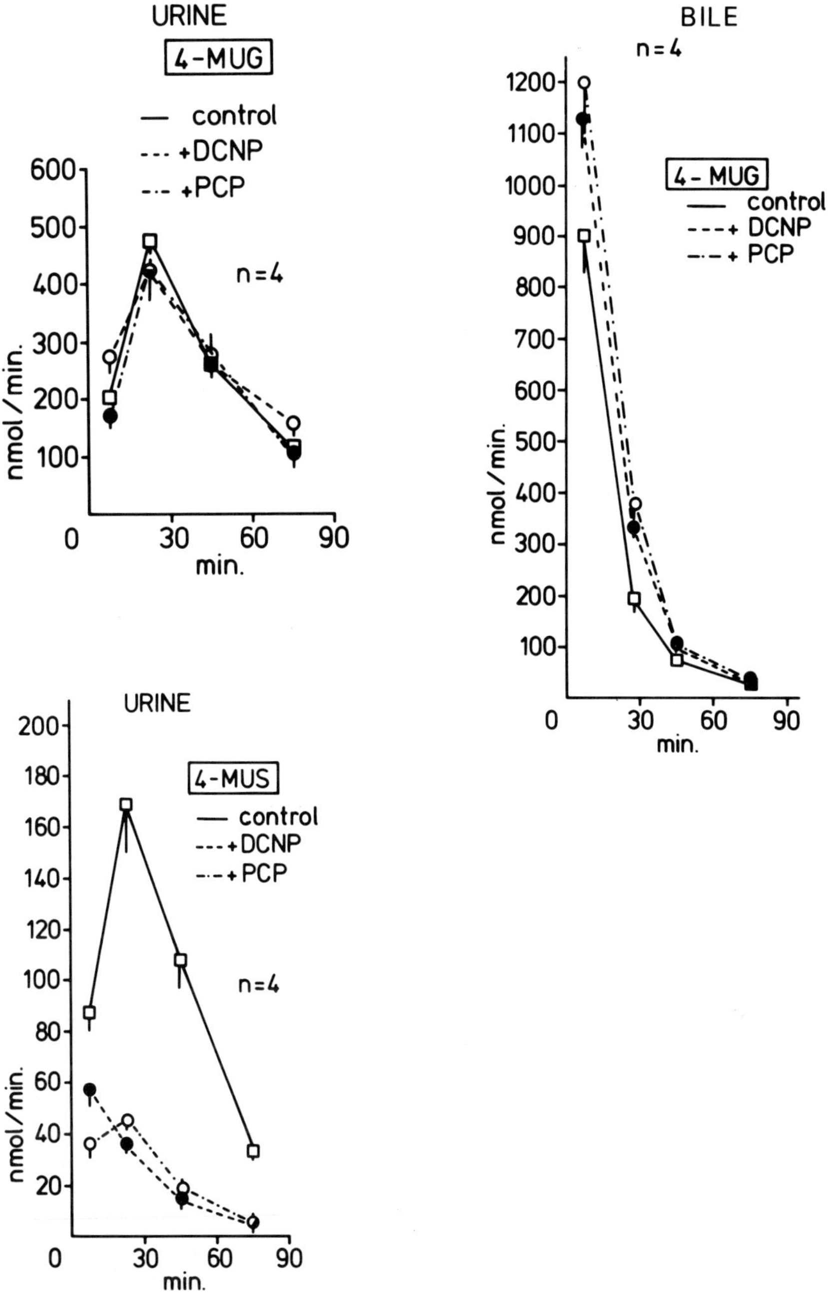

Figure 3.3 Effect of inhibition of sulphation by 2,6-dichloro-4-nitrophenol (DCNP) and pentachlorophenol (PCP) on the time course of excretion of 4-methylumbelliferone conjugates in urine and bile. For details on dose etc., see legend to Table 3.1. 4-MUS is the sulphate conjugate, and 4-MUG the glucuronide conjugate

PHARMACOKINETICS OF GLUCURONIDATION OF 4-MU

4-MU is a very good substrate for conjugation. Thus, it is rapidly cleared from the blood after a single injection: a biphasic blood disappearance curve is observed, with a $t^{\alpha}_{\frac{1}{2}}$ of approximately 5 minutes, and a $t^{\beta}_{\frac{1}{2}}$ of approximately 13 minutes. The volume of distribution (V^{ss}_{d}) of this lipid-soluble compound[24] was around 350 ml/kg. During steady-state infusion experiments the arterial blood concentration increases linearly with the infusion rate of 4-MU over the range of 1 to 12 μmol min^{-1} kg^{-1}, indicating linear kinetics of conjugation at the blood concentrations reached. A very high rate of glucuronidation can be reached *in vivo*. When an infusion of 23 μmol min^{-1} kg^{-1} was given to the rat in the jugular vein, the rate of excretion of the glucuronide in bile and urine combined was 15 μmol min^{-1} kg^{-1}, which means that 15 μmol UDPGA min^{-1} kg^{-1} was being consumed. In the liver of a 300 g rat the UDPGA concentration is 0.3 μmol/g liver[4], so that approximately 12 μmol UDPGA/kg body weight is available (in the liver). If glucuronidation of 4-MU at these high infusion rates occurs mainly in the liver (see below), the turnover of UDPGA would be so high that every minute the total amount present is utilized and resynthesized; previously, in the isolated perfused rat liver, a similar, high UDPGA turnover was measured with harmol as the substrate[25].

The clearance of 4-MU at steady-state was approximately 45 ml min^{-1} kg^{-1}, which is below total liver flow. Therefore, either the liver is the sole conjugating organ, or extraction of 4-MU by the liver *in situ* is much less than 100%, and extrahepatic organs contribute to the clearance of 4-MU.

SITE OF CONJUGATION OF 4-MU AND HARMOL

An answer to the question of a potential extrahepatic contribution to the metabolism of 4-MU came from a study on the extraction of 4-MU by the liver in the rat *in vivo*, when we measured blood levels of 4-MU in the carotid artery and the portal vein. The concentration of 4-MU in portal blood was 40% below that in arterial blood; the missing substrate was recovered in the form of the conjugates in the portal blood, the conclusion being that the gastrointestinal area had conjugated 40% of the 4-MU in arterial blood, before it could enter the liver[26]. Both in the single-pass perfused rat liver, and in an *in vivo* pharmacokinetic approach we found approximately 60% extraction of 4-MU by the liver. This seems to indicate that 4-MU entering the gastrointestinal region will be cleared to about 70–80% during single-pass by the gut and the liver, at least as long as the 4-MU concentration remains below 400 μmol/l, the highest concentration that we have used in this study. It also suggests that 4-MU is mainly conjugated in the liver at the doses used in the infusion experiments, since hepatic blood flow in the rat[2] is approximately 60 ml min^{-1} kg^{-1}, while steady-state clearance of 4-MU is 45 ml min^{-1} kg^{-1}.

For harmol we found a different pattern. In this case a clearance of approximately 200 ml min^{-1} kg^{-1} was found in the rat, which greatly exceeds liver blood flow. Moreover, it was calculated that the extraction by the liver *in situ* of harmol was only 70%, so that at low infusion rates of harmol, extrahepatic conjugation was responsible for approximately 77% of the harmol metabolism[31]. In these experiments, the conjugation of harmol was compared during infusion either in the jugular vein, or in the portal vein. When a high infusion is given in the portal vein, glucuronidation increases, presumably because a much higher concentration of harmol is presented to the liver[25].

NON-HOMOGENEOUS DISTRIBUTION OF GLUCURONIDATION AND SULPHATION ACROSS THE LIVER LOBULE

Glucuronidation and sulphation seem to occur in different zones. In the past, certain findings had suggested that sulphation had its highest activity in the zone 1 (periportal) area of the liver: toxicity of *N*-hydroxy-2-acetylaminofluorene which is due to its sulphation is located exclusively[27] in zone 1, and the pharmacokinetics of paracetamol (acetaminophen) sulphation after its generation from phenacetin, as observed during normal and retrograde perfusion of the liver, clearly indicated that paracetamol sulphation was located anterior to phenacetin oxidation (in zone 3 predominantly)[28]. Recent work with harmol as substrate in the perfused rat liver has confirmed this, and also seems to suggest that sulphation is located anterior to glucuronidation. Pang *et al.*[12] compared glucuronidation and sulphation of harmol during perfusion in the normal and retrograde flow direction, and noted a shift from sulphation to glucuronidation upon change of the flow direction from normal to retrograde. Recent experiments at various flow rates in the single-pass perfused rat liver indicate that overall glucuronidation activity seems to be rather homogeneously distributed along the liver lobule, from zone 1 to zone 3, while sulphation of harmol is mainly located in the zone 1 area (Dawson, Mulder, Pang, Stillwell, submitted).

ABERRANCIES IN CONJUGATION KINETICS IN THE INTACT CELL

When, as is the case with harmol, sulphation and glucuronidation compete for conjugation of the substrate, utilizing a common substrate pool, aberrancies from Michaelis–Menten kinetics may be observed. This occurs when the K_m for sulphation is much lower than that for glucuronidation, and when the rate of conjugation is high as compared to the rate of diffusion of the substrate into the cell[10]. When the extracellular substrate concentration (C_e) under these conditions is increased, sulphation becomes saturated and, as a consequence, the intracellular substrate concentration (C_i) increases at a higher rate with C_e than before saturation. Thus, the substrate concentration for glucuronidation (C_i) increases with C_e also at a different rate from then on; there appears to be a 'lag-phase' in glucuronidation at low extracellular (or blood) substrate concentration (Figure 3.4)[10]. These kinetic anomalies disappear (as expected) when sulphation is inhibited completely by DCNP[29].

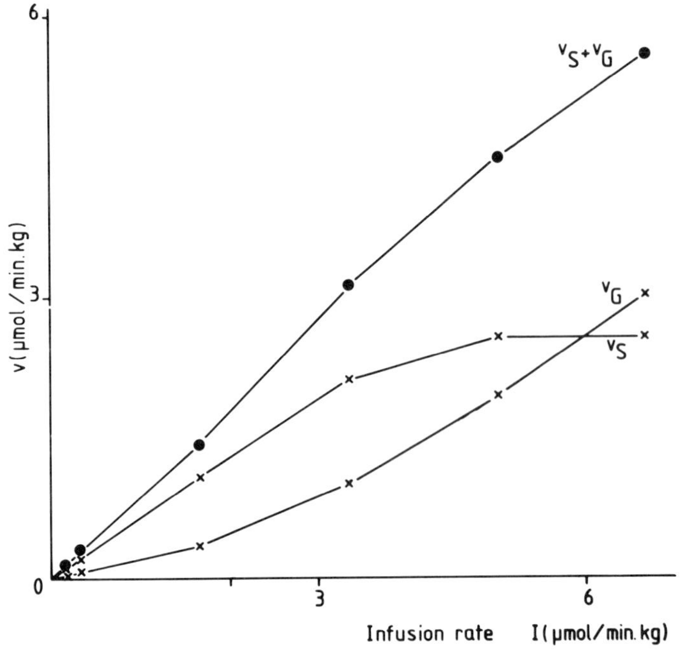

Figure 3.4 'Lag phase' of glucuronidation for a substrate of both sulphation and glucuronidation. Harmol was infused at different rates in 300 g rats, and the total excretion rate of harmol sulphate (hs) and harmol glucuronide (hg) during steady-state was determined. Data adapted from reference 30 (Table 2)

CONCLUSIONS

These results clearly demonstrate that the pharmacokinetics of harmol and 4-MU conjugation show large differences. For instance, the extrahepatic contribution to metabolism is very different. Although rate-limiting steps have not been identified, it is clear that the kinetics show deviations from 'normal' Michaelis–Menten behaviour, so that *in vitro* determined enzyme kinetic constants cannot be used to predict the kinetic behaviour *in vivo* or in other intact cell preparations.

ACKNOWLEDGEMENT

This work was supported by a NATO grant RG 35/82 (with Dr K. Sandy Pang, Toronto, Canada).

References

1. Pang, K. S. (1983). Fate of xenobiotics: physiologic and kinetic considerations. In Caldwell, J., Bend, J. and Jakoby, W. B. (eds.). *The Biological Basis of Detoxication*. pp. 213–50, (New York: Academic Press)
2. Boxenbaum, H. (1980). Interspecies variation in liver weight, hepatic blood flow, and antipyrine intrinsic clearance: extrapolation of data to benzodiazepines and phenytoin. *J. Pharmacokin. Biopharmac.*, **8,** 165–76
3. Meijer, D. K. F., Neef, C. and Groothuis, G. M. M. (1983). Carrier-mediated transport in the handling of drugs by the liver. In Breimer, D. D. and Speiser, P. (eds.). *Topics in Pharmaceutical Science*, pp. 167–89. (Amsterdam: Elsevier Science Publ.)
4. Dutton, G. J. (1980). *Glucuronidation of Drugs and Other Compounds*. (Boca Raton: CRC Press)
5. Thurman, R. G., Reinke, L. A., Belinsky, S., Evans, R. K. and Kauffman, F. C. (1981). Co-regulation of the mixed-function oxidation of *p*-nitroanisole and glucuronidation of *p*-nitrophenol in the perfused rat liver by carbohydrate reserves. *Arch. Biochem. Biophys.*, **209,** 137–42
6. Thurman, R. G. and Kauffman, F. C. (1980). Factors regulating drug metabolism in intact hepatocytes. *Pharmacol. Rev.*, **31,** 229–51
7. Mulder, G. J., Temmink, T. J. M. and Koster, H. J. (1982). The effect of fasting on sulphation and glucuronidation in the rat *in vivo*. *Biochem. Pharmacol.*, **31,** 1941–44
8. Eriksson, G. and Stråth, D. (1981). Decreased UDP-glucuronic acid in rat liver after ether narcosis. An isotachophoretic study. *FEBS Letters*, **124,** 39–42
9. Gregus, Z., Watkins, J. B., Thompson, T. N. and Klaassen, C. D. (1983). Depletion of hepatic uridine diphosphoglucuronic acid decreases the biliary excretion of drugs. *J. Pharmacol. Exp. Ther.*, **225,** 256–62
10. Koster, H. and Mulder, G. J. (1982). Apparent aberrancy in the kinetics of intracellular metabolism of a single substrate by two enzymes. An alternative explanation for anomalies in the kinetics of sulphation and glucuronidation. *Drug Metabol. Disp.*, **10,** 330–5
11. Mulder, G. J., Dawson, J. R. and Pang, K. S. (1984). Competition between sulphation and glucuronidation in the rat *in vivo*: enzyme kinetics and pharmacokinetics of conjugation. *Biochem. Soc. Trans.*, **12,** 17–20
12. Pang, K. S., Koster, H., Halsema, I. C. M., Scholtens, E., Mulder, G. J. and Stillwell, R. N. (1983). Normal and retrograde perfusion to probe the zonal distribution of sulfation and glucuronidation activities of harmol in the perfused rat liver. *J. Pharmacol. Exp. Ther.*, **224,** 647–53
13. Ullrich, D., Fischer, G., Katz, N. and Bock, K. W. (1984). Intra-lobular distribution of UDP-glucuronosyltransferase in livers from untreated, 3-methylcholanthrene- and phenobarbital-treated rats. *Chem. Biol. Interact.*, **48,** 181–90
14. Robinson, D., Smith, J. N. and Williams, R. T. (1953). β-glucuronidase and arylsulphatase in the crop fluid of locusts. *Biochem. J.*, **53,** 125–9
15. Mulder, G. J. (1973). The rate-limiting step in the biliary elimination of some substrates of uridine diphosphate glucuronyl-transferase in the rat. *Biochem. Pharmacol.*, **22,** 1751–63
16. Hirvonen, T. (1966). Fetal and postnatal development of glucuronide formation in mammalian tissue slices. *PhD Thesis*, University of Turku, Finland
17. Mulder, G. J. and Scholtens, E. (1977). Phenol sulphotransferase and uridine diphosphate glucuronyltransferase from rat liver *in vivo* and *in vitro*. *Biochem. J.*, **165,** 553–9
18. Mulder, G. J. (1984). Sulfation – metabolic aspects. In Bridges, J. W. and Chasseaud, L. F. (eds.). *Progress in Drug Metabolism*, Vol. 8, pp. 35–100. (London: Taylor & Francis)
19. Ahotupa, M., Hietanen, E. and Nienstedt, W. (1981). Drug metabolizing enzyme activities in rats exposed to chlorinated phenols. In Mozsik, G., Hänninen, O. and Javor, T. (eds.). *Advances in Physiological Sciences*, Vol. 29, pp. 421–31. (Oxford: Pergamon Press)
20. Mulder, G. J. (1974). On non-specific inhibition of rat liver microsomal UDP glucuronyltransferase by some drugs. *Biochem. Pharmacol.*, **23,** 1283–91
21. Lilienblum, W., Walli, A. K. and Bock, K. W. (1982). Differential induction of rat liver microsomal UDP-glucuronosyltransferase activities by various inducing agents. *Biochem. Pharmacol.*, **31,** 907–13

22. Ahotupa, M. and Mäntylä, E. (1983). Comparison of the inducibilities of UDP-glucuronosyltransferase and polysubstrate mono-oxygenase activities in mice exposed to 20 model xenobiotics. *Biochem. Pharmacol.*, **32,** 2612–5
23. Suolinna, E. M. and Mäntylä, E. (1980). Glucuronide and sulphate conjugation in isolated liver cells from control and phenobarbital- or PCB-treated rats. *Biochem. Pharmacol.*, **29,** 2963–8
24. Mulder, G. J. (1974). Heterogeneity of hepatic microsomal uridine diphosphate glucuronyltransferase: a critical evaluation. *Biochem. Soc. Trans.*, **2,** 1172–6
25. Pang, K. S., Koster, H., Halsema, I. C. M., Scholtens, E. and Mulder, G. J. (1981). Aberrant pharmacokinetics of harmol in the perfused rat liver preparation: sulfate and glucuronide conjugations. *J. Pharmacol. Exp. Ther.*, **219,** 134–40
26. Mulder, G. J. (1984). High-rate intestinal conjugation of 4-methylumbelliferone during intravenous infusion in the rat *in vivo*. *Biochem. Pharmacol.*, **33,** 2341–4
27. Meerman, J. H. N. and Mulder, G. J. (1981). Prevention of the hepatotoxic action of *N*-hydroxy-2-acetylaminofluorene in the rat by inhibition of *N-O*-sulfation by pentachlorophenol. *Life Sci.*, **28,** 2361–5
28. Pang, K. S. and Terrell, J. A. (1981). Retrograde perfusion to probe the heterogeneous distribution of hepatic drug metabolizing enzymes in rats. *J. Pharmacol. Exp. Ther.*, **216,** 339–46
29. Koster, H., Halsema, I., Scholtens, E., Pang, K. S. and Mulder, G. J. (1982). Kinetics of sulfation and glucuronidation of harmol in the perfused rat liver preparation. Disappearance of aberrancies in glucuronidation kinetics by inhibition of sulfation. *Biochem. Pharmacol.*, **31,** 3023–8
30. Koster, H., Halsema, I., Scholtens, E., Knippers, M. and Mulder, G. J. (1981). Dose-dependent shifts in the sulfation and glucuronidation of phenolic compounds in the rat *in vivo* and in isolated hepatocytes. The role of saturation of phenol sulfotransferase. *Biochem. Pharmacol.*, **30,** 2569–75
31. Mulder, G. J. *et al.* (1984). *Biochem. Pharmacol.*, **33,** 3081–7

Section 2
Multiple Forms of UDP-Glucuronosyltranferases

Chairman: I. M. Arias

4
UDP-Glucuronyltransferase: problems within a biological 'family'

J. ROY CHOWDHURY, N. ROY CHOWDHURY, P. M. NOVIKOFF, A. B. NOVIKOFF AND I. M. ARIAS

Cytochrome P-450, glutathione-s-transferase (GSHTase) and uridine diphosphate glucuronyltransferase (UDPGTase) constitute the three major drug metabolizing systems in mammalian liver, and are also found in fish. From an evolutionary point of view, they have been around for a long time and, therefore, are likely to have high survival value as well as biologic adaptation. Each was discovered as a biochemical activity which initially served as the basis for nomenclature and function. Initially, each was assumed to constitute a group of enzymes which could be functionally separated by substrate specificity; much later, purification of specific enzymes demonstrated that this conclusion was invalid. Eventually individual proteins were purified within each functional group. Because GSHTases are soluble enzymes, this accomplishment preceded similar observations with P-450s and UDPGTases which are intrinsic membrane proteins; their purification had to await development of techniques for solubilizing and reconstituting the activities of membrane proteins. As shown in Table 4.1, each of the three functions has now been shown to reflect participation of

Table 4.1 Summary of published data regarding the multiplicity of hepatic cytochrome P-450, GSHTase and UDPGTase

Name	P-450	GSHTase	UDPGT
Site	ER	Cytosol	ER
Number	13	6 (Yaa, Ycc, Yac Ybb, Yb′b′, Ybb′)	6
Structure	*Monomer*	*Dimer*	*Oligomer*
MW (native)	45–60 000	45–60 000	?
mRNA	? 13	4 (Ya, Yb, Yc, Yb′)	1
Cloned genes	3	Ya	

ER, endoplasmic reticulum; Y subscript designations for GSHTase refer to purified monomeric subunits a family of enzymes. The data in Table 4.1 represent the current status; new members of the families are continuously being identified on the basis of protein structure, mRNA sequencing and gene cloning. Like most biological families, there are certain similarities between members which, in these three families, are:

(1) There is overlapping substrate specificity within each family.
(2) The individual native enzymes or their subunits have similar size and are usually separable on the basis of charge; nevertheless, whenever protein structure has been examined, there are major differences in primary structure as well as considerable homology.
(3) When studied in terms of enzymatic function or individual proteins, the apparent halflife for each member of each family is approximately 24 hours.
(4) Each family is regulated by increased synthesis (induction) as, for example after administration of phenobarbital and other drugs, and by reduced degradation (stabilization) which is usually hormonally and/or nutritionally mediated. These factors and the relative abundance of each of the three families permit large variations in concentration within various cells and tissues as required by metabolic need.
(5) There is a relatively similar pattern for the development of enzyme activity within each group in comparing the three groups. With few exceptions, enzymatic activity is very low in fetal liver and matures postnatally within a few days.

It is likely that there are numerous mutations which affect members of these three families in view of their multiplicity, evolutionary preservation and structural similarities; however, detection of such mutants depends on their phenotypic manifestations. Two inheritable defects in P-450s have been described after observing adverse drug reactions in animal or human patients. Defective P-450-mediated hydroxylation of the 4-position of debrisoquine potentiates hypotensive effects of the drug and has been described in approximately 15% of the population. No naturally occurring phenotypic manifestation of this defect has been described and, therefore, without the observation of potentiated drug action, the defect would probably not be known.

The situation is different with respect to defects in UDPGTases – at least for the enzyme which is involved in the conversion of bilirubin to a glucuronide conjugate. Deficiency in this function produces non-haemolytic unconjugated hyperbilirubinaemia which is usually severe enough to produce clinical jaundice and is, therefore, readily detected.

Deficient hepatic UDPGT activity has been demonstrated in six pathobiologic states: (1) Gunn rats[1], (2) Crigler–Najjar syndrome (Type 1) patients[2], (3) Crigler–Najjar syndrome (Type 2) patients[3], (4) Gilbert's syndrome in man[4], (5) Gilbert's syndrome in Bolivian squirrel monkeys[5,6], and the most common form, (6) neonatal unconjugated hyperbilirubinaemia in man and monkeys[7]. In each disorder, reduced hepatic UDPGT activity was demonstrated when homogenates or microsomes were incubated with UDPGA and bilirubin or several other glucuronide acceptors.

The number and availability of these mutants and progress in UDPGTase purification[8–10] prompted our efforts to purify UDPGT(s) from the liver of normal and mutant rats, squirrel monkeys and man. Our goals are to determine the structure of these enzymes and develop probes to characterize their regulation, development and molecular manipulation. Based upon the accomplishments of Tukey and Tephly[8], Weatherill and Burchell[9,10], Gorski and Kasper[11], Burchell[12], Bock[13] and collaborations with Burchell and Tephly and their associates, we have made progress toward these aims.

MATERIALS AND METHODS

Congeneic homozygous normal and mutant (UDPGTase deficient) rats were bred by Dr A. D. Moscioni, Department of Pediatrics, University of Chicago, USA. An existing strain of Gunn rats was bred with an inbred RHA strain and backcrossed at several generations; inbreeding was continued for 35 generations. Homozygous normal and mutant rats equally accepted skin grafts. These animals were prepared to avoid strain differences in UDPGTase activities within different isoforms.

A method was developed for isolation of UDPGTase isoforms from liver microsomes of mutant (Gunn) and congeneic normal controls. Details have been submitted for publication[14,15]; however, a brief description follows.

Microsomes were prepared from decapitated male Wistar or Gunn rats following liver perfusion and homogenization with 150 mmol/l KCl, and centrifugation (900 *g* for 10 min, 12 000 *g* for 15 min and 105 000 *g* for 1 h). Solubilization was with Emulgen 911 and, following centrifugation (105 000 *g*) the supernatant was chromatofocused (pH 9.4–6.0) on PBE 94. Fractions which eluted at pH 8.9 were pooled and fractionated after UDP-hexanolamine-sepharose 4B chromatography (sequential elution with 30 mmol/l KCl, 50 μmol/l UDPGA and 5 mmol/l UDPGA). Fractions were eluted at pH 8.4 (peak III), 7.8 (peak IV) and 7.5 (peak V) and were concentrated and purified by h.p.l.c.[15].

Fractions of chromatographic eluates were assayed for UDPGT activity using testosterone, oestrone, β-oestradiol, androsterone, 1-naphthol, bilirubin, 4-nitrophenol, 4-methylumbelliferone and aniline as glucuronide receptors. For reconstitution of UDPGT activity, phosphatidylcholine liposomes were prepared. To enzyme assays of chromatographic fractions, phosphatidylcholine liposomes were added (1 mg/ml for bilirubin and 0.1 mg/ml for other substrates) to samples in Emulgen 911. Bilirubin glucuronide formation was assayed at pH 7.8, 4-nitrophenol and 4-methylumbelliferone at pH 7.4, and all other activities at pH 8.0. Enzyme concentrations were rate-limiting and glucuronide formation was linear with incubation time.

SDS-PAGE was performed with and without treatment with 2-mercaptoethanol. Potential protein bands were identified after staining with Coomassie brilliant blue, and gels were also stained with periodic acid Schiff (PAS) stain to identify glycoproteins.

Purified UDPGTases from various chromatographic peaks were labelled with ^{125}I and digested with staphylococcal V8 for 4 h followed by electrophoresis on a 10–26% gradient SDS-PAGE gel for 16 h with 75 V at 11°C. Detection was by radioautography.

Amino acid analysis was performed in a Beckman analyser after hydrolysis of protein in gel slices in 6 mmol/l HCl at 110°C for 16 h.

Molecular weights of purified non-denatured UDPGTases were determined by comparison with markers of known molecular weight in terms of elution from a Biogel A 1.5 m column equilibrated with 25 mmol/l ethanolamine acetate (pH 8.0) containing 0.05% Emulgen 911. Results were not corrected for detergent.

In collaboration with Dr Jung, SUNY, Buffalo, NY, target analysis was utilized to estimate molecular weights of native UDPGTases in microsomal membranes[15]. The principle of this procedure is that when a macromolecule is hit by high energy radiation, it disintegrates. The probability of being hit increases with increasing molecular size. Thus, the minimum 'functional size' of a molecule can be determined by an empirical formula from the dose required to reduce the biological activity of a molecule to 37% of its activity in the normal state (D_{37}).

A suspension of rat liver microsomes in Tris-HCl (0.1 mmol/l, pH 8.0) was layered on aluminum trays to a thickness of 1.25 mm and flash-frozen in liquid nitrogen. Radiation doses ranging from 0.5–21 megarads were delivered by a van de Graffe generator. Following radiation, the samples were thawed and UDPGTase activities for various substrates were determined using UDP-*N*-acetylglucosamine as an activator. In preliminary experiments, we determined that the required concentration of the activator was not affected by the radiation dose. Rates of glucuronidation were linear with time and microsomal protein concentration. The 'functional molecular size' was determined (Kempner) from the following formula:

$$\text{Functional molecular weight} = (6.6/D_{37}) \times 100\,000$$

A polyvalent rabbit antiserum against rat liver UDPGTase (Isoform III) was coupled with horseradish peroxidase and is being utilized (P. Novikoff and A. B. Novikoff) for light and electron microscopic studies of tissue and subcellular localization.

RESULTS

Six enzymically active peaks were eluted after chromatofocusing of the microsomal fraction of Wistar rat livers. The following elution pH peaks were observed: pH 8.9 (peak I), 8.4 (peak II), pH 8.0 (peak III), pH 7.8 (peak IV), pH 7.5 (peak V) and pH 6.5 (peak VI). Peak I was subfractionated into peaks Ia, Ib and Ic by affinity chromatography on UDP-hexanolamine-sepharose 4B. Enzymatically active peaks were concentrated and purified by h.p.l.c. to apparent homogeneity. SDS-PAGE revealed single protein bands for each of UDPGTase isoform, except Peak III which had two closely migrating bands; apparent molecular weights ranged from 50 000 to 56 000. Protein migration was not altered by prior treatment by 2-mercaptoethanol. UDPGTase activities for different substrates in purified isoforms from congeneic and Gunn rat liver are shown in Table 4.2.

In UDPGTase isoforms from normal rat liver, with the exception of peak Ic isoform of UDPGTase for which we currently lack a natural metabolite as substrate, each isoform had activity toward one or more endogenous substrate. Peaks II and III isoforms had activity for the 17-OH steroids, testosterone and β-oestradiol. Peak IV isoform had activity for the 3-OH androgenic steroid, androsterone. Peak VI was active toward the 3-OH steroids, oestrone and β-oestradiol. Oestradiol was glucuronidated in the 17-OH position by the peak II isoform and in the 3-OH position by the peak VI isoform. The peak V isoform was distinct in that it appeared specific for bilirubin glucuronidation.

In comparable studies of the UDPGTase isoforms from Gunn rat liver, peak Ic enzyme had already reduced activity for 4-nitrophenol (20%), 1-naphthol (10%) and 4-methylumbelliferone (10%). When the assay was performed in 15 mmol/l diethylnitrosamine, activities for 4-nitrophenol and 4-methylumbelliferone increased to normal levels; activity for 1-naphthol increased to 50%. Activities in peaks II, III, IV and VI were the same as in comparable preparations from normal rat liver. A major finding was the inability to detect bilirubin glucuronidation by peak V protein; an enzymically inactive protein was eluted at the pH and elution volume of the normal peak V isoform. This protein comigrated with normal peak V UDPGTase (53 000) on SDS-PAGE and was immunologically identified as UDPGT by 'Western blotting'.

In normal and Gunn rat liver preparations, proteins from chromatofocusing peaks Ib, II, III, IV and V were PAS-positive; peak Ia was PAS-negative, and peak Ic was too small to analyse. These observations suggest that most of the UDPGTase isoforms in normal and Gunn rat liver are glycoproteins.

As determined by agarose column chromatography in non-denaturing conditions, the apparent molecular weight of peak II, III and V isoforms in normal and Gunn rat liver preparations was approximately 310 000; however, no correction for detergent binding or complex formation was made. Radiation target analysis of normal and mutant Gunn rat liver microsomes revealed estimated molecular weights ranging from 100 000 to 116 000 suggesting that the native UDPGTases may exist as dimers which have subunits of 50 000–56 000 (Table 4.2). Although the results of target analysis are probably significant, they require confirmation by other analytical methods before the precise oligomeric structure of the isoforms can be established.

By immunodiffusion and immunoelectrophoresis using antiserum prepared against purified isoform III from normal rat liver, single lines of immunologic identity were observed with each of the purified isoforms from normal and Gunn rat liver.

Even though the various isoforms from normal and Gunn rat liver had similar subunit size and immunologic cross-reactivity, they apparently have different primary structures because amino acid analysis revealed a lack of identity among individual isoforms, and limited proteolysis produced different peptide maps for each isoform.

Immunomorphologic studies have, thus far, been performed in normal rat liver and kidney. In liver, immunoperoxidase localization was restricted to hepatocytes; plasma membrane and cytoplasm were negative, and all visible

Table 4.2 Elution pH, substrate specificity and estimated molecular weights of isoforms of UDP-glucuronosyltransferase purified from congeneic normal and Gunn rat liver microsomes

	Isoforms						
	Ia and b	*Ic*	*II*	*III*	*IV*	*V*	*VI*
Elution pH	8.9	8.9	8.4	8.0	7.8	7.5	6.5
Congeneic normal rats (JJ)	4-NP 1-naphthol 4-MUF 3-OH and 17-OH aromatic steroids	4-NP 1-napthol 4-MUF	17-OH-steroids; testosterone and oestradiol	same as II plus aniline	3-OH-androgens: androsterone and aetiocholonalone	bilirubin	3-OH aromatic oestrone and oestradiol
			4-NP 1-naphthol 4-MUF	*4-MUF*	*4-MUF*		
Mutant Gunn rats (jj)	normal	reduced to 10% of normal; activated to normal levels by DEN	normal	normal	normal	inactive	normal
Estimated isoform molecular weight for JJ and jj ($\times 10^3$)	50.52	56	52	52.53	53	53	several bands
Estimated native molecular weight (radiation target analysis) for JJ and jj ($\times 10^3$)	116	116	100	—	110	115	—

Isoforms were separated and purified, and enzyme activities were assayed after reconstitution with phosphatidylcholine liposomes.
Abbreviations: UDPGTase, UDP glucuronyltransferase; UDPGA, UDP glucuronic acid; SDS-PAGE, sodium dodecyl sulphate polyacrylamide-gel electrophoresis; UDPNAG, UDP-*N*-acetyl glucosamine; 4-NP, 4-nitrophenol; 4-MUF, 4-methylumbelliferone; DEN, diethylnitrosamine; PAS, periodic acid Schiff stain; JJ, homozygous normal; jj, homozygous mutant

reaction was associated with the perinuclear membrane and structures which, by light microscopy, appear to be endoplasmic reticulum. In the kidney, a similar subcellular localization was observed only in proximal convoluted tubular cells and, to a lesser degree, in distal convoluted tubular cells. Additional studies are in progress.

Although the several isoforms have some specificity, which is reminiscent of that observed with cytochrome P-450s and GSH-s-transferases, it is relative for some substrates. Additional studies are necessary to relate these observations to possible differences in tissue, cellular and subcellular localization of the various isoforms.

The findings with Gunn rat liver require special comment. The inheritable defect in Gunn rats is transmitted with the characteristics of an autosomal recessive trait, which has generally been viewed as resulting from a change in the primary structure of a specific UDPGTase. The problem may be more complex in view of defective glucuronidation of various phenolic aglycones associated with isoform Ic. In addition, DEN 15 mmol/l corrected the enzymatic defect on addition to isoform Ic, but did not restore bilirubin glucuronidation on addition to isoform V. There are several possible explanations for these findings: (1) Species and strain differences in UDPGTase may be responsible, as has been previously described for this enzyme(s) and others[16,17]. This possibility is unlikely because special efforts were made to inbreed normal and Gunn rats such that the control animals were congeneic with the Gunn rats. (2) UDPGTases may be hetero-oligomers (? dimers); *in vivo* the various isoforms may form a family of enzymes with distinct but partially overlapping functions; Ic and V may have a common subunit which is defective in the mutant. Confirmation of this hypothesis requires additional structural information and analysis of specific mRNAs. (3) Other possibilities include modification of Ic during purification and membrane lipid effects which can alter expression of enzyme activity.

Despite these problems, identificaton of six isoforms of UDPGTase in normal rat liver and the selective defects in Gunn rat liver clarify the results of many assays of UDPGTase, which used various substrates *in vivo* and *in vitro* in normal and Gunn rats. In particular, 4-methylumbelliferone and other phenols form glucuronides at reduced rates in Gunn rats whereas aniline and steroid hormone glucuronidation are normal.

We are using these methods to study UDPGTase isoforms in disorders characterized by non-haemolytic unconjugated hyperbilirubinaemia and defective glucuronide formation. Studies in Brazilian and Bolivian squirrel monkeys are in progress; similar studies will be performed when human biopsy tissue is available.

ACKNOWLEDGEMENTS

This research was partially supported by grants from the USPHS (AM 2019 and AM 17702). One of us (J.R.C.) is a recipient of a Research Career Development Award (AM 1016).

References

1. Arias, I. M. (1959). A defect in microsomal function in nonhemolytic acholuric jaundice. *J. Histochem. Cytochem.*, **7**, 250–2
2. Wolkoff, A. W., Roy Chowdhury, J. and Arias, I. M. (1977). Hereditary jaundice and disorders of bilirubin metabolism. In Stanbury, J. B., Wyngaarden, J. B., Fredrickson, D. S., Goldstein, J. L. and Brown, M. S. (eds.). *The Metabolic Basis of Inherited Diseases*, 5th Edn., pp. 1385–440. (New York: McGraw-Hill)
3. Arias, I. M., Gartner, L. M., Cohen, M., Ben-Ezzer, J. and Levi, A. J. (1969). Chronic nonhemolytic unconjugated hyperbilirubinemia with glucuronyl transferase deficiency: Clinical, biochemical, pharmacological and genetic evidence for heterogeneity. *Am. J. Med.*, **47**, 395–409
4. Arias, I. M. and London, I. M. (1957). Bilirubin glucuronide formation in *in vitro*: Demonstration of a defect in Gilbert's disease. *Science*, **126**, 563-4
5. Roy Chowdhury, J., Portman, O. W., Roy Chowdhury, N., Alexander, M., Cornelius, C. E. and Arias, I. M. (1982). Mechanism of fasting hyperbilirubinemia: Studies in Bolivian squirrel monkeys. *Hepatology*, **2**, 723
6. Roy Chowdhury, N., Portman, O., Roy Chowdhury, J., Arias, I. M. and Cornelius, C. E. (1982). A primate model of Gilbert's syndrome. *Gastroenterology*, **82**, 1225
7. Gartner, L. M., Lee, K., Vaisman, S., Land, D. and Zarafu, I. (1977). Development of bilirubin transport and metabolism in the newborn Rhesus monkey. *J. Pediatr.*, **90**, 513–31
8. Tukey, R. H. and Tephly, T. R. (1981). Purification and properties of rabbit liver estrone and *p*-nitrophenol UDP-glucuronyltransferases. *Arch. Biochem. Biophys.*, **209**, 565–78
9. Weatherill, P. J. and Burchell, B. (1978). Reactivation of a pure defective UDP-glucuronyltransferase from homozygous Gunn rat liver. *FEBS Lett.*, **87**, 207–11
10. Weatherill, P. J. and Burchell, B. (1980). The separation and purification of rat liver UDP-glucuronyltransferase activities towards testosterone and oestrone. *Biochem. J.*, **189**, 377–80
11. Gorski, J. P. and Kasper, C. B. (1977). Purification and properties of microsomal UDP-glucuronyltransferase from rat liver. *J. Biol. Chem.*, **252**, 1336–443
12. Burchell, B. (1978). Substrate specificity and properties of uridine diphosphate glucuronyltransferase purified to apparent homogeneity from phenobarbital-treated rat liver. *Biochem. J.*, **173**, 749–57
13. Bock, K. W., Josting, D., Lillienblum, W. and Pfeil, H. (1979). Purification of rat liver microsomal UDP-glucuronyltransferase. Separation of two enzyme forms inducible by 3-methylcholanthrene or phenobarbital. *Eur. J. Biochem.*, **98**, 19–26
14. Roy Chowdhury, J., Roy Chowdhury, N., Falany, C. N., Tephly, T. R. and Arias, I. M. (1982). Is there a specific UDP-glucuronyltransferase (UDPGT) for bilirubin? Purification and characterization of multiple forms of UDPGT. *Hepatology*, **2**, 722
15. Roy Chowdhury, J., Roy Chowdhury, N., Falany, C. N., Tephly, T. R. and Arias, I. M. (????). Isolation and characterization of multiple forms of rat liver uridine diphosphoglucuronate glucuronosyltransferase. (submitted)
16. Kempner, E. S. and Schlegel, W. (1979). Size determination of enzymes by radiation inactivation. *Anal. Biochem.*, **92**, 2–10
17. Matsui, M. and Watanabe, H. K. (1982). Classification and genetic expression of Wistar rats with high and low hepatic microsomal UDP-glucuronosyltransferase activity towards androsterone. *Biochem. J.*, **202**, 171–4

5
Comparison of rat and rabbit liver UDP-glucuronosyltransferase activities

C. N. FALANY, R. B. KIRKPATRICK AND T. R. TEPHLY

INTRODUCTION

Our laboratory has studied UDP-glucuronosyltransferase (UDPGT) activities isolated from rabbit liver, and has identified and characterized a *p*-nitrophenol (PNP)-UDPGT and an oestrone UDPGT[1,2]. Our knowledge of separation methodology, substrate specificities and physical–chemical characteristics of these enzymes has increased substantially. Recently, we have begun investigating the heterogeneity of UDPGT in livers of female Sprague-Dawley rats and have uncovered numerous differences between rat and rabbit liver UDPGT activities[3,4]. Substrates of physiologic (steroids) and pharmacologic nature have been used to assess the qualitative and quantitative differences in hepatic UDPGT activities in rat and rabbit liver. This paper summarizes similarities and differences that exist between UDPGT activities as isolated from rat and rabbit liver.

MATERIALS AND METHODS

Materials

[4-^{14}C]oestrone (57 mCi/mmol), [4-^{14}C]testosterone (50 mCi/mmol), [1,2-^{3}H]androsterone (40–60 mCi/mmol), [1-^{14}C]naphthol (4.3 mCi/mmol), [4-^{14}C]β-oestradiol (50 mCi/mmol) and [glucuronyl-U-^{14}C]uridine diphosphate glucuronic acid (180 mCi/mmol) were purchased from New England Nuclear, Boston, MA. *p*-Nitro[U-^{14}C]phenol (24 mCi/mmol) was obtained from California Bionuclear Corporation, Sun Valley, CA. [*N*-methyl-^{14}C]Morphine hydrochloride (40 mCi/mmol) was obtained from Amersham, Arlington Heights, IL. L-α-Phosphatidylcholine (egg yolk Type XI-E), UDP-glucuronic acid, oestrone β-oestradiol, *p*-nitrophenol, testosterone, 1-naphthol and 4-methylumbelliferone were purchased from Sigma Chemical Company, St. Louis, MO. Morphine sulphate was obtained from Mallinckrodt Chemical Works, St. Louis, MO. Lithocholic acid (5β-cholanic acid-3α-ol) and chenodeoxycholanic acid (5β-cholic acid-3α,7α-diol) were obtained from Calbiochem–Behring, La Jolla, CA. Chromatofocusing® materials were obtained from Pharmacia Fine Chemicals, Piscataway, NJ. Emulgen 911 was purchased from Kao Atlas Ltd, Tokyo, Japan. Bio-Rad dye protein assay reagent was obtained from Bio-Rad Laboratories, Richmond, CA. All other chemicals were of analytical grade. UDP-Hexanolamine Sepharose 4B affinity resin was prepared as previously described[1].

Assays

Oestrone, β-oestradiol, *p*-nitrophenol, 1-naphthol, androsterone and aetiocholanolone UDP-glucuronosyltransferase activities were determined using radiolabelled aglycone substrates in the assays as previously reported[3]. Bile acid glucuronidation activity was assayed utilizing [^{14}C]UDPGA as previously described[5]. All reactions were performed at 37°C with 5 mmol/l UDP-glucuronic acid in the presence of 100 μg of phosphatidylcholine. However, when alternate substrates were used, 10 mmol/l UDP-glucuronic acid was utilized. All reactions were linear with respect to time and protein concentration. Protein concentrations were determined using the Bio-Rad protein assay originally developed by Bradford[6].

Glucuronidation of epitestosterone, epiandrosterone and 17α-OH progesterone was determined using [^{14}C]UDPGA with a modification of the assay conditions described for determining the site of β-oestradiol glucuronidation[3]. The reactions were stopped and extracted with 10 ml dichloromethane, and the labelled steroid glucuronide in aqueous phase was identified as described previously for the β-oestradiol glucuronides[3].

Separation and characterization of rabbit liver estrone and *p*-nitrophenol UDP-glucuronosyltransferases

The procedure for the purification of oestrone and *p*-nitrophenol UDPGT from untreated female New Zealand rabbit liver microsomes has been previously described[2]. Briefly, liver microsomes were solubilized with 0.5 mg of Emulgen 911/mg of microsomal protein. Oestrone and *p*-nitrophenol UDPGT activities were separated by chromatography on DE-52. The oestrone and *p*-nitrophenol UDPGT activities were applied to UDP-hexanolamine Sepharose 4B columns. Both UDPGT activities were adsorbed to the UDP-hexanolamine Sepharose 4B and specifically eluted with UDPGA[2].

Separation and purification of rat liver *p*-nitrophenol 3α-OH steroid and 17β-OH steroid UDP-glucuronosyltransferases

The procedure for purification of *p*-nitrophenol, 3α-OH steroid (androsterone) and 17β-OH steroid (testosterone) UDP-glucuronosyltransferases has been previously described[4]. Liver microsomes were solubilized with 0.5 mg of Emulgen 911/mg of microsomal protein. The UDP-glucuronosyltransferase activities were separated by a chromatofocusing procedure from pH 9–7. The fractions obtained from the chromatofocusing procedure which contained UDP-glucuronosyltransferase activity were further separated and purified by chromatography on UDP-hexanolamine Sepharose 4B.

SDS-polyacrylamide gel electrophoresis

Polyacrylamide slab gel electrophoresis was performed in the presence of sodium dodecyl sulphate (SDS) in a Hoefer Scientific Model 600 apparatus and using the buffer system described by Laemmli[7]. Samples were pretreated by the addition of β-mercaptoethanol and SDS to final concentrations of 5 and 1%, respectively, and placed in a boiling-water bath for 10 min. Following electrophoresis, the slabs were stained for 2 h in a mixture of isopropanol : acetic acid : H_2O (25 : 10 : 65, v/v) which contained 0.1% Coomassie G-250 and destained with isopropanol : acetic acid : water (10 : 10 : 80, v/v). Minimum subunit molecular weights were estimated by comparison to commercial standards (Pharmacia).

Determination of isoelectric points of rat and rabbit liver UDP-glucuronosyltransferase activities

The pI values were determined for rabbit liver oestrone and *p*-nitrophenol UDP-glucuronosyltransferase activities by both polyacrylamide isoelectric focusing and chromatofocusing. The procedure for polyacrylamide isoelectric focusing of purified oestrone and *p*-nitrophenol UDP-glucuronosyltransferases has been described[1]. The pI values for oestrone and *p*-nitrophenol UDP-glucuronosyltransferase activities were obtained during chromatofocusing of solubilized rabbit liver microsomes utilizing a pH 9–6 gradient. Chromatofocusing of solubilized rabbit liver microsomes was performed identically to the procedure utilized for solubilized rat liver microsomes. Both polyacrylamide isoelectric focusing and chromatofocusing gave very similar pI values for oestrone and *p*-nitrophenol UDP-glucuronosyltransferase activities.

The pI values for rat liver UDP-glucuronosyltransferase activities were obtained following chromatofocusing of solubilized microsomes utilizing a pH 9–7 gradient. However, when UDP-hexanolamine affinity purified UDP-glucuronosyltransferase activities were chromatofocused, the pI values were very similar to those obtained when solubilized microsomes were used.

RESULTS

A comparison for rat and rabbit liver PNP-UDPGT is shown in Table 5.1. Rat liver PNP-UDPGT represents that isoenzyme which was resolved by chromatofocusing and purified by elution of the UDP-hexanolamine affinity column with high UDPGA[4]. The PNP-UDPGT does not appear to react with any known physiological substrates. It can be seen that, although subunit

Table 5.1 Comparison of rat and rabbit *p*-nitrophenol UDP-glucuronosyltransferase activities

	Rabbit	*Rat*
Subunit molecular weight[a]	57 000	56 000
pI value	6.8[b]	9.0[c]
K_m (PNP)	1.5 mmol/l	0.3 mmol/l
K_m (UDPGA)	2.0 mmol/l	0.3 mmol/l
Affinity column elution[d]	high UDPGA (1–5 mmol/l)	high UDPGA (1 mmol/l)
Induction by 3-methylcholanthrene[e]	−	+

[a] Subunit molecular weight determined following SDS-polyacrylamide gel electrophoresis in 10% acrylamide by the method of Laemmli[7]
[b] pI value determined by chromatofocusing of solubilized rabbit liver microsomes and polyacrylamide slab gel isoelectric focusing[1]
[c] pI value determined by chromatofocusing
[d] The concentration of UDPGA used to specifically elute the *p*-nitrophenol UDP-glucuronosyltransferase activities from the UDP-hexanolamine affinity column
[e] Indicates an increase in microsomal *p*-nitrophenol UDP-glucuronosyltransferase activity and in the purified *p*-nitrophenol UDP-glucuronosyltransferase following treatment of rats for 3 days with 3-methylcholanthrene (40 mg/kg in corn oil)

molecular weights are similar (57 000 vs. 56 000), the rat liver enzyme is induced by pretreatment of animals with 3-methylcholanthrene. The rabbit liver enzyme is not induced. Other differences are observed in pI values, Michaelis constants (K_m) for PNP and UDPGA. Each protein, as adsorbed by the UDP-hexanolamine affinity chromatographic procedures, is eluted with relatively high concentrations of UDPGA.

The substrate specificity of rabbit and rat liver PNP-UDPGT is indicated in Table 5.2. Both rat and rabbit liver PNP-UDPGT activities readily employ

Table 5.2 Substrate specificity of *p*-nitrophenol rat and rabbit UDP-glucuronosyltransferase activity

Substrates	*Rabbit*	*Rat*
p-Nitrophenol	++	++
1-Naphthol	++	++
4-Methylumbelliferone	++	++
Oestrone	±	−−
β-Oestradiol	±	−−
Testosterone	−−	−−
Androsterone	−−	−−
Morphine	−−	−−

PNP, 1-naphthol and 4-methylumbelliferone as substrates. Oestrone and β-oestradiol also appear to be glucuronidated to a very slight degree by the rabbit liver enzyme, but these substrates are not glucuronidated by the rat liver PNP-UDPGT. Neither enzyme conjugates testosterone, androsterone or morphine.

Although only one PNP-UDPGT has been identified so far in rabbit liver, when resolving rat liver PNP-UDPGT activities, it was possible to demonstrate two different PNP-UDPGT activities. One PNP-UDPGT activity eluted from the chromatofocusing column at pH 9.0 and a second at pH 8.5. As discussed above, the PNP-UDPGT which eluted at pH 9.0 did not react with any of the physiological substrates tested; whereas the second PNP-UDPGT readily employs steroids as substrates provided that they possess a 17β-hydroxy group. Therefore, we have termed the second PNPGT 17-OH steroid UDP-glucuronosyltransferase. These proteins can be dissociated by a number of physio–chemical characteristics as well as by kinetic properties. Subunit molecular weights, pI values, K_m values for PNP, substrate specificity, elution characteristics from the UDP-hexanolamine affinity column and inducibility with 3-methylcholanthrene display marked differences between these proteins (Tables 5.3 and 5.4). Limited proteolysis using *Staphylococcus aureus* protease yielded

Table 5.3 Comparison of *p*-nitrophenol UDP-glucuronosyltransferase activities in liver isolated from female Sprague-Dawley rats

	PNPGT	*Steroid 17-OH GT (PNP)*
Subunit molecular weight[a]	56 000	50 000
pI value[b]	9.0	8.5
K_m PNP[c]	0.3 mmol/l	1.7 mmol/l
K_m UDPGA[c]	0.3 mmol/l	0.3 mmol/l
Affinity column elution[d]	high UDPGA (1 mmol/l)	low UDPGA (<50 μmol/l)
Inducibility with 3-methylcholanthrene[e]	+	−

[a] Subunit molecular weight determined following SDS-polyacrylamide gel electrophoresis in 10% acrylamide by the method of Laemmli[7]
[b] pI value determined by chromatofocusing
[c] Calculated from double reciprocal plots of velocity vs. substrate concentrations in the presence of high concentrations of the non-variable substrate
[d] The concentration of UDPGA used to specifically elute the *p*-nitrophenol UDP-glucuronosyltransferase activities from the UDP-hexanolamine affinity column
[e] Indicates an increase in microsomal *p*-nitrophenol UDP-glucuronosyltransferase activity and in the purified *p*-nitrophenol UDP-glucuronosyltransferase following treatment of rats for 3 days with 3-methylcholanthrene (40 mg/kg in corn oil)

Table 5.4 Substrate specificity of *p*-nitrophenol and 17-OH steroid UDP-glucuronosyltransferase activities

Substrates	*PNP-UDPGT*	*17-OH Steroid UDPGT*
PNP	+	+
1-Napthol	+	+
4-Methylumbelliferone	+	−
Testosterone	−	+
β-Oestradiol	−	+
Oestrone	−	−
Androsterone	−	−
Aetiocholanolone	−	−
Morphine	−	−
Lithocholic acid	−	−
Chenodeoxycholic acid	−	−

different peptide maps. The substrate specificities of PNP-UDPGT and 17β-OH steroid UDPGT are shown in Table 5.4. The PNP-UDPGT from rat liver reacts with PNP, 1-naphthol and 4-methylumbelliferone. The 17β-OH steroid UDPGT glucuronidates testosterone and the 17β-OH position of β-oestradiol, and also reacts with PNP and 1-naphthol. However, the 17-OH steroid UDPGT does not utilize 4-methylumbelliferone as a substrate. Furthermore, the 4-methylumbelliferone does not exert inhibition of testosterone or PNP glucuronidation as catalysed by 17β-OH steroid UDPGT. In contrast, 4-methylumbelliferone exerts competitive inhibition of *p*-nitrophenol glucuronidation catalysed by PNP-UDPGT. Also, the K_m for *p*-nitrophenol is 0.3 mmol/l and 1.7 mmol/l for the PNP-UDPGT and 17β-OH steroid UDPGT, respectively. The 17β-OH steroid UDPGT does not catalyse the glucuronidation of oestrone, androsterone, aetiocholanolone, morphine, lithocholic acid or chenodeoxycholic acid.

Chromatofocusing and UDP-hexanolamine affinity chromatographic procedures have also allowed for the separation and purification of another steroid UDPGT. This transferase has been termed 3α-OH steroid UDPGT because it appears to be capable of catalysing the glucuronidation of 3α-OH androgenic steroids, such as androsterone and aetiocholanolone (Table 5.5). It also catalyses the glucuronidation of the 3α-OH position of lithocholic acid, chenodeoxycholic acid and other bile acids possessing a 3α-OH moiety[5]. The transferase was named for its reaction with androgenic steroid substrates since reactivity with the androgenic substrates is greater than that for bile acids. Furthermore, bile acid substrates are only glucuronidated to a substantial degree in pathologic conditions[8–10].

Table 5.5 Substrate specificity of steroid UDP-glucuronosyltransferase activities isolated from female Sprague-Dawley rat liver

Substrate	*17-OH Steroid UDPGT*	*3-OH Androgen UDPGT*
Testosterone	+	−
Epitestosterone	−	−
β-Oestradiol	+	−
5α-Androstan-17β-ol-3-one	+	−
Oestrone	−	−
17α-OH Progesterone	−	−
Androsterone	−	+
Aetiocholanolone	−	+
Lithocholic acid	−	+
Chenodeoxycholic acid	−	+
Lithocholic acid-24-methyl ester	−	+
Epiandrosterone	−	−

We should note that the steroid UDPGT activities are specific for configuration as well as the position of the hydroxyl on the steroid nucleus. The 17β-OH steroid UDPGT glucuronidates testosterone and β-oestradiol. In addition, 5α-androstan-17β-ol-3-one is also utilized as substrate (Table 5.5). However, steroids with α-substituted hydroxyl moieties at the 17-position are not glucuronidated, i.e. epitestosterone and 17α-hydroxy progesterone (Table 5.5). We have also determined that the 3α-OH steroid UDPGT is incapable of catalysing the glucuronidation of 3β-hydroxy substituted steroids, i.e. epiandrosterone

(Table 5.5). It is interesting to note that, when the 24-methyl ester of lithocholic acid is employed as substrate, it serves as a better substrate than lithocholic acid; thus indicating that not only is the carboxylic not glucuronidated but, when that carboxylic acid is esterified, lithocholic acid appears to be a more reactive substrate. Also, the presence of the 24-methyl ester shifts the pH maxima for lithocholic acid from 6.9 to 8.0, which is the pH maxima for androsterone glucuronidation[5].

Table 5.6 Comparison of steroid UDP-glucuronosyltransferase activities isolated from Sprague-Dawley rat liver

	17β-OH Steroid UDPGT	*3α-OH Steroid Bile/acid UDPGT*
Subunit molecular weight[a]	50 000	52 000
pI value[b]	8.5	7.8
K_m[c]		
Testosterone	13 μmol/l	–
β-Oestradiol	25 μmol/l	–
PNP	1.7 mmol/l	–
UDPGA	0.3 mmol/l	0.3 mmol/l
Androsterone	–	10 μmol/l
Aetiocholanolone	–	5 μmol/l
Lithocholic acid	–	50 μmol/l
Chenodeoxycholic acid	–	100 μmol/l
Competitive inhibitors[d]		
Epitestosterone (50 μmol/l)	+	+
17α-OH Progesterone (50 μmol/l)	+	+
Epiandrosterone (50 μmol/l)	+	+

[a] Subunit molecular weight determined following SDS-polyacrylamide gel electrophoresis in 10% acrylamide by the method of Laemmli[7]
[b] pI value determined by chromatofocusing
[c] Calculated from double reciprocal plots of velocity vs. substrate concentrations in the presence of high concentrations of the non-variable substrate
[d] Tested as inhibitors using testosterone glucuronidation activity of the 17β-OH steroid UDPGT and androsterone glucuronidation activity of the 3α-OH steroid/bile acid UDPGT

Other comparisons of the 3α-OH and 17β-OH steroid UDPGT activities obtained from Sprague-Dawley rats are shown in Table 5.6. Subunit molecular weights, pI values and kinetic constants all attest to the differences between these transferase activities. In addition, epitestosterone, 17α-OH progesterone and epiandrosterone, although not glucuronidated by either enzyme, can serve as competitive inhibitors of the glucuronidation of other substrates which react with these steroid UDPGT activities. Limited proteolysis using *Staph. aureus* protease generates different peptide maps as determined by SDS-polyacrylamide gel electrophoresis.

DISCUSSION

It would appear that rat liver possesses UDPGT activities which are quantitatively and qualitatively different from those observed in rabbit liver. We have been able to separate only one PNP-UDPGT activity from rabbit liver, whereas several occur in rat liver. Rat liver PNP-UDPGT activities are seen with different substrate specificities, inducibility to 3-methylcholanthrene, pI values and affinity for PNP. Terminology, as suggested by a recent workshop[11], has been assigned based on the utilization of physiologic substrates for one of the PNPGT activities, that is, the 17β-OH steroid UDPGT.

The 17β-OH steroid UDPGT appears not to react with 4-methylumbelliferone, although it does react with PNP and 1-naphthol. In addition, there appears to be marked specificity for the 17β-OH vs. the 17α-OH configuration of the steroid. Thus, it would appear that these enzymes which react with steroids have marked specificity for the steroid, although they appear to be capable of utilizing drug substrates in a far less specific fashion.

Bile acid glucuronidation, where the 3α-OH position is present, was expected to react with the 3-OH androgen UDPGT. Our studies demonstrated this[5]. Previous work suggested that testosterone and chenodeoxycholate glucuronidations were catalysed by the same protein[12]. Since the 17β-OH steroid UDPGT appeared to be quite specific toward the 17β-OH position and the 3α-OH steroid UDPGT appeared to be quite specific for the 3α-OH position, it is possible that previous work represents a mixture of these two proteins. We have also found similar results when ion exchange chromatography procedures were employed, and only through the use of chromatofocusing was it possible to separate these UDPGT activities.

ACKNOWLEDGEMENTS

These authors wish to acknowledge the assistance of Mrs Birgit Coffman, Elizabeth Swain and Jaime Puig in this research, which was supported by NIH grant GM26221.

References

1. Tukey, R. H. and Tephly, T. R. (1981). Purification and properties of rabbit liver estrone and *p*-nitrophenol UDP-glucuronyltransferases. *Arch. Biochem. Biophys.*, **209**, 565–78
2. Tukey, R. H., Robinson, R., Holm, B., Falany, C. N. and Tephly, T. R. (1982). A procedure for the rapid separation and purification of UDP-glucuronosyltransferases from rabbit liver microsomes. *Drug Metab. Dispos.*, **10**, 97-101
3. Falany, C. N., Chowdhury, J. R., Chowdhury, N. R. and Tephly, T. R. (1983). Steroid 3- and 17-OH UDP-glucuronosyltransferase activities in rat and rabbit liver microsomes. *Drug Metab. Dispos.*, **11**, 426–32
4. Falany, C. N. and Tephly, T. R. (1983). Separation, purification and characterization of three isoenzymes of UDP-glucuronyltransferase from rat liver microsomes. *Arch. Biochem. Biophys.*, **227**, 248–58
5. Kirkpatrick, R. B., Falany, C. N. and Tephly, T. R. (1984). Glucuronidation of bile acids by rat liver 3-OH androgen UDP-glucuronyltransferase. *J. Biol. Chem.*, **259**, 6176–80

6. Bradford, M. (1976). A rapid and sensitive method for the quantification of microgram quantities of protein utilizing the principle of protein–dye binding. *Anal. Biochem.*, **72,** 248–53
7. Laemmli, U. K. (1970). Cleavage of structural proteins during the assembly of the head of *Bacteriophase T4. Nature*, **227,** 680–5
8. Fröhling, W. and Stiehl, A. (1976). Bile salt glucuronides: Identification and quantitative analysis in the urine of patients with cholestasis. *Eur. J. Clin. Invest.*, **6,** 67–74
9. Back, P. (1976). Bile acid glucuronides, II: Isolation and identification of a chenodeoxycholic acid glucuronide from human plasma in intrahepatic cholestasis. *Hoppe Seylers Z. Physiol. Chem.*, **357,** 213–7
10. Back, P. (1976). Bile acid glucuronides. In Bianchi, L., Gerok, W. and Sickinger, K. (eds.). *Liver and Bile*, pp. 121–8. (Baltimore: University Park Press)
11. Bock, K. W., Burchell, B., Dutton, G. J., Hänninen, O., Mulder, G. J., Owens, I., Siest, G. and Tephly, T. R. (1983). UDP-Glucuronyltransferase activities: Guidelines for consistent interim terminology and assay conditions. *Biochem. Pharmacol.*, **32,** 953–5
12. Matern, H., Matern, S. and Gerok, W. (1982). Isolation and characterization of rat liver microsomal UDP-glucuronyltransferase activity towards chenodeoxycholic acid and testosterone as a single form of enzyme. *J. Biol. Chem.*, **257,** 7422–9

6
Immunochemical studies on a 3-methylcholanthrene-inducible UDP-glucuronosyltransferase of rat liver

K. W. BOCK AND W. LILIENBLUM

ABSTRACT

Our studies were aimed at elucidating functional and molecular properties of various isoenzymes of UDP-glucuronosyltransferase.

Studies with xenobiotic inducers suggested the presence of a 3-methylcholanthrene-inducible isoenzyme of UDP-glucuronosyltransferase (GT_{MC}) in rat liver. This isoenzyme, involved in the conjugation of planar phenols, may play a major role in the detoxication of carcinogenic aromatic hydrocarbons. The isoenzyme appears to be remarkably regioselective. For example, administration of 3-methylcholanthrene increased (5-fold) the conjugation of 3-hydroxy- but not of 9-hydroxybenzo(a)pyrene. In addition, diglucuronide formation of benzo(a)pyrene-3,6-quinol was increased 40-fold. The latter finding raises the possibility that more than one 3-methylcholanthrene-inducible isoenzyme of UDP-glucuronosyltransferase exists in liver microsomes.

GT_{MC} was purified to apparent homogeneity from livers of 3-methylcholanthrene-treated rats, and antibodies were raised in rabbits. Immunochemical studies suggested both some selectivity of the antibody for GT_{MC} and immunochemical similarities between various isoenzymes. Immunoblot analysis of purified GT_{MC} and of rat liver microsomes from variously pretreated rats revealed 54 000 and 56 000 polypeptides as the major components of GT_{MC}. However, other polypeptides were also stained by the antibody. The staining pattern was different when variously pretreated rat liver microsomes, microsomes from rat hepatoma cells, rat kidney and human liver were analysed. Further work is needed to characterize the different polypeptides stained by the antibody.

INTRODUCTION

Conjugation with glucuronic acid is a major pathway in the metabolism of lipid-soluble drugs and endogenous compounds such as bilirubin and steroids[1]. This reaction greatly facilitates their detoxication and elimination. Glucuronidation is catalysed by a family of closely related isoenzymes with different but overlapping substrate specificities[2–5]. Studies on the effects of xenobiotic inducers of UDP-glucuronosyltransferase (GT)[6–10] and on its perinatal development[11] indicated functional heterogeneity between groups of GT activities. In particular a 3-methylcholanthrene (MC)-inducible group of GT activities, operationally termed GT_1 activities, corresponded well with a late-fetal cluster of activities. This correspondence was suggestive of an independently regulated isoenzyme. The isoenzyme appeared to be particularly interesting for two reasons:

(1) The enzyme appears to be regulated by the so-called Ah locus which controls the synthesis of a cytosolic receptor protein for planar aromatic inducing agents, for which 3-methylcholanthrene is a prototype[12,13]. Following the translocation of the inducer–receptor complex into the nucleus, numerous structural genes are activated in a pleiotropic response, for example those of certain isoenzymes of cytochrome P-450[12,13] and of GT[13,14]. Interestingly the induced isoenzymes, e.g. P_1-450* and GT_{MC}* are primarily involved in the metabolism of planar aromatic compounds. They are genetically linked in their regulation by the Ah locus and functionally linked in their metabolism of aromatic hydrocarbons. For example, benzo(a)pyrene is oxidized by P_1-450 to 3-hydroxybenzo(a)pyrene which is subsequently conjugated with glucuronic acid by GT_{MC}.

(2) Following initiation of hepatocarcinogenesis in rats GT_{MC} is permanently increased in preneoplastic rat liver[15–18] (*see* Chapter 33).

Recently our laboratory was involved in studies on the functional and molecular properties of GT_{MC}. The following summarizes some recent advances in characterizing the substrate specificity and immunochemical properties of this isoenzyme.

REGIOSELECTIVITY OF GT_{MC} IN THE CONJUGATION OF BENZO (a) PYRENE-PHENOLS AND -QUINOLS

Major substrates of GT_{MC} are planar aromatic phenols such as 3-hydroxybenzo(a)pyrene 1-naphthol and 4-nitrophenol[7]. Several lines of evidence sug-

* Terminology for isoenzymes of cytochromes P-450 (P-450) and UDP-glucuronosyltransferase (GT) is inadequate at present. As defined by Nebert, P_1-450 is used as the polycyclic aromatic-inducible P-450, most closely associated with the polycyclic aromatic-inducible aryl hydrocarbon hydroxylase activity (calibrated by the fluorescence of 3-hydroxybenzo(a)pyrene)[12,13]. Similarly GT_1 or GT_{MC} is used as the polycyclic aromatic-inducible isoenzyme of GT most closely associated with the polycyclic aromatic-inducible conjugation of 3-hydroxybenzo(a)pyrene.

gest that GT_{MC} plays a major role in the detoxication of carcinogenic aromatic hydrocarbons. For example, (1) addition of UDP-glucuronic acid to the Ames test reduces benzo(a)pyrene mutagenicity[19,20]; (2) inhibition of glucuronidation leads to enhanced cytotoxicity caused by redox-cycles between quinones and quinols[21,22].

Besides the preference for planar phenols the isoenzyme shows a remarkable regioselectivity. For example, the conjugation of 3-hydroxybenzo(a)pyrene is enhanced 5-fold in liver microsomes from 3-methylcholanthrene-treated rats, whereas the conjugation of 9-hydroxybenzo(a)pyrene is only moderately enhanced (1.6-fold)[23]. Quite distinct from the so-called group 1 activities which are increased 3- to 5-fold, the conjugation of benzo(a)pyrene-3, 6-quinol to the diglucuronide is enhanced 40-fold in rat liver microsomes after the administration of 3-methylcholanthrene (Table 6.1). This dramatic increase of V_{max}

Table 6.1 UDP-glucuronosyltranferase activity toward benzo(a)pyrene- 3,6-quinol in liver microsomes from untreated controls and 3-methylcholanthrene-treated rats.

Under anaerobic conditions benzo(a)pyrene-3,6-quinone was first reduced (>95%) to the corresponding quinol in the presence of NADPH and microsomes. Thereafter glucuronidation was started by the addition of UDP-glucuronic acid. Diglucuronide formation was measured fluorimetrically

Treatment	K_m, *Quinol* (mmol/l)	*Kinetic constants* K_m, *UDPGA* (mmol/l)	V_{max} (nmol min^{-1} mg^{-1} protein)
None	0.05	2.1	0.17
3-Methylcholanthrene	0.04	1.4	6.4

substantiated previous observations[24]. In line with enhanced enzyme activity glucuronide formation was also increased more than 10-fold in isolated hepatocytes from 3-methylcholanthrene-treated rats compared with untreated controls[22].

To obtain accurate K_m values for the conjugation of the quinol several precautions had to be taken. Due to its instability the quinol is not available. Therefore, benzo(a)pyrene-3,6-quinone was reduced under anaerobic conditions to prevent autoxidation. Benzo(a)pyrene-3,6-quinol can be conjugated at the 6-OH and/or 3-OH position (Figure 6.1). The resulting glucuronides can be distinguished by their fluorescence spectra[22]. In this way it could be shown that it is the conjugation at the 3-OH position which is enhanced by 3-methylcholanthrene-treatment. Recent studies with UDP-[^{14}C]glucuronic acid and separation of two glucuronides by thin-layer chromatography showed that conjugation at the 3-OH position occurs mostly after conjugation at the 6-OH position. In other words, 3-methylcholanthrene-treatment appears to stimulate diglucuronide formation.

There are several explanations for the observation that conjugation of benzo(a)pyrene-3,6-quinol to the diglucuronide is increased 40-fold whereas conjugation of known GT_1 substrates is only increased 3- to 5-fold: (1) The quinol monoglucuronide may be a more selective substrate for GT_{MC} than simple phenols which have been shown to be overlapping substrates for several isoenzymes[4,5]. (2) There may be more than one 3-methylcholanthrene-indu-

Microsomes from tissues other than liver and from other species were also analysed (Figure 6.2**B**).

Rat hepatoma cells

Rat hepatomas are known to contain high levels of GT activities, in particular GT_1 activities[15,31]. Therefore, we analysed microsomal proteins of a permanent hepatoma cell line (H4IIE) derived from a rat hepatoma[32,33]. These hepatoma cells and isolated hepatocytes from untreated rat liver contain similar levels of GT activity toward 1-naphthol. To our surprise a 61 000 polypeptide of hepatoma microsomes was the major protein stained by our antibody. A corresponding 61 000 polypeptide is also stained in rat liver microsomes when larger quantities of microsomal protein (>10 μg) are analysed. This polypeptide is also retained during purification of GT_{MC} on UDP-hexanolamine Sepharose[30]. It can be separated from GT_{MC} by eluting the affinity column first with 0.1 mmol/l UDP-glucuronic acid. Subsequently the 61 000 polypeptide is eluted with 0.5 mmol/l UDP-glucuronic acid. These observations suggest that the 61 000 polypeptide may also represent an isoenzyme of GT. However, further work is needed to prove this, and to elucidate whether the different polypeptides represent different gene products or post-translational modifications of a com-

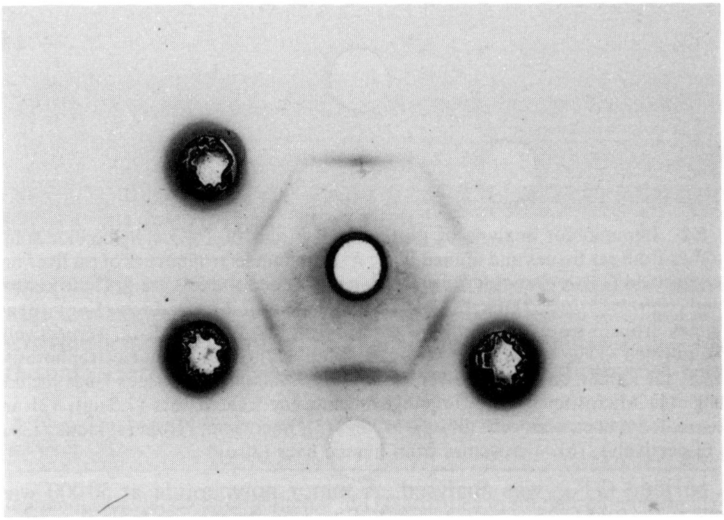

Figure 6.3 Ouchterlony double-diffusion analysis of rat liver and hepatoma UDP-glucuronosyltransferases. Central well: anti-GT_{MC}-IgG (600 μg). Dark wells: hepatoma microsomes (20 μg). White wells: purified GT_{MC} (2 μg)

mon gene product. As shown in Figure 6.3, Ouchterlony double-diffusion analysis shows lines of identity between purified GT_{MC} (white wells) and hepatoma proteins (dark wells). However, the occurrence of spurs between GT_{MC} and hepatoma microsomes indicates only partial identity, in line with the results of immunoblot analysis.

Rat kidney

Rat kidney microsomes contain high GT activity toward 1-naphthol[34]. When kidney microsomes were analysed immunochemically a high molecular weight polypeptide (at 60 000) was preferentially stained.

Human liver

In microsomes from several human beings GT_1 activities were highly correlated, whereas the correlation between GT_1 activities and other GT activities was poor[35]. This observation raised the possibility that isoenzymes exist in human liver similar to those delineated in rat liver. It was, therefore, of interest to see whether human GT is recognized by the antibody against rat liver GT_{MC}. No immunochemical reaction could be detected in Ouchterlony double-diffusion analysis[26]. However, with the more sensitive immunoblot analysis polypeptides of human liver microsomes in the range of 54 000 were stained by the antibody. Similar polypeptides were enriched in enzyme purification of the human liver enzyme[30]. A more detailed analysis of the immunochemical similarity between the rat and human liver enzymes will be presented elsewhere[30].

Immunoblot analysis adds a new dimension to the immunochemical analysis of GT. Further work on the isolation of GT isoenzymes is needed to identify the different polypeptides recognized by our antibody and their biogenetic relationship. Immunochemical techniques would be greatly improved by the availability of monospecific antibodies. *Note that even monoclonal antibodies may not be monospecific*. Nevertheless immunoblot analysis will greatly facilitate further progress in this field.

ACKNOWLEDGEMENTS

We thank Mrs U. Jongepier and R. Blume for expert technical assistance, Dr F. Wiebel for kindly providing H4IIE-cells and the Deutsche Forschungsgemeinschaft for financial support.

References

1. Dutton, G. J. (1980). *Glucuronidation of drugs and other compounds*. (Boca Raton, Florida: CRC Press)
2. Burchell, B. (1981). Identification and purification of multiple forms of UDP-glucuronosyltransferase. In Hodgson, E., Bend, J. R. and Philpot, R. M. (eds.) *Reviews in Biochemical Toxicology*. Vol. 3, pp. 1–32 (New York: Elsevier/North Holland).
3. Bock, K. W., Burchell, B., Dutton, G. J., Hänninen, O., Mulder, G. J., Owens, I. S., Siest, G. and Tephly, T. R. (1983). UDP-glucuronosyltransferase: Guidelines for consistent interim terminology and assay conditions. *Biochem. Pharmacol.*, **32,** 953–5
4. Falany, C. N. and Tephly, T. R. (1983). Separation, purification and characterization of three isoenzymes of UDP-glucuronyltransferase from rat liver microsomes. *Arch. Biochem. Biophys.*, **227,** 248–58
5. Roy Chowdhury, J., Roy Chowdhury, N. and Arias, I. M. (1984). UDP-glucuronosyltransferase deficiency in man and animals. *Biochem. Soc. Transact.*, **12,** 81–3

7
Isolation of a bile acid glucosyltransferase from human liver microsomes. Characterization of a lipid intermediate-dependent glucoside conjugation

H. MATERN, S. MATERN AND W. GEROK

INTRODUCTION

Sugar nucleotides have been described as the only source of carbohydrate in glycoside conjugation[1]. However, glycoside formation of various aglycones such as *p*-nitrophenol[2], bilirubin[3], or oestrogens[4] was also shown to occur in the absence of added sugar nucleotides when washed liver microsomes from animal species were used as the enzyme source. From these results the existence of a lipid-soluble microsomal sugar donor was postulated reacting as an intermediate in sugar transfer from sugar nucleotides to an aglycone[1,3,4]. Attempts, however, failed to demonstrate a glycolipid capable of aglycone glycosylation[1,5].

The present study demonstrates the existence of a sugar nucleotide-independent glucosyltransferase in human liver microsomes catalysing the transfer of glucose from lipophilic alkyl-β-D-glucopyranosides or dolichol monophosphate glucose to bile acids. Sugar nucleotides are not utilized as a carbohydrate donor by the purified glucosyltransferase. Furthermore, the present study shows, that in addition to the known mechanisms of bile acid conjugation such as amino acid conjugation[6], sulphation[7] and glucuronidation[8], glucosidation may represent a novel pathway of bile acid conjugation in man.

MATERIALS AND METHODS

Sources of chemicals and of human liver autopsy samples were the same as described in a previous paper[9].

Conjugation of 0.1 mmol/l [^{14}C]chenodeoxycholic acid (4 μCi/μmol) with glucuronic acid[10] or with glucose[9] was estimated according to published procedures. Octyl-β-D-glucopyranoside (1 mmol/l) was used as donor substrate for the assay of bile acid glucosyltransferase activity, if not otherwise stated. All assays were performed in the presence of sonicated dispersions of 50 μg of egg yolk L-α-phosphatidylcholine prepared as described elsewhere[11]. Units of enzyme activities are expressed as nanomoles of aglycone substrate conjugated per minute.

Methods of protein determination, disc gel electrophoresis in the presence of sodium dodecyl sulphate, identification of chenodeoxycholic acid glucoside, and purification of glucosyltransferase activity toward chenodeoxycholic acid were performed as described elsewhere[9].

RESULTS AND DISCUSSION

Purification of glucosyltransferase activity toward chenodeoxycholic acid

Conjugation of bile acids with glucuronic acid was hitherto known as the only glycoside conjugation mechanism of bile acids in man which is catalysed by a microsomal UDP-glucuronosyltransferase[12–14]. The results of the present study demonstrate the existence of a bile acid glucosyltransferase in human liver microsomes in addition to the known bile acid UDP-glucuronosyltransferase.

As shown in Figure 7.1, bile acid UDP-glucuronosyltransferase and bile acid glucosyltransferase represent two different forms of enzymes since separation of both enzyme activities was achieved on a DEAE–Trisacryl column. Whereas bile acid UDP-glucuronosyltransferase was not retained on the column, and was eluted before a salt gradient was applied, bile acid glucosyltransferase was eluted within a linear gradient from 0 to 0.15 mol/l NaCl. No further glycoside

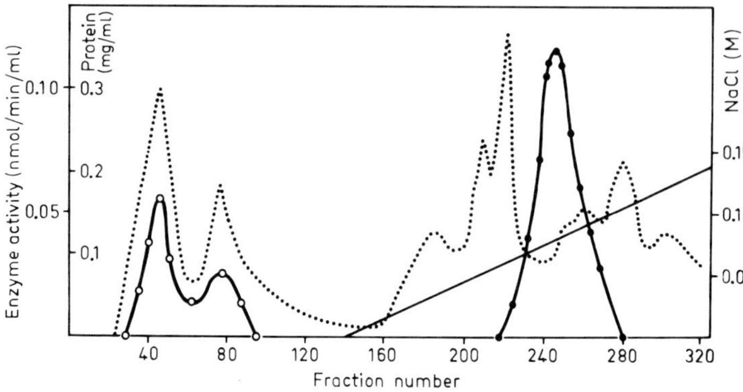

Figure 7.1 DEAE-Trisacryl chromatography of bile acid UDP-glucuronosyltransferase (○) and bile acid glucosyltransferase (●) activities. A polyethylene glycol-fractionated preparation of enzyme (total activities towards the bile acid chenodeoxycholic acid, 25 units of UDP-glucuronosyltransferase and 14 units of glucosyltransferase) was chromatographed on a DEAE-Trisacryl column as previously described[9]. ···, protein; —— NaCl gradient; fraction volume = 3 ml

conjugating activity toward chenodeoxycholic acid could be eluted from the column when the concentration of NaCl was raised to 1 mol/l.

Glucosyltransferase activity towards chenodeoxycholic acid was purified about 900-fold from the solubilized microsomal preparation with the aid of polyethylene glycol fractionation, anion exchange chromatography on DEAE–Trisacryl and on Mono Q, chromatofocusing on Mono P, and hydrophobic chromatography on ethylagarose (Table 7.1). The final purified preparation exhibited a single band in disc gel electrophoresis in the presence of sodium dodecyl sulphate[9]. The subunit molecular weight of the enzyme was determined by this method to be about 56 000[9].

Table 7.1 Purification of glucosyltransferase activity towards chenodeoxycholic acid

Step	*Total protein* (mg)	*Specific activity*
Solubilized microsomes	551	0.053
Polyethylene glycol fractionation	129	0.108
DEAE-Trisacryl	8.6	0.97
Mono Q FPLC	0.57	11.7
Mono P FPLC*	0.047	38.3
Ethylagarose*	0.012	48.3

* Data are given for the activity peak eluting at pH 5.0 of Mono P chromatography[9]. FPLC, fast protein, peptide and polynucleotide liquid chromatography. The specific activity is expressed as units per mg of protein

Identification of chenodeoxycholic acid glucoside

The product of the reaction of the isolated glucosyltransferase with chenodeoxycholic acid and octyl-β-D-glucopyranoside (octyl glucoside) was identified as chenodeoxycholic acid glucoside as shown in Figure 7.2. After treatment of the purified reaction product with β-glucosidase the radioactive material labelled in the bile acid moiety gave one radioactive spot in thin-layer chromatography with the same mobility as authentic chenodeoxycholic acid (Figure 7.2A,B), whereas in the region corresponding to the reaction product before treatment with β-glucosidase (Figure 7.2E) no radioactivity was detectable (Figure 7.2B). When the β-glucosidase hydrolysis was performed in the presence of 10 mmol/l of the β-glucosidase inhibitor glucono-1·5-lactone (not shown) or when the reaction product was treated with yeast α-glucosidase or bovine liver β-glucuronidase the radioactivity corresponding to the reaction product was preserved (Figure 7.2C–E). The sensitivity of the reaction product to β-glucosidase hydrolysis and the inhibition of hydrolysis by the β-glucosidase inhibitor glucono-1·5-lactone indicate that β-linked chenodeoxycholic acid glucoside is formed as a product of the reaction of chenodeoxycholic acid and octyl glucoside. Furthermore, the glucose moiety of the reaction product was identified by thin-layer chromatography after mild acid hydrolysis of the purified reaction product[9].

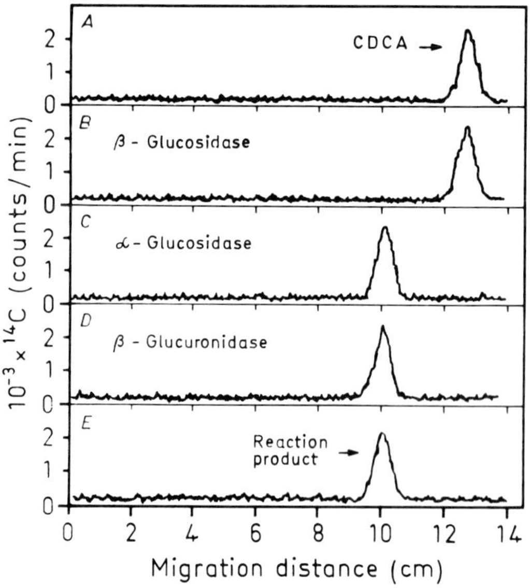

Figure 7.2 Identification of chenodeoxycholic acid glucoside. The reaction product labelled in the bile acid moiety was treated with β-glucosidase, α-glucosidase or β-glucuronidase, and analysed on silica gel plates in n-butanol : acetic acid : water (50 : 5 : 10, v/v) (B, C, D). A, reference [^{14}C]chenodeoxycholic acid (CDCA); E, untreated reaction product

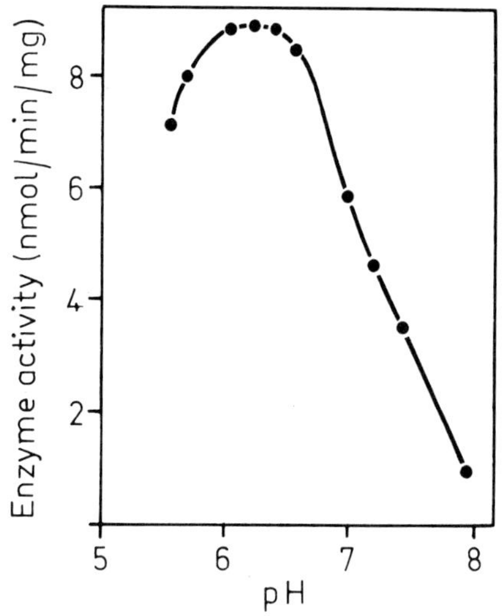

Figure 7.3 pH-Dependence of glucosyltransferase activity toward chenodeoxycholic acid. The transfer of glucose from octyl glucoside (1 mmol/l) to chenodeoxycholic acid (10 μmol/l) was estimated in a mixture of 0.1 mol/l concentrations of MES (morpholinoethane sulphonic acid), ACES (*N*-(2-acetamido)-2-aminoethane sulphonic acid) and HEPPS (*N*-2-hydroxyethyl-piperazine-N′-propane-sulphonic acid) as buffers

Characterization of bile acid glucosyltransferase

Catalytic properties

The effect of pH on the transfer of glucose from octyl glucoside to chenodeoxycholic acid as catalysed by the pure enzyme is shown in Figure 7.3. Enzyme activity was optimal between pH 6.0 and 6.5.

Double reciprocal plots of initial rates of enzyme activity as a function of varying concentrations of chenodeoxycholic acid at several fixed concentrations

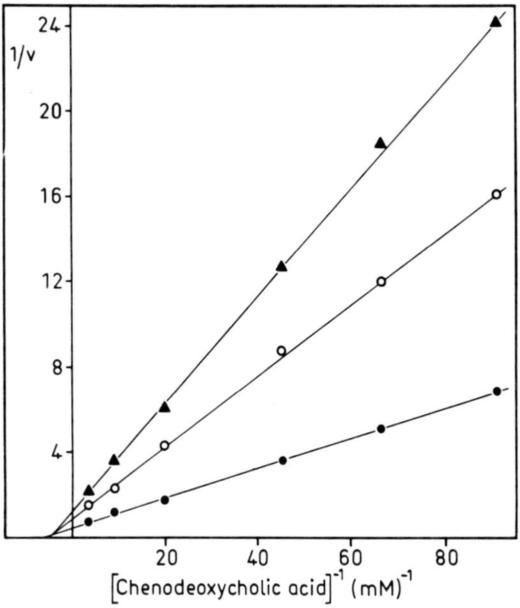

Figure 7.4 Double reciprocal plots of initial rates of glucosyltransferase activity as a function of the concentration of chenodeoxycholic acid at different concentrations of octyl glucoside which were held fixed at either 33 μmol/l (▲), 77 μmol/l (○) or 660 μmol/l (●). The enzyme preparation used was obtained after DEAE-Trisacryl chromatography (*see* Table 7.1) and contained 0.2% (w/v) CHAPS (3-[(3-cholamidopropyl)-dimethylammonio]-1-propane sulphonate) as detergent. v = units per mg of protein

of octyl glucoside are shown in Figure 7.4. The apparent K_m for chenodeoxycholic acid was calculated from the intersection of the straight lines to be 210 μmol/l. The intersecting pattern observed in the present kinetic study (Figure 7.4) indicates that a sequential mechanism[15] applies to the enzyme-catalysed formation of chenodeoxycholic acid glucoside.

Substrate specificity

Studies on the bile acid substrate specificity of the pure glucosyltransferase showed that the enzyme was able to utilize deoxycholic and ursodeoxycholic acids as aglycone substrates in addition to chenodeoxycholic acid. In the presence of 50 μmol/l concentrations of these bile acids and 1 mmol/l octyl glucoside as donor substrate the rates of bile acid glucoside formation were estimated to be 30 nmol of chenodeoxycholic acid, 25 nmol of ursodeoxycholic acid and 68 nmol of deoxycholic acid conjugated per min per mg of protein, respectively. No synthesis of bile acid glucosides was detectable when incubations were performed in the presence of a heat-denatured enzyme, indicating that a spontaneous formation of bile acid glucosides can be excluded.

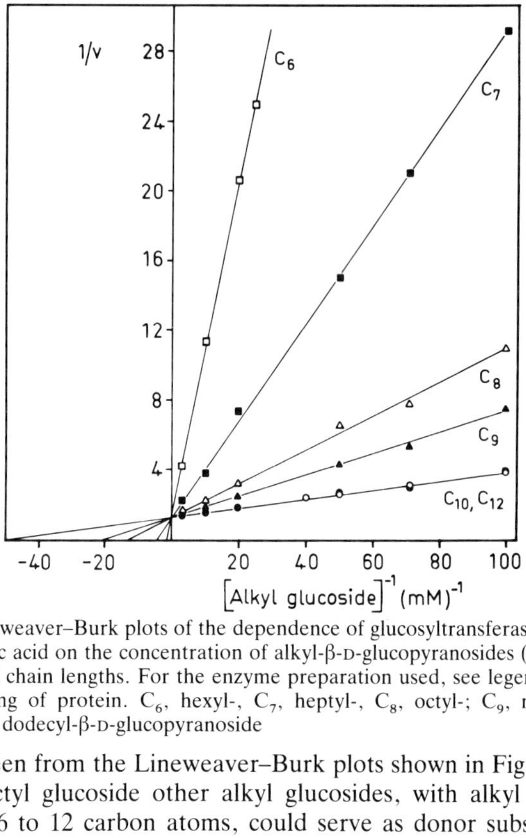

Figure 7.5 Lineweaver–Burk plots of the dependence of glucosyltransferase activity toward chenodeoxycholic acid on the concentration of alkyl-β-D-glucopyranosides (alkyl glucosides) of different alkyl chain lengths. For the enzyme preparation used, see legend to Figure 7.4. v = units per mg of protein. C_6, hexyl-, C_7, heptyl-, C_8, octyl-; C_9, nonyl-; C_{10} (●), decyl-; C_{12} (○), dodecyl-β-D-glucopyranoside

It may be seen from the Lineweaver–Burk plots shown in Figure 7.5 that in addition to octyl glucoside other alkyl glucosides, with alkyl chain lengths varying from 6 to 12 carbon atoms, could serve as donor substrates for the purified enzyme in the formation of chenodeoxycholic acid glucoside. It is evident from the data shown in Figure 7.5 that the affinity of alkyl glucosides to the enzyme increased with increasing alkyl chain length up to a chain length of 10 carbon atoms. The apparent K_m values decreased from 680 μmol/l for hexyl-β-D-glucopyranoside to 20 μmol/l as estimated for decyl- and dodecyl-β-D-glucopyranoside. In contrast to the various alkyl glucosides studied dodecyl-β-D-maltoside (1 mmol/l) did not act as donor substrate for the purified glucosyltransferase in bile acid glycoside formation, suggesting that the purified enzyme is specifically involved in glucosyl transfer.

Since the results shown in Figure 7.5 indicate that the enzyme exhibits a requirement towards lipophilic donor substrates the naturally occurring glucolipid dolichol monophosphate glucose, known as a source of glucose in glycoprotein biosynthesis[16], was estimated to act as carbohydrate donor for the purified glucosyltransferase. The purified enzyme (*see* legend to Figure 7.4) was able to catalyse the transfer of glucose from [^{3}H]dolichol monophosphate glucose (0.15 μmol/l, 6.5 Ci/mmol) to chenodeoxycholic acid (0.3 mmol/l) with a reaction rate of 0.02 nmol of chenodeoxycholic acid glucoside formed per min per mg of protein. These results indicate that in addition to the known role of dolichol monophosphate glucose as a glucosyl donor in glycoprotein biosynthesis[16], this glucolipid is also involved as a donor substrate in glucoside conjugation.

In contrast to dolichol monophosphate glucose, 10 mmol/l concentrations of sugar nucleotides, such as UDP-glucuronic acid, UDP-glucose, ADP-glucose, CDP-glucose, GDP-glucose or TDP-glucose or of free glucose, did not cause measurable formation of chenodeoxycholic acid glucoside by the purified glucosyltransferase (*see* legend to Figure 7.4). Thus, the enzymatic formation of bile acid glucosides described in the present study represents a sugar nucleotide-independent glucoside conjugation that is, therefore, distinct from the known mechanisms of glycoside conjugation.

ACKNOWLEDGEMENTS

This work was supported by the Deutsche Forschungsgemeinschaft (SFB 154-84) and by the Fritz Thyssen-Stiftung. H.M. is the recipient of a Heisenberg award from the Deutsche Forschungsgemeinschaft.

References

1. Dutton, G. J. and Burchell, B. (1977). Newer aspects of glucuronidation. *Prog. Drug Metab.*, **2,** 1–70
2. Dutton, G. J. (1966). The biosynthesis of glucuronides. In Dutton, G. J. (ed.), *Glucuronic Acid, Free and Combined*, pp. 185–299. (New York: Academic Press)
3. Heirwegh, K. P. M., Van de Vijver, M. and Fevery, J. (1972). Assay and properties of digitonin-activated bilirubin uridine diphosphate glucuronyltransferase from rat liver. *Biochem. J.*, **129,** 605–18
4. Williamson, D. G., Polakowa, A. and Layne, D. S. (1971). Estrogen glucosides and galactosides: Formation by rabbit liver microsomes *in vitro*. *Biochim. Biophys. Res. Commun.*, **42,** 1057–62
5. Puhakainen, E. and Hänninen, O. (1974). Lipid acceptor in UDP-glucuronic acid metabolism in rat liver microsomes. *FEBS Lett.*, **39,** 144–8
6. Killenberg, P. G. and Jordan, J. T. (1978). Purification and characterization of bile acid–CoA: amino acid *N*-acyltransferase from rat liver. *J. Biol. Chem.*, **253,** 1005–10
7. Palmer, R. H. (1967). The formation of bile acid sulfates: a new pathway of bile acid metabolism in humans. *Proc. Natl. Acad. Sci. USA*, **58,** 1047–50
8. Back, P., Spaczynski, K. and Gerok, W. (1974). Bile salt glucuronides in urine. *Hoppe-Seyler's Z. Physiol. Chem.*, **355,** 749–52
9. Matern, H., Matern, S. and Gerok, W. (1984). Formation of bile acid glucosides by a sugar nucleotide-independent glucosyltransferase isolated from human liver microsomes. *Proc. Natl. Acad. Sci. USA*, **81,** in press
10. Matern, H., Matern, S. and Gerok, W. (1983). A rapid and sensitive method for the assay of UDP-glucuronosyltransferase activity toward bile acids. *Anal. Biochem.*, **133,** 417–24
11. Matern, H., Matern, S. and Gerok, W. (1982). Isolation and characterization of rat liver microsomal UDP-glucuronosyltransferase activity toward chenodeoxycholic acid and testosterone as a single form of enzyme. *J. Biol. Chem.*, **257,** 7422-9

12. Matern, H., Matern, S., Schelzig, Ch. and Gerok, W. (1980). Bile acid UDP-glucuronyltransferase from human liver. Properties and studies on aglycone substrate specificity. *FEBS Lett.*, **118,** 251–4

13. Matern, H., Matern, S. and Gerok, W. (1981). Characterization of bile acid UDP-glucuronyltransferase from human liver. In Paumgartner, G., Stiehl, A. and Gerok, W. (eds.). *Bile Acids and Lipids*, pp. 111–6. (Lancaster: MTP Press)

14. Matern, S., Matern, H., Farthmann, E. H. and Gerok, W. (1984). Hepatic and extrahepatic glucuronidation of bile acids in man. Characterization of bile acid uridine 5′-diphosphate-glucuronosyltransferase in hepatic, renal, and intestinal microsomes. *J. Clin. Invest.*, **74,** 402–10

15. Cleland, W. W. (1970). In Boyer, P. D. (ed.). *The Enzymes*, 3rd. Edn. Vol. 2, pp. 1–65. (New York: Academic Press)

16. Parodi, A. J. and Leloir, L. F. (1979). The role of lipid intermediates in the glycosylation of proteins in the eucaryotic cell. *Biochim. Biophys. Acta*, **559,** 1–37

8
Processing of mouse and rat nascent UDP-glucuronosyltransferase

P. I. MACKENZIE AND I. S. OWENS

ABSTRACT

Rat liver UDP-glucuronosyltransferase activity is shown to cross-react with anti-mouse transferase γ-globulin. Three forms of transferase ranging in molecular weights from 49 000 to 52 000 were immunoadsorbed from control and phenobarbital-treated microsomes and analysed by SDS-polyacrylamide gel electrophoresis. Four transferase forms ranging from 51 000 to 57 000 were similarly immunoadsorbed from 3-methylcholanthrene-treated microsomes. The intensity of the electrophoretic bands indicated that at least two transferase forms were increased by each inducer. Under similar conditions the antibody immunoadsorbed about 70–90% of the transferase activities toward 4-nitrophenol, 1-naphthol, 3-hydroxybenzo(a)pyrene, 9-hydroxybenzo(a)pyrene and 4-methylumbelliferone from rat liver microsomes.

Using poly (A) RNA isolated from either control, phenobarbital- or 3-methylcholanthrene-treated rats, *in vitro* translated products immunoadsorbed by the antibody showed only a 52 000 protein by SDS-polyacrylamide gel electrophoresis. Inclusion of dog pancreatic microsomes during translation resulted in the appearance of a new 50 000 protein, in addition to the 52 000 species.

In a similar *in vitro* translation study with mouse poly (A) RNA it was shown that a 50 000 protein was converted to a mature form of 51 000 by glycosylation and possibly cleavage. These results indicate that processing of nascent polypeptides by cleavage and/or glycosylation occurs for at least one category of membrane-bound drug metabolizing enzymes.

INTRODUCTION

UDP-glucuronosyltransferase (EC 2.4.1.17) is a family of integral membrane enzymes which catalyses the glucuronidation of many endogenous and exogenous lipophilic compounds. The glucuronide products have enhanced water solubilities and excretion rates. Several forms of transferase with distinct but overlapping substrate specificities are shown to conjugate a wide range of substrates, such as steroids, biogenic amines, bile salts, bilirubin, as well as, pesticides, drugs, food additives and environmental pollutants.

The transferases are integrally associated with the endoplasmic reticulum (ER) requiring detergent solubilization to isolate and purify the different forms[1–4]. An important question concerns the biochemical events leading to the insertion of proteins into the ER. It has been proposed that during biosynthesis of membrane-bound proteins co- and/or post-translational modifications occur whereby an amino terminal signal sequence is proteolytically cleaved during membrane insertion[5]. Further evidence exists indicating that certain proteins are glycosylated on the luminal surface of the ER[5] after insertion. Although many integrally associated proteins of the ER are presumed to undergo similar biosynthetic processing[6] as described for several plasma membrane proteins[6,7], it has not yet been demonstrated that proteolytic cleavage occurs during insertion into the membrane for any of the microsomal drug metabolizing enzymes (*cf.* Reference 8).

In this study, UDP-glucuronosyltransferase synthesized *in vitro* from isolated poly (A) RNA was shown to produce a 52 000 protein on SDS-polyacrylamide gel electrophoresis. This band which represented transferase was processed by the inclusion of dog pancreatic microsomes in the translation assay and produced in addition to the 52 000 transferase, a new band with increased electrophoretic mobility. These results are consistent with the post-translational cleavage of at least one form of UDP-glucuronosyltransferase during the process of membrane insertion.

MATERIAL AND METHODS

Preparation of transferase and transferase antibody

Anti-serum to purified mouse transferase was raised in goats and subjected to ammonium sulphate fractionation as previously described[9].

Immunoadsorption of rat transferase activity with anti-mouse transferase γ-globulin

Liver microsomes were prepared from phenobarbital-treated Sprague-Dawley rats and solubilized[9] with CHAPS (Calbiochem). Increasing concentrations of partially purified[9] anti-transferase γ-globulin were incubated with a constant amount of solubilized microsomes for 1 h at 4°C. Purified preimmune γ-globulin was added to the mixture to equalize the total protein concentration in all mixtures. Immune complexes were pelleted with protein A-Sepharose and transferase activities were measured in the supernatant.

Transferase activities were assayed using 4-methylumbelliferone, 4-nitrophenol, 1-naphthol, 3-hydroxybenzo(a)pyrene and 9-hydroxybenzo(a)pyrene as already described[10].

Tritiation of microsomal proteins

Microsomal proteins were tritiated *in vitro* with $NaB(^3H)_4$ by the method of Kreibich[11] as modified by Negishi[12]. Transferase was immunoadsorbed and analysed by SDS-polyacrylamide (7.5%) gels as already described[13].

Isolation of mRNA

Male Sprague-Dawley rats were treated with phenobarbital or 3-methylcholanthrene as already described[10]. Total mRNA was isolated by the method of Chirgwin *et al.*[14], and poly(A) RNA was isolated according to the method of Aviv and Leder[15].

In vitro *synthesis and immunoadsorption of UDP-glucuronosyltransferase*

Poly(A) RNA was translated *in vitro* in a micrococcal nuclease-treated rabbit reticulocyte lysate in the presence of (^{35}S)methionine (Amersham) for 90 min at 25°C, and analysis of immunoadsorbed products on SDS-polyacrylamide (7.5%) gels were as previously described[13].

Digestion with endoglycosidase H

Immune complexes of tritiated transferase and antibody, bound to protein A-Sepharose, were treated with endoglycosidase H as reported[13]. Polyacrylamide gel electrophoresis was carried out in the presence of SDS according to Laemmli[16].

RESULTS

Rat hepatic microsomal UDP-glucuronosyltransferase activity was examined for cross-reactivity with anti-mouse transferase γ-globulin in order to study molecular aspects of the rat transferase system, and to compare these results with that of the mouse. It can be seen in Figure 8.1 that increasing concentrations of antibody to microsomal protein up to a ratio of 20 : 1 progressively immunoadsorbed 60–90% of the transferase activities toward 4-nitrophenol, 1-naphthol, 3-hydroxybenzo(a)pyrene, 9-hydroxybenzo(a)pyrene, and 4-methylumbelliferone. Transferase activity was not adsorbed by preimmune γ-globulin.

Ouchterlony double-diffusion analysis showed a precipitin line between solubilized rat microsomes and anti-mouse transferase γ-globulin (results not shown).

In order to determine the number of electrophoretically distinct rat transferase forms which react with the antibody, transferase in tritiated microsomes prepared after treatment of rats with either phenobarbital or 3-methylcholanthrene was immunoadsorbed and analysed by SDS-polyacrylamide gel electrophoresis as described under 'Materials and Methods'. It can be seen in Figure 8.2 (lanes 1 and 2) that the antibody recognized at least three transferase forms

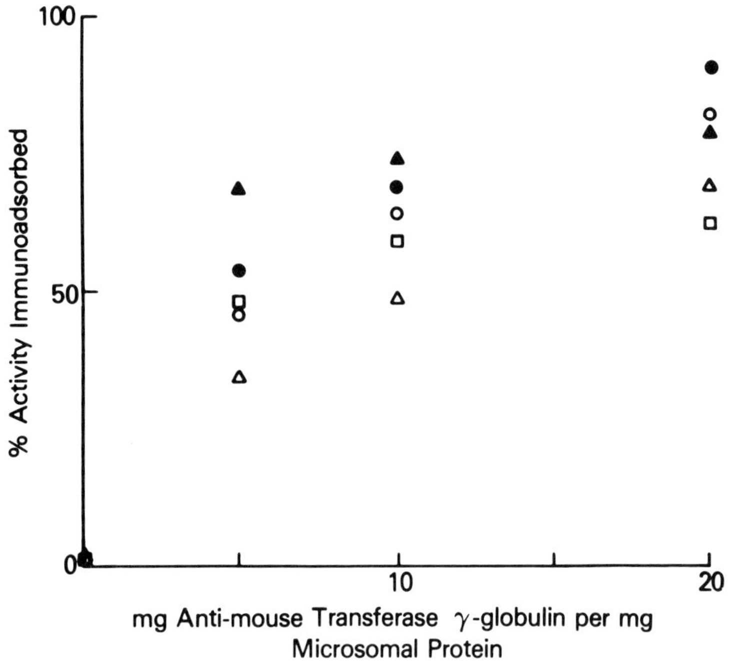

Figure 8.1 Immunoadsorption of rat UDP-glucuronosyltransferase activity with anti-mouse transferase γ-globulin. Microsomes from phenobarbital-treated rats were solubilized and incubated with antibody as described under 'Materials and Methods'. Transferase activities towards 4-nitrophenol (●), 1-naphthol (○), 3-hydroxybenzo(a)pyrene (△), 9-hydroxybenzo-(a)pyrene (▲), and 4-methylumbelliferone (□) were assayed in the supernatant after immune complexes were pelleted with protein A-Sepharose. The activities immunoadsorbed are expressed as a percentage of the total activity determined on the sample which contained 100% preimmune γ-globulin. (Reproduced with permission from American Society of Biological Chemists)

in control microsomes, and that after phenobarbital treatment (lane 3) the levels of two of these forms were markedly increased. The molecular weights of the bands representing transferase ranged from 49 000 to 52 000. On the other hand, the antibody immunoadsorbed at least four transferase forms after 3-methylcholanthrene treatment (lane 4) which ranged in molecular weights from 51 000 to 57 000. The intensity of at least two of the bands representing transferase was increased by 3-methylcholanthrene treatment.

To investigate further the reactivity of the antibody with rat transferase, immunoadsorbed *in vitro* translation products were compared with immunoadsorbed microsomal product as shown in Figure 8.3. The immunoadsorbed translation products of both control (lane 1) and phenobarbital-induced (lane 4) poly(A) RNA showed only one electrophoretic band of approximately 52 000, whereas the three bands were again observed in control (lane 2) and phenobarbital-treated (lane 5) microsomes. Both translation products and microsomal material were mixed for control (lane 3) and for phenobarbital-treated samples (lane 6). The results showed no discernible effect of 'loading' on the electrophoretic mobility of the translation product.

Figure 8.2 Immunoadsorption of rat transferase from tritiated microsomes with anti-mouse tranferase γ-globulin. Liver microsomes from control (lanes 1 and 2), phenobarbital- (lane 3) and 3-methylcholanthrene-treated (lane 4) rats were tritiated, solubilized, immunoadsorbed with anti-mouse transferase γ-globulin and analysed by SDS-polyacrylamide gel electrophoresis as described under 'Materials and Methods'. (Reproduced with permission from Academic Press)

This difference in the number of bands representing transferase between the *in vitro* translation system and the microsomes was explored further by comparing the translation product in the absence and in the presence of dog pancreatic microsomes (Figure 8.4). The translation products for both phenobarbital- (lane 3) and 3-methylcholanthrene-induced (lane 5) poly(A) RNA showed two transferase forms due to processing by the microsomes. In each case a lower molecular weight protein of approximately 50 000 appeared compared to the unprocessed transferase (lanes 2 and 4 for phenobarbital and 3-methylcholanthrene, respectively). The highest molecular weight protein in each lane is due to some protein which binds non-specifically to either protein-A-Sepharose or preimmune serum (lane 1 for phenobarbital-induced poly(A) RNA and lane 6 for 3-methylcholanthrene-induced poly(A) RNA). An electrophoretic band at 52 000 representing transferase remained at that position and was presumed not to undergo any type of processing.

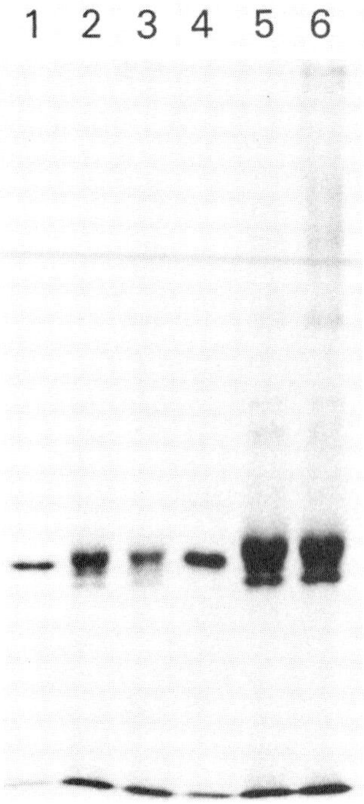

Figure 8.3 Comparison of rat immunoadsorbed proteins from an *in vitro* translation assay and from tritiated microsomes using anti-mouse transferase γ-globulin. *In vitro* translation products using either control (lane 1) or phenobarbital-induced (lane 4) poly(A) RNA were immunoadsorbed with anti-transferase γ-globulin; either control (lane 2) or phenobarbital-treated (lane 5) tritiated microsomes were similarly immunoadsorbed. Both samples were analysed by SDS-polyacrylamide gel electrophoresis described under 'Materials and Methods'. Lane 3 contained a mixture of the samples placed on lanes 1 and 2, and lane 6 contained a mixture of the samples in lanes 4 and 5. (Reproduced with permission from Academic Press)

The *in vitro* translated transferase generated by rat poly(A) RNA was compared with that for mouse in Figure 8.5. Phenobarbital- (lanes 2, 3, 7 and 8) and 3-methylcholanthrene-induced (lanes 4, 5, 9 and 10) poly(A) RNA-dependent protein synthesis was compared after immunoadsorption of the rat (lanes 1–6) and mouse (lanes 7–11) translation products in the same experiment. As already noted for the rat at least part of the 52 000 transferase is cleaved to 50 000 (lanes 3 and 5). On the contrary, the antibody immunoadsorbed two transferase forms generated by either phenobarbital- (lane 7) or 3-methylcholanthrene-induced (lane 9) poly(A) RNA for the mouse. The proteins immunoadsorbed were 50 000 and 54 000 compared to that from mouse microsomes[13] of 51 000 and 54 000. The inclusion of dog pancreatic microsomes in the *in vitro* translation system supported by mouse poly(A) RNA showed that the 50 000 protein (lower band, lanes 7 and 9) increased in molecular weight to 51 000 for both phenobarbital- (lane 8) and 3-methylcholanthrene-induced (lane 10) poly(A) RNA. Also, a small amount of a protein of approximately 49 000 appeared in the processed translation product (lower bands, lanes 8 and 10).

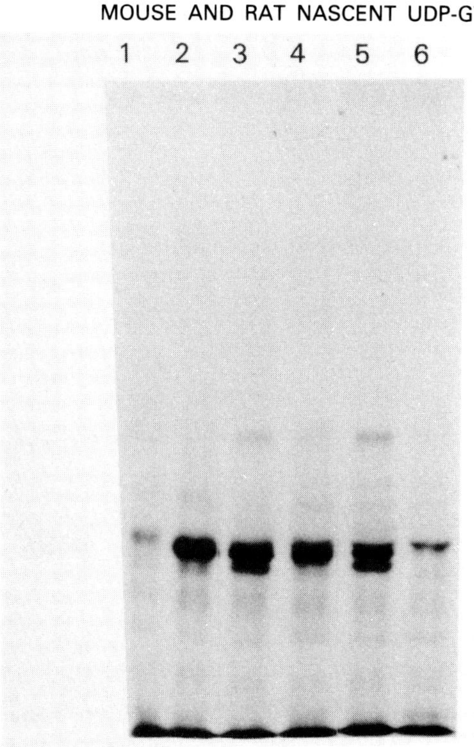

Figure 8.4 *In vitro* translation of rat liver poly(A) RNA in the absence and presence of dog pancreatic microsomes. Poly(A) RNA isolated from phenobarbital- (lanes 1–3) and 3-methylcholanthrene-treated (lanes 4–6) rats were translated *in vitro* in the absence (lanes 2 and 4) and in the presence (lanes 3 and 5) of 1 μl of dog pancreatic microsomes. Lanes 1 and 6 contained material which non-specifically bound to protein A-Sepharose or preimmune γ-globulin. (Reproduced with permission from Academic Press)

By comparison only the 51 000 and 54 000 proteins are observed in mouse microsomes. The result suggests that the 51 000 form is glycosylated by the dog pancreatic microsomes.

Further evidence that the 51 000 mouse transferase form is glycosylated is shown in Figure 8.6. It can be seen that endoglycosidase H (lane 1) caused a shift of the 51 000 form of transferase to a lower molecular weight compared to untreated transferase (lane 2). The increased electrophoretic mobility of the 51 000 form, and not the 54 000 form, is consistent with the removal of sugar moieties from the 51 000 form by endoglycosidase H.

DISCUSSION

In studying the cross-reactivity of anti-mouse transferase γ-globulin with rat transferase it was shown that at least three proteins were immunoadsorbed from control and phenobarbital-treated microsomes. The molecular weights ranged from 49 000 to 52 000. Four transferase forms were immunoadsorbed

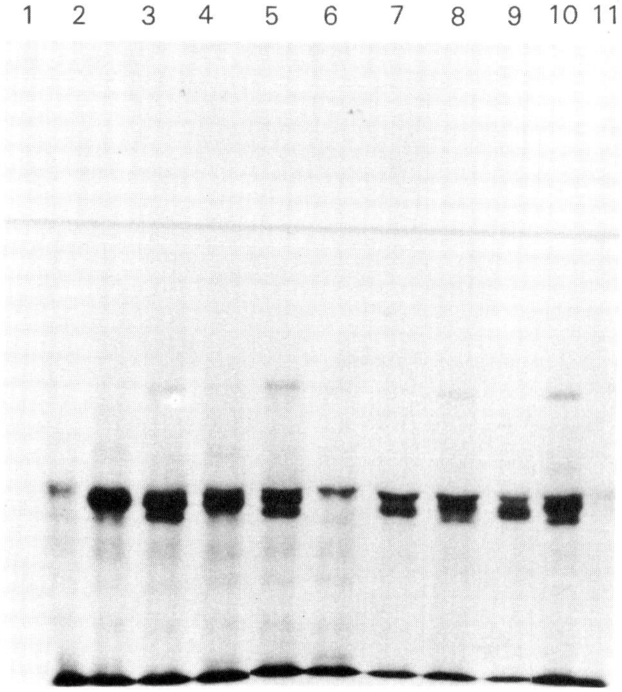

Figure 8.5 *In vitro* translation products of rat and mouse liver poly(A) RNA in the absence and presence of dog pancreatic microsomes. Poly(A) RNA was isolated from phenobarbital-treated rats (lanes 1–3) and C57BL/6N mice (lanes 7 and 8) or from 3-methylcholanthrene-treated rats (lanes 4–6) and mice (lanes 9–11). *In vitro* translated product was synthesized in the absence (lanes 2, 4, 7 and 9) or presence of 1 μl of dog pancreatic microsomes (lanes 3, 5, 8 and 10). The translation products were immunoadsorbed with anti-mouse γ-globulin (lanes 2–11) or preimmune γ-globulin (lanes 1 and 11) as described in Figures 8.3 and 8.4. The rats and mice were treated with the inducers as already described[13]

from 3-methylcholanthrene-treated microsomes ranging in molecular weights from 51 000 to 57 000. The levels of at least two proteins were increased by either inducer. Similar immunoadsorption studies with unlabelled microsomes removed 60–90% of the glucuronidating activities toward 1-naphthol, 4-nitrophenol, 3-hydroxybenzo(a)pyrene, 9-hydroxybenzo(a)pyrene and 4-methylumbelliferone. These results are consistent with the existence of at least one common determinant between two forms of mouse[9] and a minimum of four forms of rat transferase. Since transferase represents a family of membrane-bound proteins all catalysing glucuronidation, a common determinant may exist at the enzymatic active site, phospholipid binding site or a transmembrane site.

A central question relates to the mechanism for inserting integral membrane proteins into the ER, i.e. whether there are cleavable[17] and/or non-cleavable[17–20] signal sequences and, ultimately, whether the cleaved proteins are all glycosylated[17]. In this study it is shown for the first time that a drug metabolizing enzyme, UDP-glucuronosyltransferase, is cleaved by dog

Figure 8.6 Endoglycosidase H treatment of mouse labelled microsomal transferase. Tritiated microsomal transferase from phenobarbital-treated microsomes were immunoadsorbed and either undigested (lane 2) or digested with endoglycosidase H (lane 1) before SDS-polyacrylamide gel electrophoresis as described in 'Materials and Methods'. (Reproduced with permission from Academic Press)

pancreatic microsomes such that the molecular weight is reduced by about 2000 for a transferase form made *in vitro* with poly(A) RNA isolated after treatment with either phenobarbital or 3-methylcholanthrene. Based on no further change in mobility of this form under prolonged incubation with dog pancreatic membranes, it does not appear that subsequent glycosylation takes place. This processed form of about 50 000 is consistent with the molecular weight of transferase forms seen in rat native microsomes (Figure 8.3). Since some of the *in vitro* transferase forms after 3-methylcholanthrene treatment that were recognized by this antibody (Figure 8.2) had molecular weights at least 5000 greater than the corresponding *in vitro* translation product of 52 000, it is postulated that some of these forms of rat transferase require glycosylation. It is possible that the dog pancreatic microsomes in the *in vitro* system do not efficiently glycosylate the 3-methylcholanthrene-inducible transferase forms.

A second possibility is that the *in vitro* system was not optimized to translate all of the 3-methylcholanthrene-induced transferase specific poly(A) RNAs. In the same experiment the *in vitro* translation product for mouse showed processing of the 50 000 protein band to a higher molecular weight as previously shown[13]. This increase in molecular weight is consistent with glycosylation[13] to generate the mature form of 51 000 seen in native microsomes[13]. The small amount of the 49 000 band seen in the processed system may indicate that the glycosylated 51 000 form is first cleaved and then glycosylated, since such a low molecular weight form is not immunoadsorbed from mouse native microsomes. These results with rat and mouse *in vitro* synthesis of transferase show that cleavage is required for at least one form in rat, and that glycosylation, and possibly cleavage, are required for at least one form in mouse for the process of inserting transferase into the endoplasmic reticulum.

It has been shown that two other integral ER membrane proteins, ribophorins, are cleaved and glycosylated as insertion into the membrane occurs[21]. Ribophorins are involved in the binding of ribosomes to membranes[21]. The requirement for cleavage or glycosylation of certain transferase forms indicates that processing of nascent polypeptides occurs for at least one category of membrane-bound drug metabolizing enzymes.

References

1. Gorski, J. P. and Kasper, C. B. (1977). Purification and properties of microsomal UDP-glucuronosyltransferase from rat liver. *J. Biol. Chem.*, **252,** 1333–43
2. Burchell, B. (1977). Purification of UDP-glucuronosyltransferase from untreated rat liver. *FEBS Lett.*, **78,** 101–4
3. Bock, K. W., Josting, D., Lilienblum, N. and Pfiel, H. (1979). Purification of rat liver microsomal UDP-glucuronosyltransferase. *Eur. J. Biochem.*, **98,** 19–26
4. Tukey, R. H. and Tephly, T. R. (1981). Purification and properties of rabbit liver estrone and *p*-nitrophenol UDP-glucuronosyltransferase. *Arch. Biochem. Biophys.*, **209,** 565–78
5. Blobel, G. and Dobberstein, B. (1975). Transfer of proteins across membranes: Presence of proteolytically processed and unprocessed nascent immunoglobulin light chains on membrane-bound ribosomes of murine myeloma. *J. Cell Biol.*, **67,** 835–51
6. Lingappa, V. R., Katz, F. N., Lodish, H. and Blobel, G. J. (1978). A signal sequence for the insertion of a transmembrane glycoprotein. *J. Biol. Chem.*, **253,** 8667–70
7. Dobberstein, B., Garoff, H. and Warren, G. (1979). Cell-free synthesis and membrane insertion of mouse H-2D^d histocompatibility antigen and β_2-microglobulin. *Cell*, **17,** 759–69
8. Kreibich, G., Sabatini, D. D. and Adesnik, M. (1983). Biosynthesis of hepatocyte endoplasmic reticulum proteins. *Meth. Enzymol.*, **96,** 530–42
9. Mackenzie, P. I., Hjelmeland, L. M. and Owens, I. S. (1984). Purification and immunochemical characterization of a low pI form of UDP-glucuronosyltransferase from mouse liver. *Arch. Biochem. Biophys.*, **231,** 487–97
10. Mackenzie, P. I. and Owens, I. S. (1983). Differences in UDP-glucuronosyltransferase activities in congenic inbred rats homozygous and heterozygous for the jaundice locus. *Biochem. Pharmacol.*, **32,** 3777–81
11. Kreibich, G., Hubbard, A. L. and Sabatini, D. D. (1974). On the spatial arrangement of proteins in microsomal membranes from rat liver. *J. Cell Biol.*, **60,** 616–27
12. Negishi, M., Jensen, N. M., Garcia, G. S. and Nebert, D. W. (1981). Structural gene products of the murine *Ah* locus. Differences in ontogenesis, membrane location, and glucosamine incorporation between liver microsomal cytochromes P_1-450 and P-448 induced by polycyclic aromatic compounds. *Eur. J. Biochem.*, **115,** 585–94
13. Mackenzie, P. I., Gonzalez, F. J. and Owens, I. S. (1984). Cell-free translation of mouse

liver mRNA coding for two forms of UDP-glucuronosyltransferase. *Arch. Biochem. Biophys.*, **230,** 676–80

14. Chirgwin, J. M., Przybyla, A. E., McDonald, R. J. and Rutter, W. J. (1979). Isolation of biologically active ribonucleic acid from sources rich in ribonuclease. *Biochemistry*, **18,** 5294–9
15. Aviv, H. and Leder, P. (1972). Purification of biologically active globin mRNA by chromatography on oligothymidylic acid cellulose. *Proc. Natl. Acad. Sci. USA*, **69,** 1408–22
16. Laemmli, U. K. (1970). Cleavage of structural proteins during the assembly of the head of bacteriophage T_4. *Nature*, **227,** 680–5
17. Bar-Nun, S., Kreibich, G., Adesnik, M., Alterman, L., Negishi, M. and Sabatini, D. D. (1980). Synthesis and insertion of cytochrome P-450 into endoplasmic reticulum membranes. *Proc. Natl. Acad. Sci. USA*, **77,** 965–9
18. Okada, Y., Frey, A. B., Guenthner, T. M., Oesch, F., Sabatini, D. D. and Kreibich, G. (1982). Studies on the biosynthesis of microsomal proteins: Site of synthesis and mode of insertion of cytochrome b_5, cytochrome b_5 reductase, cytochrome P-450 reductase, and epoxide hydrolase. *Eur. J. Biochem.*, **122,** 393–402
19. Gonzalez, F. J. and Kasper, C. B. (1980). Phenobarbital induction of NADPH-cytochrome c (P-450) oxidoreductase messenger ribonucleic acid. *Biochemistry*, **19,** 1790–6
20. Gonzalez, F. J. and Kasper, C. B. (1980). *In vitro* translation of epoxide hydratase messenger RNA. *Biochem. Biophys. Res. Commun.*, **93,** 1254–8
21. Kreibich, G., Marcantonio, E. E. and Sabatini, D. D. (1983). Ribophorins I and II: Membrane proteins characteristic of the rough endoplasmic reticulum. *Meth. Enzymol.*, **96,** 520–30

Section 3
Regulation of UDP-Glucuronosyltransferase and UDP-Glucosyltransferase by Membrane Components

Chairman: G. C. Wood

9
Phosphohpid regulation of UDP-glucuronyltransferase

G. C. WOOD, G. SCOTT AND A. B. GRAHAM

Like a number of other membrane-bound enzymes, the catalytic function of liver microsomal UDP-glucuronyltransferase is regulated by interaction of the enzyme with its membrane phospholipid environment (reviewed in references 1–4). There are two mechanisms, superimposed upon one another, by which membrane phospholipids modulate the enzyme[1,2,5,6]. Firstly, the intact membrane structure of most microsomal fractions restricts enzyme activity (latency), and most experimental evidence indicates that this is due to the phospholipid bilayer acting as a substantial part of a permeability barrier between the enzyme (located deep within the membrane) and its substrates[2,6–12]. The second mechanism of membrane modulation is evident in those microsomal preparations in which latency is low, or from which latency has been removed by mild perturbation of the membrane bilayer. Removal or degradation of phospholipids from such preparations results in loss of transferase activity; full activity is restored by sonicated dispersions of microsomal phospholipids and by phosphatidylcholine[5,13,14].

Studies in our laboratory have established the phospholipid-dependence of a purified UDP-glucuronyltransferase from guinea-pig liver which catalyses the glucuronidation of 4-nitrophenol (Table 9.1). The enzyme eluted from the affinity column (UDP-glucuronosyldiaminohexanyl-Sepharose) contains sufficient phospholipid to maintain high activity; removal of most of the phospholipid by means of hydroxyapatite inactivates the enzyme but reactivation occurs when phospholipid is added back. Similar phospholipid-dependence has been demonstrated for purified or partially purified UDP-glucuronyltransferase from other species with 4-nitrophenol and other acceptors[16–21]. There have been some reports, however, that rat liver enzyme (acceptor 4-nitrophenol) can be isolated in a highly active form which is, apparently, essentially free of phospholipid[19,20,22,23].

Several mechanisms have been postulated from time to time to account for the phospholipid-dependence of membrane-bound enzymes. One way in which phospholipids might maintain the activity of UDP-glucuronyltransferase is by

Table 9.1 Purification of guinea-pig liver microsomal UDP-glucuronyltransferase

*Purification step**	*Specific activity* (units†/mg protein)	*Purification*	*Yield* (%)	*Phospholipid content* (μg of P/mg protein)
Microsomal pellet suspended in 1% Lubrol	23.5	1.0	—	33.9
Lubrol-soluble protein	25.0	1.1	100	24.6
25–60% Saturated ammonium sulphate	25.0	1.1	67	22.8
DEAE-cellulose eluate	59.9	2.5	40	16.7
DEAE-Sephadex eluate	86.3	3.7	19	19.5
UDP-glucuronosyldiaminohexanyl-Sepharose eluate	3812	162	18	112‡
Hydroxyapatite eluate	344	—	—	2.2§

* for details of purification procedure and enzyme assay see ref. 15
† 1 unit = 1 nmol *p*-nitrophenol glucuronidated/min
‡ 190 mol/mol GTase sub-unit
§ 3.7 mol/mol GTase sub-unit

constraining the enzyme protein in an active conformation in which it can bind substrates and catalyse their glucuronidation[5]. In recent preliminary work we obtained evidence from circular dichroism (CD) measurements that in highly purified guinea-pig UDP-glucuronyltransferase containing sufficient phospholipid to maintain activity, the protein has a higher α-helical content than in lipid-depleted inactive enzyme[24].

ENZYME PURIFICATION

In order to embark on further investigations of the mechanism of phospholipid-dependence it is necessary for the highly purified enzyme to be readily available in sufficient amounts to permit the systematic application of physical techniques such as CD. With these requirements in mind we have re-investigated some aspects of the purification of guinea-pig UDP-glucuronyltransferase (acceptor 4-nitrophenol) with a view to simplifying the five-stage procedure used hitherto[15], based on the procedure of Burchell[19].

The first stage in fractionation of the Lubrol 12A9-soluble microsomal protein was ammonium sulphate fractionation. By collecting the fraction precipitating between 25% and 60% saturation Burchell and co-workers[19,23] had been able to remove more than 90% of the phospholipid from rat liver microsomal UDP-glucuronyltransferase. Substantial delipidation was also achieved by ammonium sulphate fractionation of cholate-solubilized microsomes from rat[22] and rabbit[25]. In our experience with guinea-pig liver microsomes, collection of the 25-60% saturation fraction was completely ineffective in separating phospholipid and protein (Table 9.1). We now find that the use of smaller increments in the concentration of ammonium sulphate separates much of the phospholipid from the protein (the results shown in Table 9.2 are typical), so that the phospholipid content is reduced from about 25 μg phospholipid phosphorus/mg protein to 4–8 μg/mg. In spite of this partial delipidation the enzyme remains active; the activities shown in Table 9.2 were obtained without added phospholipid. Addition of egg yolk phosphatidylcholine (100 μg P/mg protein) increased the activity of the enzyme-rich fraction by only 12%. For further purification work the fraction of the Lubrol-soluble protein precipitating in the narrow range of ammonium sulphate concentration (33–48% saturation) was used in preference to the broad (25–60% saturation) fraction.

Table 9.2 Fractionation of Lubrol-soluble protein from guinea-pig liver microsomes by ammonium sulphate precipitation

Ammonium sulphate concentration (% saturation)	*Protein precipitated* (mg)	*Phospholipid content* (μg P/mg protein)	*Specific activity* (units/mg protein)
25–30	57.0	36.5	3.4
30–35	49.8	11.3	8.6
35–45	86.4	4.5	22.8
45–50	32.8	1.4	14.6
50–60	62.2	1.0	4.9

The protein fractionated (568 mg) contained 6563 μg P and 13 051 units of enzyme activity

The narrow and broad ammonium sulphate fractions behaved similarly when subjected to chromatography on DEAE cellulose (Figure 9.1). Four major fractions (I–IV) were obtained when the column was eluted by stepwise increase in the concentration of KC1 in 25 mmol/l Tris HCl buffer pH 7.4. The phospholipid content of the protein in the various fractions are markedly different, as shown in the typical data in Table 9.3. Not only are the chromatographic fractions from the broad ammonium sulphate fraction richer in phospholipid than those from the narrow ammonium sulphate fraction, but also the chromatography affords some further separation of phospholipid and protein. The specific enzyme activity is highest in fraction II from each chromatogram, and it is higher in fraction II from the narrow ammonium sulphate fraction than in the corresponding chromatographic peak from the broad ammonium sulphate fraction. The activities given in Table 9.3 are those observed after adding phosphatidylcholine which is now *required* (*see* Figure 9.2) for maximum activity in all those fractions whose phospholipid content falls below about 17 μg phospholipid phosphorus/mg protein (~30 moles of phospholipid per enzyme subunit of MW 55 000).

Fraction II from the narrow ammonium sulphate fraction provided the purest enzyme at this stage of purification, i.e. the highest reconstituted specific activity and low phospholipid content. However, because only meagre purification was given by DEAE cellulose chromatography and because recovery of enzyme activity at this stage was rather low, fraction II was not considered to be a good starting point for further purification, bearing in mind our desire to simplify purification and increase its efficiency.

In recent work we have investigated direct application of the narrow ammo-

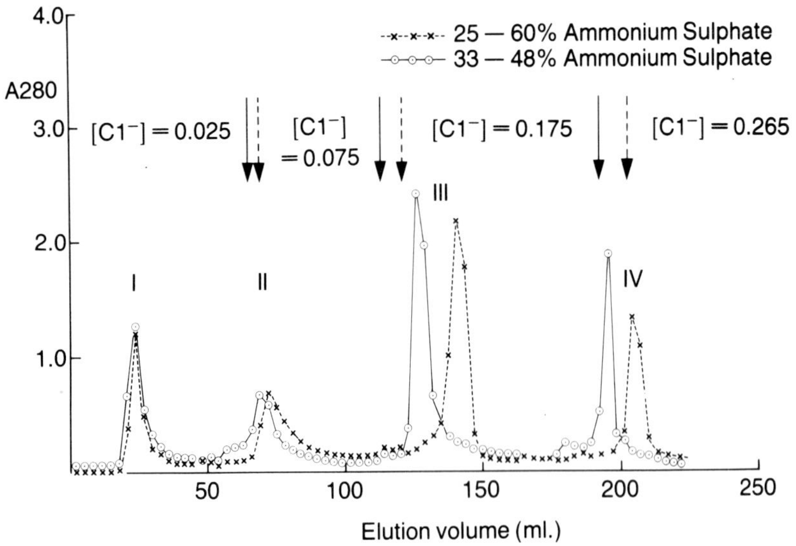

Figure 9.1 Chromatography of ammonium sulphate fractions on DEAE-cellulose. Protein samples (240 mg) precipitated by ammonium sulphate were chromatographed as described in reference 15. Fraction I was eluted with the equilibration buffer, 25 mmol/l Tris HCl buffer pH 7.4 containing 0.05% Lubrol 12A9. Subsequent fractions II-IV were eluted by stepwise additions of KCl to this buffer to give the concentrations of Cl^- indicated. The arrows indicate the steps in $[Cl^-]$

Table 9.3 Fractionation of ammonium sulphate fractions on DEAE cellulose

	Broad ammonium sulphate fraction			*Narrow ammonium sulphate fraction*		
Chromatographic fraction	*Protein content* (mg)	*Phospholipid content* (μg P/mg protein)	*Specific activity* (units/mg protein)	*Protein content* (mg)	*Phospholipid content* (μg P/mg protein)	*Specific activity* (units/mg protein)
I	20.8	51.7	10.8	19.7	14.7	21.2
II	22.8	21.2	38.2	14.9	4.8	98.9
III	38.9	5.9	27.4	32.5	1.1	16.0
IV	16.9	3.1	10.0	18.1	1.6	16.2

240 mg of protein were subjected to chromatography as described in ref. 15. Chromatographic fractions are identified in Figure 9.1

nium sulphate fraction to an affinity chromatography column (UDP-hexanolamine Sepharose 4B). Elution with 5 mmol/l UDPGA yields an enzyme fraction with low phospholipid content (20–50 moles of phospholipid per enzyme subunit of MW 55 000) and low activity (50–70 units/mg protein) in the absence of added phospholipid. The activity is markedly increased (to between 1400 and 2200 units/mg protein) by adding phosphatidylcholine (300 moles per mole of enzyme subunit). The overall yield of activity relative to the Lubrol-solubilized microsomal protein is about 25%, but on SDS polyacrylamide gel electrophore-

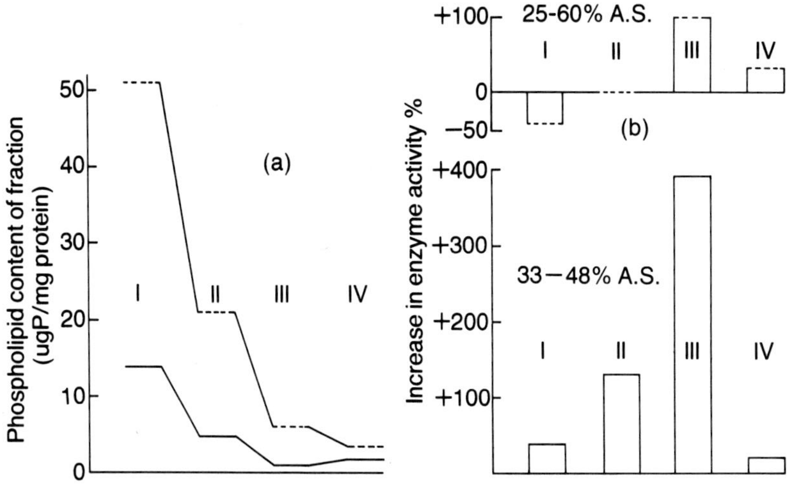

Figure 9.2 Reactivation of UDP-glucuronyltransferase in fractions from DEAE-cellulose chromatography. (a) Phospholipid content of the chromatographic fractions obtained from the broad (---) and narrow (——) ammonium sulphate fractions. (b) Increase in enzyme activity after adding phosphatidylcholine (100 μg P/mg protein) to chromatographic fractions from the broad (---) and narrow (——) ammonium sulphate fractions. Conditions of reactivation and enzyme assay are described in reference 15

sis it runs as two components with apparent molecular weights of 53 000 and 62 000, so that its purity is as yet uncertain.

EFFECT OF MEMBRANE PHOSPHOLIPIDS ON PROTEIN CONFORMATION

Consideration of those intrinsic membrane proteins which are well characterized indicates that the α-helix is the preferred conformation, at least in those parts of the proteins which traverse the membrane and are closely associated with the hydrocarbon chains of membrane phospholipids[26]; examples are glycophorin[27,28], bacteriorhodopsin[29,30] and rhodopsin[30]. With very few membrane proteins has a purified lipid-depleted protein been isolated, and the effects of added phospholipid on protein conformation studied systematically. Even more rarely has an attempt been made to relate conformational changes induced by phospholipids to the activity of phospholipid-dependent enzymes.

Hardwicke and Green[31] and LeMaire *et al.*[32] observed that inactivation of sarcoplasmic reticulum Ca^{2+}-ATPase by separation from membrane phospholipid was accompanied by changes in circular dichroism indicative of a decrease in α-helix content. Dean and Tanford[33] also proposed that a conformational change in this enzyme was induced by binding of lipid. More recently Gavilanes *et al.*[34,35] isolated a fatty acid synthetase multi-enzyme complex from the larvae of *Ceratitis capitata* as a 1 : 1 (w/w) complex of protein and lipid. Treatment with lipases, including phospholipase A2, or removal of phospholipids by incubation and gel-filtration, resulted in a progressive loss of 80% of the enzyme activity and a parallel change in conformation (from circular dichroism spectra) from 43% α-helix, 16% β to 25% α-helix, 25% β. Although the enzyme was reactivated by phosphatidylethanolamine no reversal of the conformational change was reported. In another recent study Yu and Yu[36] reported that intact mitochondrial ubiquinone-cytochrome C reductase, containing 8 μg phospholipid phosphorus/mg protein, has an α-helix content (from CD) of about 40%. Progressive removal of lipid by repeated ammonium sulphate precipitation in 0.5% cholate, gradually inactivated the enzyme system, and there was a parallel reduction in α-helix content to about 30%. Chiang and Coon[37,38] recently isolated two cytochrome P-450 isoenzymes from rat liver microsomes in highly purified form essentially free of phospholipid (< 20 mol phospholipid/mol cytochrome P-450). The α-helical content of both proteins (37% and 25%) was substantially increased (to 44% and 49%, respectively) by adding dilaurylphosphatidylcholine, and this suggested that the known enhancement of the catalytic activity of the NADPH/cytochrome P-450/cytochrome P-450 reductase system by phospholipids may result from a structural change in the cytochrome P-450.

Thus, such evidence as is available suggests that the presence of adequate phospholipid in these various membrane enzyme preparations helps to maintain their α-helix content, and that this effect might be connected with phospholipid-dependence of enzyme activity.

Our recent work with UDP-glucuronyltransferase[24] suggests that this enzyme falls into the same pattern. The CD spectrum (Figure 9.3) of highly purified guinea-pig enzyme (containing 570 moles phospholipid per protein subunit) isolated as indicated in Table 9.1, indicates that this protein has an α-helix content of about 27%. Progressive delipidation resulted in loss of activity and loss of α-helix content, and the latter was at least partially restored when the enzyme was reactivated by replacing the phospholipid. As shown in Figure 9.4, reduction of the phospholipid content below 170–200 moles/mole of protein subunit results in both a sharp fall of enzyme activity and an abrupt change in protein conformation. The circular dichroism technique gives information about the average conformation over the whole protein. It is unlikely that the conformation of the polypeptide chain in all parts of the molecule will be equally important for the properties of the active site region and, therefore, a simple relationship between α-helical content and enzyme activity is not to be expected. It was in order to investigate this relationship more fully that we embarked on the refinement of enzyme purification. While this work is incomplete, the CD spectrum of the delipidated (inactive) guinea-pig enzyme resulting from the simplified two-step fractionation of Lubrol-soluble microsomal protein has been determined. It indicates that the protein contains significant α-helix content, and this is increased significantly when the enzyme is reactivated by adding phosphatidylcholine. Further work is in progress.

ACKNOWLEDGEMENT

G.S. thanks the Science and Engineering Research Council for the award of a Research Studentship.

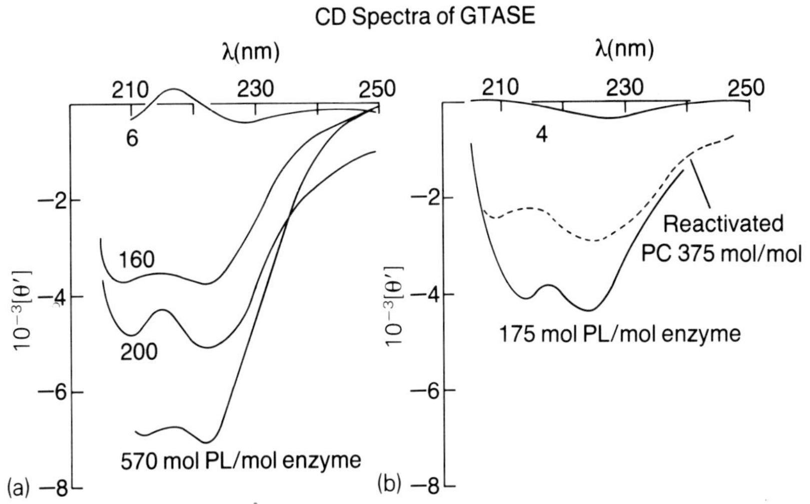

Figure 9.3 Circular dichroism spectra of purified UDP-glucuronyltransferase. (a) Spectrum of enzyme obtained from the affinity chromatography step of the purification procedure summarized in Table 9.1, containing 570 mol phospholipid/mol enzyme subunit, and spectra after delipidation to various extents by hydroxyapatite chromatography. (b) Spectrum of another enzyme preparation containing 175 mol phospholipid/mol enzyme subunit and spectra after delipidation followed by addition of egg yolk phosphatidylcholine (375 mol/mol enzyme subunit).
$[\theta']$ = mean residue ellipticity (deg. cm^2 dmol^{-1}) calculated using a mean residue weight of 115. For experimental details *see* reference 24

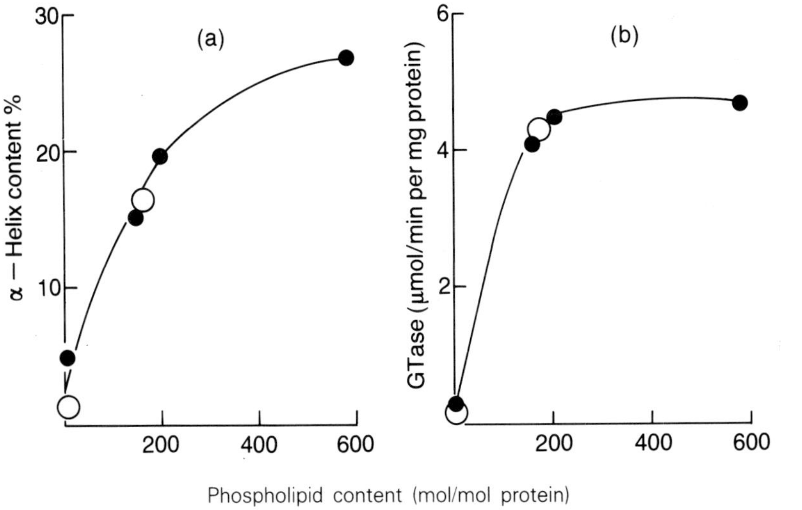

Figure 9.4 Relationship between the α-Helix content and the catalytic activity of UDP-glucuronyltransferase and its phospholipid content. α-Helix contents were calculated[39] from the CD spectra of Figure 9.3. Data from Figure 9.3a (●) and from Figure 9.3b (○)

References

1. Dutton, G. J. and Burchell, B. (1978). Newer aspects of glucuronidation. *Progr. Drug. Metab.*, **2,** 1–70
2. Dutton, G. J. (1980). *Glucuronidation of Drugs and Other Compounds.* (Boca Raton, Florida: CRC Press)
3. Kasper, C. B. and Henton, D. (1980). Glucuronidation. In Jakoby, W. B. (ed.). *Enzymatic Basis of Detoxication*, Vol. 2, pp. 3–36. (London: Academic Press)
4. Zakim, D. and Vessey, D. A. (1982). The role of the microsomal membrane in modulating the activity of UDP-glucuronyltransferase. In Martonosi, A. N. (ed.). *Membranes and Transport*, Vol. 1, pp. 269–73. (New York: Plenum Press)
5. Graham, A. B., Pechey, D. T., Wood, G. C. and Woodcock, B. G. (1974). The role of the microsomal membrane in control of UDP-glucuronyltransferase *in vitro* and *in vivo. Biochem. Soc. Trans.*, **2,** 1167-72
6. Wood, G. C., Graham, A. B. and Toogood, K. C. (1978). Membrane modulation of microsomal UDP-glucuronyltransferase. In Aitio, A. (ed.). *Conjugation Reactions in Drug Biotransformation*, pp. 203–12. (Amsterdam: Elsevier/North Holland)
7. Hallinan, T. (1978). Comparison of compartmented and of conformational phospholipid-constraint models for the intramembranous arrangement of UDP-glucuronyltransferase. In Aitio, A. (ed.). *Conjugation Reactions in Drug Biotransformation*, pp. 257–67. (Amsterdam: Elsevier/North-Holland)
8. Graham, A. B., Pechey, D. T. and Wood, G. C. (1979). Responses of microsomal UDP-glucuronyltransferase to trypsin. *Molec. Pharmacol.*, **15,** 375–85
9. Haeger, B., de Brito, R. and Hallinan, T. (1980). Diazobenzene sulphonate selectively abolishes stimulation of glucuronidation by UDP-*N*-acetylglucosamine. *Biochem. J.*, **192,** 971–4
10. Graham, A. B., Pechey, D. T. and Wood, G. C. (1978). Phospholipid phase changes affecting microsomal UDP-glucuronyltransferase activity. In Aitio, A. (ed.). *Conjugation Reactions in Drug Biotransformation*, pp. 213–22. (Amsterdam: Elsevier/North-Holland)
11. Cummings, J., Graham, A. B. and Wood, G. C. (1980). The phospholipid-dependence of UDP-glucuronyltransferase: temperature-dependence of microsomal enzyme activity (reverse reaction). *Biochem. J.*, **185,** 521–6
12. Cummings, J. and Graham, A. B. (1984). Anomalous kinetics of latent microsomal UDP-glucuronyltransferase. (In press)
13. Attwood, D., Graham, A. B. and Wood, G. C. (1971). The phospholipid-dependence of UDP-glucuronyltransferase. Reactivation of phospholipase A-inactivated enzyme by phospholipids and detergents. *Biochem. J.*, **123,** 875–82
14. Graham, A. B., Pechey, D. T., Toogood, K. C., Thomas, S. B. and Wood, G. C. (1977). The phospholipid-dependence of UDP-glucuronyltransferase. Phospholipid depletion and reactivation of guinea-pig liver microsomal enzyme. *Biochem. J.*, **163,** 117–24
15. Singh, O. M. P., Graham, A. B. and Wood, G. C. (1981). The phospholipid-dependence of UDP-glucuronyltransferase. Purification, delipidation and reconstitution of microsomal enzyme from guinea-pig liver. *Eur. J. Biochem.*, **116,** 311–6
16. Tukey, R. H. and Tephly, T. R. (1981). Purification and properties of rabbit liver estrone and *p*-nitrophenol UDP-glucuronyltransferases. *Arch. Biochem. Biophys.*, **209,** 565–78
17. Hochman, Y., Zakim, D. and Vessey, D. A. (1981). A kinetic mechanism for modulation of the activity of microsomal UDP-glucuronyltransferase. *J. Biol. Chem.*, **256,** 4783–8
18. Magdalou, J., Hochman, Y. and Zakim, D. (1982). Factors modulating the catalytic specificity of a pure form of UDP-glucuronyltransferase. *J. Biol. Chem.*, **257,** 13624–9
19. Burchell, B. (1980). Purification of UDP-glucuronyltransferase from untreated rat liver. *FEBS Letters*, **111,** 131–5
20. Weatherill, P. J. and Burchell, B. (1980). The separation and purification of rat liver UDP-glucuronyltransferase activities towards testosterone and oestrone. *Biochem. J.*, **189,** 377–80
21. Matern, H., Matern, S. and Gerok, W. (1982). Isolation and characterisation of rat liver microsomal UDP-glucuronyltransferase activity towards chenodeoxycholic acid and testosterone as a single form of enzyme. *J. Biol. Chem.*, **257,** 7422–9
22. Bock, K. W., Josting, D., Lilenblum, W. and Pfeil, H. (1979). Purification of rat liver glucuronyltransferase. Separation of two enzyme forms inducible by 3-methylcholanthrene of phenobarbital. *Eur. J. Biochem.*, **98,** 19–26

23. Burchell, B. and Hallinen, T. (1978). Phospholipid content and activity of pure UDP-glucuronyltransferase from rat liver. *Biochem. J.*, **171,** 821–4
24. Singh, O. M. P., Graham, A. B. and Wood, G. C. (1982). The phospholipid dependence of UDP-glucuronyltransferase: conformation/reactivity studies with purified enzyme. *Biochem. Biophys. Res. Commun.*, **107,** 345–9
25. Tukey, R. H., Billings, R. E., Autor, A. P. and Tephly, T. R. (1979). Phospholipid-dependence of oestrone UDP-glucuronyltransferase and *p*-nitrophenol UDP-glucuronyltransferase. *Biochem. J.*, **179,** 59–65
26. Capaldi, R. A. (1977). The structural properties of membrane proteins. In Capaldi, R. A. (ed.). *Membrane Proteins and their Interactions with Lipids*, pp. 1–19 (New York: M. Dekker)
27. Segrest, J. P. and Jackson, R. L. (1977). Molecular properties of membrane proteins. In Capaldi, R. A. (ed.). *Membrane Proteins and their Interactions with Lipids*, pp. 21–45. (New York: M. Dekker)
28. Schulte, T. H. and Marchesi, V. T. (1979). Conformation of human erythrocyte glycophorin A and its constituent peptides. *Biochemistry*, **18,** 275–80
29. Henderson, R. and Unwin, P. W. T. (1975). Three dimensional model of purple membrane obtained by electron microscopy. *Nature*, **257,** 28–32
30. Wallace, B. A. (1982). Comparison of bacteriorhodopsin and rhodopsin molecular structure. In Colowick, S. P. and Kaplan, N. O. (eds.). *Methods in Enzymology*, Vol. 88, part 1, pp. 447–62. (New York: Academic Press)
31. Hardwicke, P. M. D. and Green, N. M. (1974). The effect of delipidation on the adenosine triphosphatase of sarcoplasmic reticulum. Electron microscopy and physical properties. *Eur. J. Biochem.*, **42,** 183–93
32. LeMaire, M., Jorgensen, K. E., Røigaard-Petersen, H. and Møller, J. V. (1976). Properties of deoxycholate solubilised sarcoplasmic reticulum Ca^{2+}-ATPase. *Biochemistry*, **15,** 5805–12
33. Dean, W. L. and Tanford, C. (1978). Properties of a delipidated, detergent-activated Ca^{2+}-ATPase. *Biochemistry*, **17,** 1683–90
34. Gavilanes, J. G., Lizarbe, M. A., Municio, A. M. and Onaderra, M. (1981). Effect of phospholipids on the length of the helical segments in the fatty acid synthetase complex from *Ceratitis capitata. FEBS Letters*, **126,** 253–6
35. Gavilanes, J. G., Lizarbe, M. A., Municio, A. M. and Onaderra, M. (1981). Fatty acid synthetase complex from the insect *Ceratitis capitata*. Structural studies. *Biochim. Biophys. Acta*, **668,** 246–56
36. Yu, C. A. and Yu, L. (1980). Structural role of phospholipids in ubiquinol-cytochrome C reductase. *Biochemistry*, **19,** 5715–20
37. Chiang, Y.-L. (1978). Phospholipid interactions with cytochrome P-450. *Fed. Proc.*, **37,** 1719
38. Chiang, Y.-L. and Coon, M. J. (1979). Comparative study of two highly purified forms of liver microsomal cytochrome P-450. Circular dichroism and other studies. *Arch. Biophys. Biochem.*, **195,** 178–87
39. Chen, Y. H., Yang, J. T. and Martinez, H. M. (1972). Determination of the secondary structure of proteins by circular dichroism and optical rotatory dispersion. *Biochemistry*, **11,** 4120–31

10
Kinetic studies of latent microsomal UDP-glucuronyltransferases: Activation by UDP-*N*-acetylglucosamine and Mg^{2+}

A. B. GRAHAM, J. CUMMINGS AND G. C. WOOD

ABSTRACT

UDP-*N*-acetylglucosamine and Mg^{2+} activated latent rat and guinea-pig liver microsomal UDP-glucuronyltransferases (*p*-nitrophenol acceptor) by mechanism(s) which affected the two enzyme forms of these membranes at both *K* and *V*. Their most striking and significant effect in combination was to decrease by 10–15-fold the Michaelis constant of the high-K buried transferase form (K_2). The results provide additional support for our two-enzyme variation of the 'compartmentational' model of latency, and they suggest that the activators might increase rates of glucuronidation by increasing the affinity of a facilitated transport system for UDP-glucuronate.

INTRODUCTION

In a recent paper[1], we have proposed a model which explains the anomalous kinetics of latent microsomal UDP-glucuronyltransferases and their responses to the membrane perturbants Triton X-100 and lysophosphatidylcholine. This assessment of the kinetics of glucuronidation of *p*-nitrophenol has strengthened our contention[2,3] that there are two populations of transferase molecules in membranes exhibiting enzyme latency. A small proportion of the enzyme molecules appears to be located at or near the outer surface of the microsomal vesicle with unrestricted access to substrates, while the majority occupy locations nearer the inner membrane surface with UDP-glucuronate (UDP-GlcUA) being transported to these sites by a process with the characteristics of facilitated diffusion[1].

Proponents of the 'conformational' concept of transferase latency postulated that UDP-*N*-acetylglucosamine (UDP-Glc*N*Ac) activates *p*-nitrophenol glucuronidation by increasing specifically the 'affinity' of the latent enzyme for UDP-GlcUA, and they demonstrated that bivalent metal ions (Mg^{2+} or Mn^{2+}) enhanced activation by UDP-Glc*N*Ac[4]. The cations themselves also activated the latent transferase by a mechanism which appeared only to involve an increase in the maximum velocity of glucuronidation[5,6]. From these and other kinetic data it was argued that UDP-Glc*N*Ac is a physiological modulator of multisubunit transferases[7-9]; it was proposed that UDP-Glc*N*Ac is a positive K-type allosteric effector, and that in conjunction with metal ions it promotes efficient physiological control of the rates of glucuronide biosynthesis.

A very different interpretation of the effects of UDP-Glc*N*Ac on latent transferases has come from the supporters of the 'compartmentation' theory of latency. They have concluded that UDP-Glc*N*Ac activates merely by increasing the maximum velocity of the reaction[10], and it has been suggested that the activator in presence of metal ions stimulates a microsomal permease system which transports UDP-GlcUA to intramembrane catalytic sites[11,12].

In order to study our two-enzyme model of latency more thoroughly, we investigate, in this paper, the effects of UDP-Glc*N*Ac and Mg^{2+}, both singly and in combination, on the kinetics of latent microsomal UDP-glucuronyltransferases.

MATERIALS AND METHODS

The sources of chemicals and animals were listed previously[1]. UDP-Glc*N*Ac was from Sigma Chemical Co. Ltd., Poole, Dorset, UK. The preparation of liver microsomal membranes with 0.25 mol/l sucrose and the determinations of initial rates of *p*-nitrophenol glucuronidation were also described[1]. When Mg^{2+} was added to transferase reaction mixtures, the buffer used was 50 mmol/l. Tris-HCl (pH 7.1), and EDTA, added to inhibit the hydrolysis of UDP-GlcUA, was omitted from reactions containing rat liver microsomal membranes.

The kinetic data were fitted by computer to equation [1] by the two procedures described earlier[1];

$$v_0 = \frac{V_1 s}{K_1 + s} + \frac{V_2 s}{K_2 + s} \qquad [1]$$

v_0 is the initial velocity observed, s is the initial concentration of UDP-GlcUA, and the subscripts refer to the separate enzyme forms.

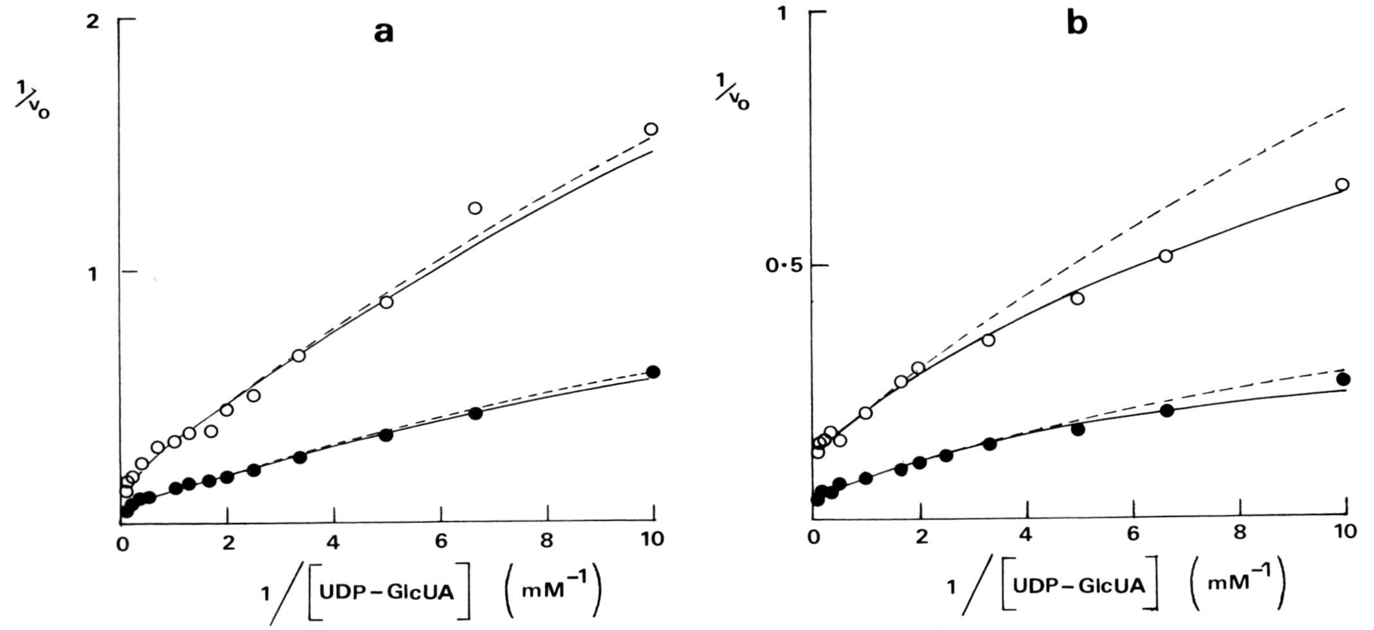

Figure 10.1 Double-reciprocal plots of the rate of glucuronidation of *p*-nitrophenol in intact microsomal membranes with UDP-GlcUA as varied substrate: the effects of UDP-Glc*N*Ac and Mg^{2+} singly and in combination.

Initial rates were determined with a fixed concentration of acceptor (0.6 mmol/l); v_0 is expressed as nmol of acceptor glucuronidated $min^{-1} mg^{-1}$ of microsomal protein. The dashed line gives the best fit obtained by the Osmundsen weighted non-linear regression method, the solid line gives the best least-squares fit[1]. (a) ○, Guinea-pig membranes with no additions; ●, guinea-pig membranes plus 2 mmol/l UDP-Glc*N*Ac. (b) ○, Guinea-pig membranes plus 5 mmol/l $MgCl_2$; ●, guinea-pig membranes plus 2 mmol/l UDP-Glc*N*Ac and 5 mmol/l $MgCl_2$. (c) ○, Rat membranes with no additions; ●, rat membranes plus 2 mmol/l UDP-Glc*N*Ac. (d) ○, Rat membranes plus 5 mmol/l $MgCl_2$; ●, rat membranes plus 2 mmol/l UDP-Glc*N*Ac and 5 mmol/l $MgCl_2$

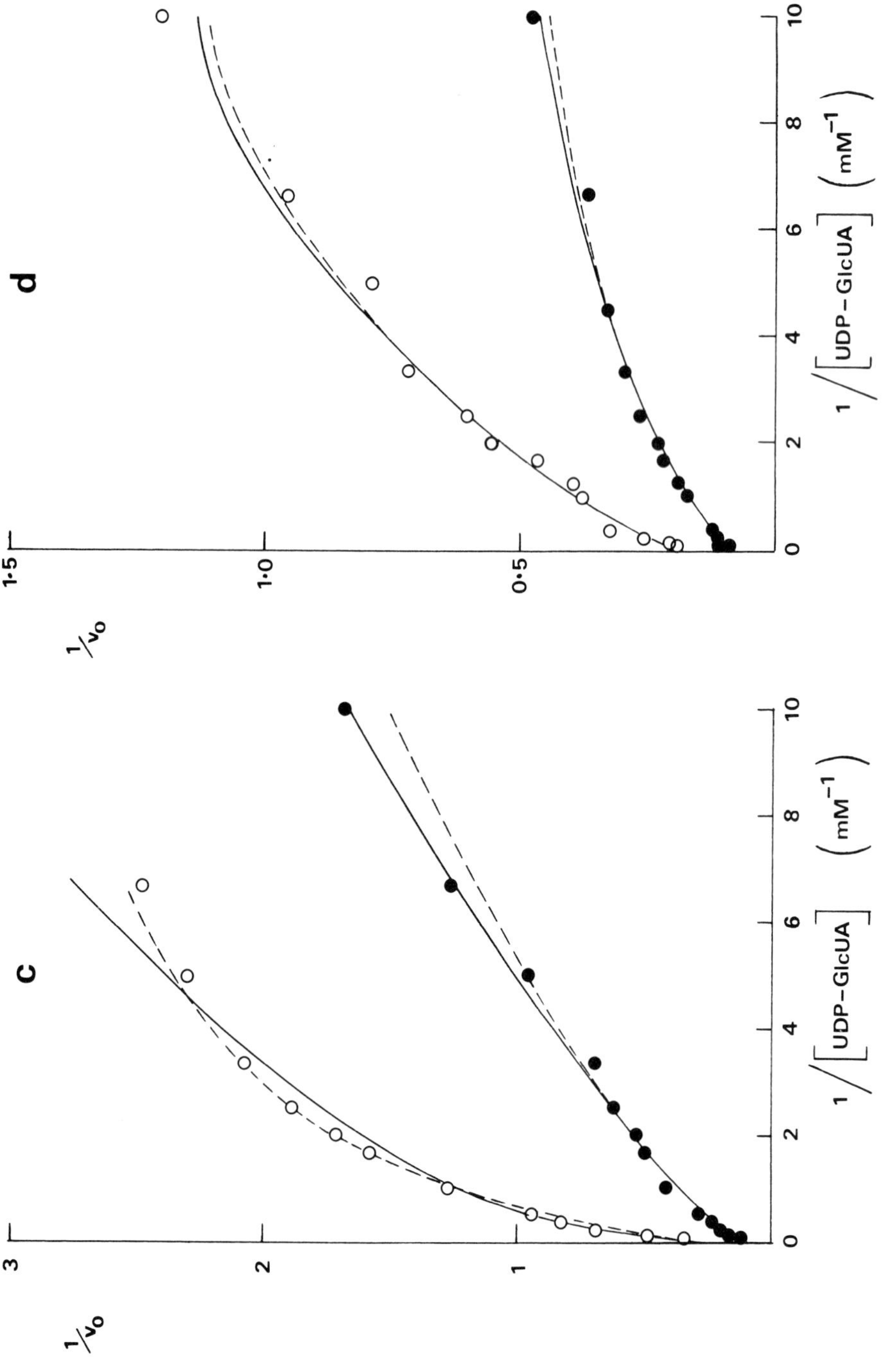

Figure 10.1 (c, d)

Table 10.1 Kinetic parameters of UDP-glucuronyltransferase forms in intact microsomal membranes: the effects of UDP-Glc*N*Ac and Mg^{2+} singly and in combination.

(**A**) Denotes experiments with guinea-pig membranes, (**B**) experiments with rat membranes; (a) signifies values of parameters calculated by the tangential approximation/least-squares method, (b) by the Osmundsen weighted non-linear regression procedure[1]. Values of K are expressed as mmol/l UDP-GlcUA, values of V as nmol of acceptor glucuronidated $min^{-1} mg^{-1}$ of microsomal protein. See text and Figure 10.1

Type of membranes	*Kinetic parameter*	*Calculation method*	*No. additions*	*UDP-GlcNAc (2 mmol/l)*	*$MgCl_2$ (5 mmol/l)*	*UDP-GlcNAc + $MgCl_2$ (2 mmol/l + 5 mmol/l)*
A	K_1	a	0.56	0.31	0.74	0.15
		b	0.64	0.48	0.56	0.14
	V_1	a	4.31	6.65	6.36	7.13
		b	4.79	9.01	7.42	5.53
	K_2	a	32.08	9.81	9.93	1.77
		b	—	19.19	—	2.09
	V_2	a	8.05	18.27	20.86	16.76
		b	—	19.78	—	21.64
B	K_1	a	0.19	0.33	0.25	0.08
		b	0.07	0.19	0.07	0.02
	V_1	a	0.73	2.13	2.63	3.20
		b	0.52	1.48	1.14	2.02
	K_2	a	30.48	6.17	9.94	2.30
		b	16.59	4.69	2.18	1.60
	V_2	a	5.50	7.00	4.34	9.77
		b	4.31	7.32	4.09	8.96

RESULTS AND DISCUSSION

When 2 mmol/l UDP-Glc*N*Ac, 5 mmol/l $MgCl_2$ and 2 mmol/l UDP-Glc*N*Ac plus 5 mmol/l $MgCl_2$ were added to reaction mixtures with guinea-pig and rat microsomal membranes prepared with sucrose (where the transferases are highly latent[1,13]), rates of glucuronidation were increased at all concentrations of UDP-GlcUA from 0.1 to 20 mmol/l, and all the double-reciprocal plots were continuously curved concave-down (Figures 10.1a–d). The kinetic parameters calculated for the two transferase forms by fitting the data to equation [1] are shown in Table 10.1. Again these results are entirely consistent with the existence of high-*K* and low-*K* forms of the enzyme in intact membranes.

With guinea-pig membranes (*see* Table 10.1), UDP-Glc*N*Ac had little or no effect on both K_1 and V_1 (the parameters of the exposed enzyme form). Its effects on the parameters of the buried form were to decrease K_2 to about one third of its value, and to increase V_2 about 2-fold. Mg^{2+} brought about very similar effects. Together, UDP-Glc*N*Ac and Mg^{2+} did not alter V_1, but decreased K_1 some 3-fold. However, their most striking and significant effect in combination was to decrease K_2 approximately 15-fold; they also almost doubled the value of V_2. Mg^{2+} and UDP-Glc*N*Ac apparently had additive effects on K_1 and K_2 but not upon V_2.

With rat membranes UDP-Glc*N*Ac altered the kinetic parameters of both enzyme forms (Table 10.1). It increased K_1 slightly and increased V_1 3-fold; it decreased K_2 5-fold and increased V_2 slightly. Mg^{2+} produced similar effects; K_1 was not affected, V_1 was increased 3-fold, K_2 was decreased 3–8-fold and V_2 was unchanged. When the activators were added together K_1 was decreased 2–3-fold, V_1 was increased 3-fold and V_2 was doubled; again their most pronounced effect was to cause a 10–15-fold decrease in the value of K_2, and as seen with guinea-pig membranes, they had additive effects on K_1 and K_2, but not upon V_1 or V_2.

According to the model of a single compartmented enzyme species[11,12], the intact structure of the microsomal membrane restricts access of UDP-GlcUA to deeply buried sites of glucuronidation, and transport of the donor substrate is facilitated by the permease system. Hallinan and co-workers[10] investigated the effect of 0.8 mmol/l UDP-Glc*N*Ac plus 4 mmol/l Mg^{2+} on the kinetics of the latent transferase in guinea-pig membranes prepared with sucrose. They used a fixed concentration of acceptor (0.4 mmol/l *p*-nitrophenol) and various concentrations of UDP-GlcUA (0.33–4 mmol/l). They observed linear double-reciprocal plots and evaluated *K* and *V* assuming Michaelis–Menten kinetics. Their data suggested that the activators selectively increased transferase activity at *V* and it was concluded that Mg^{2+} and UDP-Glc*N*Ac had stimulated the permease system specifically. However, the range of substrate concentrations selected by these workers was much too narrow. Double-reciprocal plots for the latent guinea-pig enzyme have the appearance of linearity from 0.1–2 mmol/l and 2–20 mmol/l UDP-GlcUA (Figure 10.1a, *see* also ref. 4) and bend quite sharply near 2 mmol/l UDP-GlcUA. The latent enzyme does not obey the classical rate law, and if the apparently linear portions (at low substrate concentrations) of the plots of Figure 10.1 were extrapolated to infinite substrate concentration it would indeed appear that a selective increase at *V* had occurred. Our data, from a much more extensive range of donor concentrations, show that the activators predominantly affect K_2 and do not support this simpler 'compartmentational' model of latency.

The analysis of the effects of UDP-Glc*N*Ac and bivalent metal ions by Zakim's group led to quite different conclusions. It was claimed that 2 mmol/l UDP-Glc*N*Ac altered only the value of K of the latent guinea-pig enzyme[4]. This conclusion was reached by extrapolating the apparently linear portions of curvilinear double-reciprocal plots (2.5–40 mmol/l UDP-GlcUA) to infinite substrate concentration and calculating K and V by assuming simple single enzyme Michaelis–Menten kinetics with no diffusion control. The curved portions of their plots were explained by negatively cooperative substrate binding. Using this rationale, it was claimed that Mn^{2+} affected only the value of V for a single enzyme species exhibiting negative cooperativity in the binding of low concentrations of UDP-GlcUA[5,6]. The validity of these conclusions depends upon how these anomalous kinetics are interpreted, and, as we have reasoned earlier[1], this allosteric interpretation is questionable.

Our analysis of the kinetics indicates that UDP-Glc*N*Ac and Mg^{2+} have similar effects on the parameters of the two enzyme forms of native membranes, and that they involve changes at both K and V. Their most obvious and significant effect in combination is to decrease substantially the value of K_2. Our data for the enzyme in perturbant-treated membranes indicate that form 2 is the buried species and that UDP-GlcUA crosses the membrane matrix by a process resembling facilitated transport[1]. Thus, the kinetics of the transporter are likely to affect the reactivity of the buried form. For this enzyme form in intact membranes (*see* equations 11–15 of ref. 1) we have argued that the reciprocal of the affinity of the transporter for UDP-GlcUA (K_T) is greater than the Michaelis constant of the buried enzyme form (K_b); i.e. χ (the affinity modulus) >1, and its activity is constrained (ν, the activity modulus <1). As a result, any reagent which reduces χ or increases ν would increase the activity of the buried form and activate glucuronidation. UDP-Glc*N*Ac plus Mg^{2+} decrease markedly the apparent value of K_2 (thus reducing χ) and activate glucuronidation. By increasing the affinity of the transporter (i.e. decreasing K_T) for UDP-GlcUA these activators might increase rates of glucuronidation. Nevertheless, even in the presence of these activators the activity of the buried transferase population would still be constrained to some extent by the transport system, and double-reciprocal plots for the enzyme under these conditions would be expected to be curved. Figure 10.1 shows very clearly that this is the case. By increasing the efficiency of the transporter, UDP-Glc*N*Ac and bivalent metal ions may be important physiologically in regulating rates of UDP-glucuronyltransferase reactions. The results presented here furnish additional evidence in favour of our two-enzyme variation of the 'compartmentation' model of latency.

ACKNOWLEDGEMENT

J. C. is indebted to the Glasgow Educational Trust for financial support.

References

1. Cummings, J., Graham, A. B. and Wood, G. C. (1984). Kinetic studies of latent microsomal UDP-glucuronyltransferases: kinetics of glucuronidation in intact and perturbant-treated membranes. *Biochim. Biophys. Acta*, **771**, 127–41
2. Graham, A. B., Pechey, D. T. and Wood, G. C. (1979). Responses of microsomal UDP-glucuronyltransferase to trypsin. *Mol. Pharmacol.*, **15**, 375–85
3. Onah, J. O., Graham, A. B. and Wood, G. C. (1982). Responses of latent microsomal UDP-glucuronyltransferases to trypsin. *Biochem. Soc. Trans.*, **10**, 542–3
4. Vessey, D. A., Goldenberg, J. and Zakim, D. (1973). Kinetic properties of microsomal UDP-glucuronyltransferase: evidence for cooperative kinetics and activation by UDP-*N*-acetylglucosamine. *Biochim. Biophys. Acta*, **309**, 58–66
5. Zakim, D., Goldenberg, J. and Vessey, D. A. (1973). Effects of metals on the properties of hepatic microsomal UDP-glucuronyltransferase. *Biochemistry*, **12**, 4068–73
6. Zakim, D., Goldenberg, J. and Vessey, D. A. (1973). Kinetic properties of microsomal UDP-glucuronyltransferase: regulation by metal ions. *Biochem. Biophys. Res. Commun.*, **52**, 453–8
7. Zakim, D. and Vessey, D. A. (1976). The effects of lipid–protein interactions on the kinetic parameters of microsomal UDP-glucuronyltransferase. In Martonosi, A. (ed.). *The Enzymes of Biological Membranes*. Vol. II, pp. 443–61. (New York: Plenum Press)
8. Zakim, D. and Vessey, D. A. (1977). Regulation of microsomal UDP-glucuronyltransferase: mechanism of activation by UDP-*N*-acetylglucosamine. *Biochem. Pharmacol.*, **26**, 129–31
9. Zakim, D. and Vessey, D. A. (1978). Are glucuronidation reactions compartmented? In Aitio, A. (ed.). *Conjugation Reactions in Drug Biotransformation*. pp. 247–55. (Amsterdam: Elsevier/North Holland)
10. Bingham, P., Berry, C. S. and Hallinan, T. (1978). Compartmentation of UDP-glucuronyltransferase: effect of UDP-*N*-acetylglucosamine on the apparent V of glucuronidation. *Biochem. Soc. Trans.*, **6**, 178–80
11. Berry, C. S. (1978). Critical evaluation of UDP-*N*-acetylglucosamine and product glucuronides as allosteric effectors of UDP-glucuronyltransferase. In Aitio, A. (ed.). *Conjugation Reactions in Drug Biotransformation*. pp. 233–46. (Amsterdam: Elsevier/North Holland)
12. Hallinan, T. (1978). Comparison of compartmented and of conformational phospholipid-constraint models for the intramembranous arrangement of UDP-glucuronyltransferase. In Aitio, A. (ed.). *Conjugation Reactions in Drug Biotransformation*, pp. 257–67. (Amsterdam: Elsevier/North Holland)
13. Pechey, D. T., Graham, A. B. and Wood, G. C. (1978). The phospholipid-dependence of UDP-glucuronyltransferase: temperature-dependence of microsomal enzyme activity and thermotropic changes in membrane structure. *Biochem. J.*, **175**, 115–24

11
Biotransformation, especially glucuronidation and their control by temperature in fish

O. HÄNNINEN, U. KOIVUSAARI AND P. LINDSTRÖM-SEPPÄ

INTRODUCTION

Fish are exposed to chemicals occurring in the water. The chemicals can enter their body through the skin, via gills in respired water and through the gastrointestinal tract in ingested water and food. The food (plankton, plants and other fish) is similarly exposed to chemicals in water. The lipophilic compounds would stay in fish tissues if not converted into water soluble form; fish contain lipid material as do all other living organisms. Formerly it was suggested that fish are devoid of biotransformation ability[1], but this has been proved not to be the case (for reviews see references 2–4). In fact fish were one of the first poikilothermic species in which glucuronidation was observed[5]. Later it was shown that in fish all the sites of entry of xenobiotics appear to show some biotransformation ability in addition to the liver and kidneys[6]. Several factors contribute to the control of biotransformation ability, exemplified by the sex hormones[7] and certain environmental chemicals[8–10]. In this paper the role of the seasonal cycles, as well as the water temperature, will be described and discussed: The rainbow trout (*Salmo gairdneri*) has been used as the model. It appears that in these studies one should measure the various activities both at the temperatures where the fish have been living as well as at a constant, not denaturing, temperature to get a clear picture of the adaptive phenomena.

ADAPTATION TO THE COOLING OF WATER

In boreal regions the waters cool during the autumn from the summer temperatures (close to 20°C) to freezing point. Under the ice temperatures vary from

4 to 0°C. Several adaptation phenomena occur in the tissues of fish. It appears that during water cooling several mono-oxygenase activities in the liver of rainbow trout remain the same, if measured at the temperature of the water where the fish were caught. If the measurements are carried out at a constant temperature (18°C), the mono-oxygenase activities show a several-fold increase[11]. Since the content of the cytochrome P-450 does not change, the phenomenon is due to a modification of the catalytic properties (Table 11.1). It has been demonstrated that the unsaturation of the membrane lipids takes place in fish with water cooling[12]. This contributes to the maintenance of the homeoviscosity of the membrane and of the mobility of mono-oxygenase components. Although the mono-oxygenase activities show an ideal temperature compensation pattern[13] in the rainbow trout liver microsomes, this is not the case for UDP-glucuronosyltransferase located in the same membrane

Table 11.1 The activities of 7-ethoxycoumarin-*o*-deethylase and UDP-glucuronosyltransferase in the liver microsomes of male rainbow trouts in August and November, measured at constant temperature (18°C) and at environmental temperatures (i.e. 20°C and 5°C, respectively)

	August *+18°C*	*November* *+18°C*	*August* *+20°C*	*November* *+5°C*
7-Ethoxycoumarin-*O*-deethylase mol/min × mol P-450	0.26±0.02*	0.91±0.18*	0.35±0.02	0.34±0.07
UDP-glucuronosyl-transferase nmol/min × mg protein	0.17±0.02	0.13±0.01	0.18±0.02†	0.05±0.004†

* $p<0.01$
† $p<0.001$

structure (Table 11.1) (Figure 11.1). In fact this enzyme follows the non-compensation pattern[13], i.e. if the activities are measured at the temperature of the water where the fish were caught, a drastic drop in UDP-glucuronosyltransferase is seen, whereas for the activities measured at constant temperatures (18°C) no change can be observed from summer to early winter[11]. There are also some other differences between the microsomal mono-oxygenase system and UDP-glucuronosyltransferase, since the glucuronidation is considerably more temperature resistant than mono-oxygenation *in vitro* in salmonid fish[6].

If the water cooling is simulated under laboratory conditions, 7-ethoxycoumarin-*O*-deethylase shows partial temperature compensation, but 7-ethoxyresorufin-*O*-deethylase and UDP-glucuronosyltransferase show no compensation (Table 11.2).

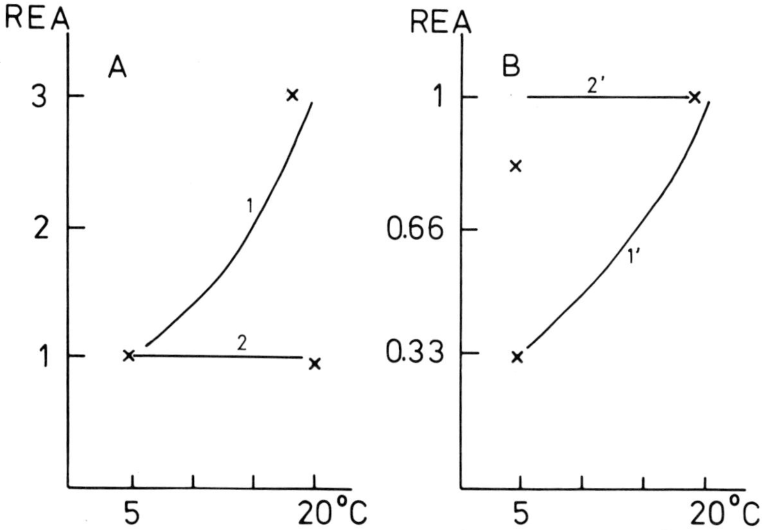

Figure 11.1 The responses of 7-ethoxycoumarin-*o*-deethylase (**A**) and UDP-glucuronosyl-transferase (**B**) in the liver microsomes of rainbow trout to the cooling of waters in autumn. Line 1 and 1′ indicate the calculated reaction rates with the change of incubation – and water temperature. Line 2 in panel (**A**) shows the calculated behaviour of an enzyme having an ideal temperature compensation, i.e. the measurable activity remains the same at the varying living environmental temperatures. Line 2′ in panel (**B**) indicates the non-compensation pattern of an enzyme obtained from fish adapted to different environmental temperatures measured at a constant *in vitro* temperature. The crosses in panel (**A**) along line 2 are observed values of 7-ethoxycoumarin-*O*-deethylase measured at temperatures where the fish have been living in August and November, and along line 1 the values observed after an incubation at 5°C and 18°C with the enzyme in cold adapted rainbow trouts. The crosses in panel (**B**) along line 2′ indicate the observed values of UDP-glucuronosyltransferase from liver samples of cold (autumn) and warm (summer) adapted fish measured at constant temperature 18°C, and along line 1′ the behaviour of the enzyme measured at environmental temperatures where the fish have been caught in August or November

Table 11.2 Microsomal 7-ethoxyresorufin-*O*-deethylase, 7-ethoxycoumarin-*O*-deethylase and UDP-glucuronosyltransferase activities in cold (in July) acclimatized juvenile rainbow trout livers

	T_A*	*Acclimatization* *from 17°C*	*to 5°C*
7-Ethoxyresorufin-*O*-deethylase	5°C	0.028±0.007	0.026±0.006
nmol/min × mg protein	16°C	0.071±0.013	0.063±0.014
7-Ethoxycoumarin-*O*-deethylase	5°C	0.019±0.001	0.030±0.004
nmol/min × mg protein	16°C	0.035±0.003	0.050±0.006
UDP-glucuronosyltransferase	5°C	0.100±0.020	0.120±0.010
nmol/min × mg protein	16°C	0.020±0.020	0.240±0.060

* T_A = assay temperature
Results are given as mean ± SEM

ADAPTATION TO THE WARMING OF WATER

The warming of waters in spring and early summer coincides with the recovery from spawning of the rainbow trout studied. During the spawning period several mono-oxygenase activities, as well as the cytochrome P-450 levels, of the liver are much depressed especially in female rainbow trout[11]. In contrast to the behaviour of the mono-oxygenase system the hepatic UDP-glucuronosyltransferase activities tend to increase during the preparation to spawning[11]. After spawning the cytochrome P-450 level and mono-oxygenase activities rise. Therefore, in mature fish the adaptation to the warming of water is difficult to see[14]. In juvenile fish the effects of reproductive changes do not shadow the effects of the warming-up of water. In these immature fish partial temperature compensation can be seen in the mono-oxygenase activities (Table 11.3). In juvenile fish the UDP-glucuronosyltransferase appears to follow the pattern of the mono-oxygenase system[15].

Table 11.3 Hepatic mono-oxygenase and UDP-glucuronosyltransferase activities in juvenile (1+ years old) rainbow trout in April and in June

Experimental temp.	*April 10°C*	*June 10°C*	*April 3°C*	*June 16°C*
7-Ethoxyresorufin-*O* deethylase nmol/mg protein × min	0.50±0.08	0.41±0.07	0.12±0.02‡	0.55±0.08‡
7-Ethoxycoumarin-*O* deethylase nmol/mg protein × min	0.087±0.006†	0.063±0.004†	0.051±0.004‡	0.093±0.007‡
Benzo(a)pyrene hydroxylase nmol/mg protein × min	0.043±0.004†	0.026±0.003†	0.024±0.003*	0.038±0.004*
UDP-glucuronosyl-transferase nmol/mg protein × min	0.22±0.03	0.18±0.01	0.21±0.03†	0.32±0.02†

* $p<0.05$
† $p<0.01$
‡ $p<0.001$

WATER TEMPERATURE AND INDUCTION OF BIOTRANSFORMATION ENZYMES

Certain chemicals also appear to be able to induce the biotransformation enzymes in fish[9,10,16,17]. The response seems to be modified by the environmental temperature. Thus β-naphthoflavone administration increases mono-oxygenase activities several-fold within a day at the environmental temperature of 17°C, but the increase is only seen after a lag phase when administered at the environmental temperature of 5°C. In both cases the relative activity increase is, however, similar. UDP-glucuronosyltransferase is induced less and the induction rate is slower (Figure 11.2).

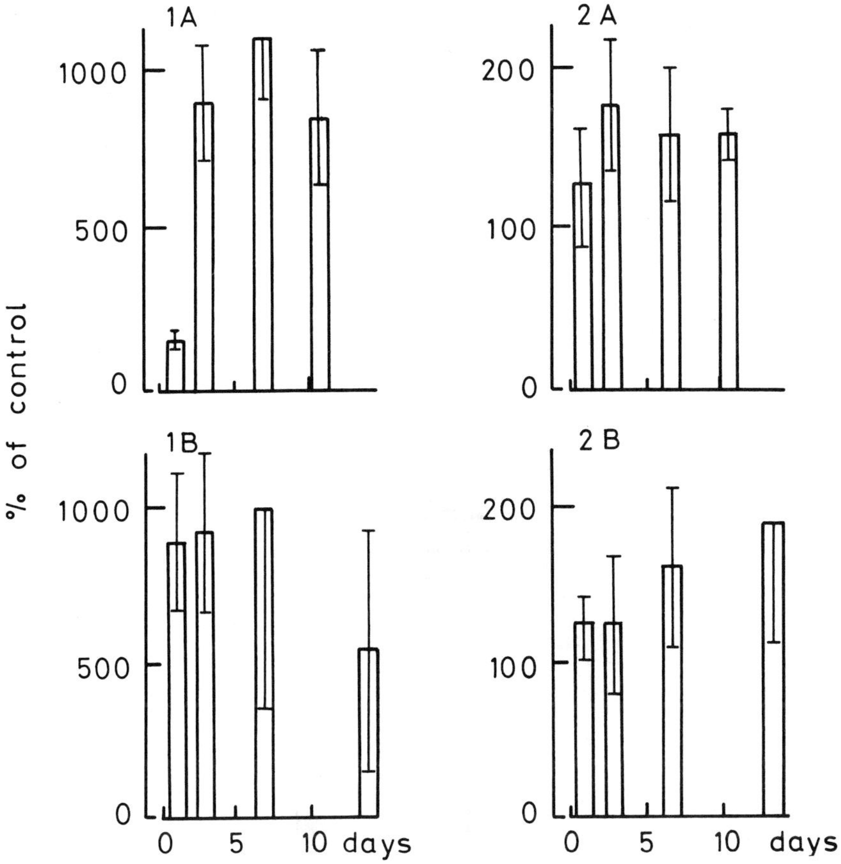

Figure 11.2 The induction of 7-ethoxycoumarin-*O*-deethylase (panels 1) and UDP-glucuronosyltransferase (panels 2) in the liver microsomes of rainbow trouts by β-naphthoflavone (i.p. 100 mg/kg) at environmental temperatures 5°C (**A**) and 17°C (**B**)

SUMMARY

The biotransformation enzymes, exemplified by hepatic microsomal mono-oxygenase and UDP-glucuronosyltransferase, of the rainbow trout vary considerably through seasons with temperature oscillation. During water cooling the mono-oxygenase activity shows an ideal temperature compensation pattern, whereas UDP-glucuronosyltransferase shows a non-compensation pattern. During water warming both enzyme systems show a partial temperature compensation response in juvenile fish. In mature fish the recovery from spawning overshadows the adaptation to temperature shift in the environment. The induction rate of the mono-oxygenase system to β-naphthoflavone appears to be temperature sensitive. UDP-Glucuronosyltranferase is also induced, although not to the same degree.

ACKNOWLEDGEMENT

This work was supported by the Academy of Finland (project 40).

References

1. Brodie, B. B. and Maickel, R. P. (1962). Comparative biochemistry of drug metabolism. *Proc. Int. Pharmacol. Meet. 1st.*, **6,** 299–324
2. Dewaide, J. H. (1971a). Metabolism of xenobiotics. Comparative and kinetic studies as a basis for environmental pharmacology, *PhD Thesis*, University of Nijmegen, Netherlands
3. Ahokas, J. T. (1977). Cytochrome P-450 and mixed function oxidase of trout, *Salmo trutta lagustris. PhD Thesis, Acta Universitasis Ouluensis*, Series D Medica 20
4. Bend, J. R. and James, M. O. (1978). Xenobiotic metabolism in marine and freshwater species. In Malins, D. C. and Sargent, J. R. (eds.). *Biochemical and Biophysical Perspectives in Marine Biology*. Vol. 4, pp. 125–88. (New York: Academic Press)
5. Dutton, G. J. and Montgomery, J. P. (1958). Glucuronide synthesis in fish and the influence of temperature. *Biochem. J.*, **70,** 17
6. Lindström-Seppä, P., Koivusaari, U. and Hänninen, O. (1981). Extrahepatic xenobiotic metabolism in North-European freshwater fish. *Comp. Biochem. Physiol.*, **69C,** 259–63
7. Hansson, T. (1981). Studies on hepatic steroid metabolism in rainbow trout, *Salmo gairdneri. PhD Thesis,* University of Göteborg
8. Förlin, L. and Lidman, U. (1978). Effects of clophen A50, 2,5, 2, 5,-tetra- and 2, 4, 5, 2, 4, 5-hexachlorobiphenyl on the mixed function oxidase system of rainbow trout (*Salmo gairdneri Rich.*) liver. *Comp. Biochem. Physiol.*, **60C,** 193–7
9. Elcombe, C. R. and Lech, J. J. (1979). Induction and characterization of hemoprotein(s) P-450 and mono-oxygenation in rainbow trout (*Salmo gairdneri*). *Toxicol. Appl. Pharmacol.*, **439,** 437–50
10. Vodicnik, M. J., Elcombe, C. R. and Lech, J. J. (1981). The effect of various types of inducing agents in hepatic microsomal mono-oxygenase activity in rainbow trout. *Toxicol. Appl. Pharmacol.*, **59,** 364–74
11. Koivusaari, U., Harri, M. and Hänninen, O. (1981). Seasonal variation of hepatic biotransformation in female and male rainbow trout (*Salmo gairdneri*). *Comp. Biochem. Physiol.*, **70C,** 149–57
12. Sellner, P. A. and Hazel, J. R. (1982). Time course of changes in fatty acid composition of gills and liver from rainbow trout (*Salmo gairdneri*) during thermal acclimation. *J. Exp. Zool.*, **221,** 159–68
13. Precht, H. (1973). The normal temperature range: constant systems. In Precht, H., Christopherson, J., Hausel, H. and Larcher, W. (eds.). *Temperature and Life*, pp. 302–53. (Berlin: Springer Verlag)
14. Koivusaari, U. (1983). Thermal acclimatization of hepatic polysubstrate mono-oxygenase and UDP-glucuronosyltransferase of mature rainbow trout (*Salmo gairdneri*). *J. Exp. Zool.*, **227,** 35–42
15. Koivusaari, U. and Andersson, T. (1984). Partial temperature compensation of hepatic biotransformation enzymes in juvenile rainbow trout (*Salmo gairdneri*) during the warming of water in spring. *Comp. Biochem. Physiol.*, **78B,** 223–6
16. Elcombe, C. R., Franklin, R. B. and Lech, J. J. (1979). Induction of hepatic microsomal

enzymes in rainbow trout. In. Khan, M. A. Q., Lech, J. J. and Menn, J. J. (eds.). *Pesticides and Xenobiotic Metabolism in Aquatic Organisms*, pp. 319–37. (Washington: ACS Symposium Series 99)

17. Stegeman, J. J. (1979). Temperature influence on basal activity and induction of mixed function oxygenase activity in *Funduluc heteroclitus*. *J. Fish. Res. Board Can.*, **36,** 1400–5

Section 4
Development and Induction of UDP-Glucuronosyltransferases

Chairman: H. Remmer

12
Development of hepatic UDP-glucuronyltransferase activities in rats and rhesus monkeys

J. E. A. LEAKEY

INTRODUCTION

UDP-glucuronyltransferase is absent from early fetal liver, but activities towards many of its endogenous and xenobiotic substrates develop perinatally in most species and in man; delayed development of the transferase activity towards bilirubin may contribute to postnatal jaundice[1]. It is now well established that in the rat, hepatic UDP-glucuronyltransferase activities develop differentially, in two clusters, which differ in substrate specificity. Activities belonging to Cluster 1 surge towards adult values during late gestation, whereas those belonging to Cluster 2 remain low until birth and then rise neonatally[2].

Evidence suggests that the development of Cluster 1 activities is triggered by corticosterone[3], which surges in concentation in the fetal plasma concurrently with this cluster[4]. The mechanism controlling the development of Cluster 2 activities is more complex, but glucocorticoids could be involved here also, because pretreatment of neonatal rats with glucocorticoids, such as dexamethasone, increases UDP-glucuronyltransferase activity towards bilirubin, which develops[5,6] in Cluster 2.

Hepatic UDP-glucuronyltransferase exists in multiple forms in the rat[7], and forms glucuronidating bilirubin, testosterone, oestrone and androsterone all of which have been separately isolated from adult rat liver[8–10]. However, activities towards all of these substrates develop postnatally in the rat[1,6], and it is, therefore, probable that an additional form exists which is responsible for the Cluster 1 activities *in utero*. Unfortunately, the commonly used assays for Cluster 1 UDP-glucuronyltransferase activities utilize xenobiotic substrates such as 2-aminophenol, and these may be glucuronidated by more than one form of the transferase[7].

We have, therefore, further investigated the effects of glucocorticoid on the development of UDP-glucuronyltransferase in liver microsomes from perinatal rats, using activities towards endogenous substrates because these substrates may be more specific for individual forms of the enzyme than xenobiotic substrates. We have assayed UDP-glucuronyltransferase activity towards 5-hydroxytryptamine (a Cluster 1 activity), and activities towards bilirubin, testosterone, oestradiol and oestrone (which all develop in Cluster 2) to determine whether or not more than one form of the transferase is stimulated by glucocorticoid treatment.

In addition, we report preliminary results on the effects of glucocorticoids on these activities in liver from rhesus monkey fetuses; we have previously shown that UDP-glucuronyltransferase also develops in two clusters in the rhesus monkey, and that these clusters have analogous constituent activities to those of the rat[11].

METHODS

Time-mated, pregnant Wistar rats were injected (i.p.) with 10 mg dexamethasone in sesame oil per kg body weight either on the 14th, 15th and 16th days of gestation or on the 17th, 18th and 19th days of gestation. In each case the rats were sacrificed 15 h after the last injection. Term in this strain of rat is between 21 and 22 days gestation. The fetuses were removed, decapitated and their livers pooled together, so that all the fetuses from a single litter made up each sample. Neonatal rat pups were similarly injected with 10 mg dexamethasone per kg body weight on days 1, 2 and 3 *post partum* and they were sacrificed on day 4. Livers from four pups were pooled from each sample. Control rats or rat pups received injections of equivalent volumes of sesame oil to their dexamethasone-treated counterparts. Microsomal UDP-glucuronyltransferase activities in these controls did not differ significantly from those of untreated litter mates.

Rhesus monkey fetuses (*Macaca mulatta*) were used at gestational ages ranging from 142 to 146 days. Term in this species is at 165±5 days. The pregnant rhesus monkeys were injected with 10 μg dexamethasone per kg body weight 3, 2 and 1 days before surgery. The fetuses were removed by caesarian section, killed by exsanguination and their livers collected. Duplicate samples of 1.5–2.5 g were used from each fetus.

Liver samples were homogenized at 0–4°C in 8.5 ml of 10 mmol/l Tris/HCl buffer pH 7.6 containing 0.25 mol/l sucrose, 1 mmol/l dithiothreitol, 0.5 mmol/l EDTA, 25 mmol/l KCl, 0.1 g/100ml phenylmethanesulphonyl fluoride and 5 g/100 ml glycerol. Microsomal suspensions were prepared from these homogenates by centrifugation as described by Leakey *et al.*[11]. These suspensions could be stored for up to 48 h in ice at 0–4°C without significant loss of activity, and this allowed sufficient time for all the assays of UDP-glucuronyltransferase activity. The microsomal protein content was measured by the method of Lowry *et al.*[12].

UDP-glucuronyltransferase activities towards 2-aminophenol, bilirubin and 5-hydroxytryptamine were assayed by the methods of Dutton *et al.*[13], Van Roy and Heirwegh[14] and Leakey[15] respectively, whereas activities toward oestradiol, oestrone and testosterone were assayed by the method of Rao *et al.*[16]. Assay incubation times and amounts of microsomal suspensions added were adjusted to give maximum sensitivity while retaining linear rates of UDP-glucuronyltransferase activity towards all six substrates. The final concentration of UDP-glucuronic acid in the incubation mixtures was 2 mmol/l in all cases except the assay of activity towards 5-hydroxytryptamine where it was 4 mmol/l. Maximally activated activities were obtained by assaying over a range of digitonin concentrations (0.05–0.5/100 ml in the assay mixture) or, for the steroid substrates, over a range of Brij-58 (polyoxyethylene 20-cetyl ether) concentrations (0.005–0.05/100 ml in the assay mixture).

The assay substrates, UDP-glucuronic acid, digitonin, Brij-58, dexamethasone, phenylmethanesulphonyl fluoride and sesame oil were obtained from Sigma Chemical Co., Poole, Dorset, UK and the ^{14}C-labelled steroids were obtained from Amersham International, Amersham, UK.

RESULTS

Effect of dexamethasone pretreatment on microsomal UDP-glucuronyltransferase activities in fetal rat liver

Table 12.1 shows the effects of dexamethasone pretreatment on maximally activated UDP-glucuronyltransferase activities in fetal rat liver microsomes. At 17 days gestation, control activities towards 2-aminophenol and 5-hydroxytryptamine, which belong to Cluster 1, are just beginning to develop, whereas activities towards bilirubin and the steroid substrates are below the limits of accurate detection for their respective assays. Pretreatment with dexamethasone produced large increases in the Cluster 1 activities, but no increases in the Cluster 2 activities could be detected.

By 20 days gestation, significant amounts of the Cluster 1 activities have already developed in liver from the control fetuses, and low activities towards bilirubin, oestradiol and testosterone are also detectable. Dexamethasone pretreatment increased the existing UDP-glucuronyltransferase activities towards 2-aminophenol and 5-hydroxytryptamine still further, but did not significantly increase the low activities towards bilirubin, oestradiol and testosterone. UDP-glucuronyltransferase activity towards oestrone was also not increased by dexamethasone pretreatment in 20-day fetal liver microsomal preparations (R. Forest, unpublished data, not shown in Table).

Effect of dexamethasone pretreatment on microsomal UDP-glucuronyltransferase activities in neonatal rat liver

In Wistar rats, the Cluster 1 activities of UDP-glucuronyltransferase fall following birth, whereas the Cluster 2 activities rapidly develop to approach adult values by 3–4 days *post partum*[1,6]. Table 12.2 shows the effect of dexamethasone pretreatment on native (i.e. unactivated) and maximally activated UDP-glucuronyltransferase activities in liver microsomal suspensions from 4-day-old rat pups. UDP-glucuronyltransferase activities towards bilirubin, oestradiol, testosterone and 2-aminophenol were increased to 1.5–3 times

Table 12.1 Effect of dexamethasone pretreatment on microsomal UDP-glucuronyltransferase activities in fetal rat liver

Age	*No.**	*Treatment*	*UDP-glucuronyltransferase activity†* (nmol/min per mg of protein)				
			Bilirubin	*Oestradiol*	*Testosterone*	*2-Aminophenol*	*5-Hydroxytryptamine*
17	3	Control	<0.001	<0.015	<0.011	0.05±0.02	0.22±0.05
17	3	Dexamethasone	<0.001	<0.015	<0.011	1.96±0.45	3.67±0.18
	% of Control		—	—	—	3920	1668
20	4	Control	0.010±0.002	0.09±0.02	0.10±0.01	2.61±0.57	5.96±1.16
20	4	Dexamethasone	0.011±0.002	0.10±0.02	0.08±0.01	6.22±0.70	9.32±0.48
	% of Control		110	104	82	238	156

* No. of pools of livers
† Maximally activated with digitonin or Brij-58

their control values in both the native and maximally activated microsomal preparations.

However, UDP-glucuronyltransferase activity towards oestrone was not increased by dexamethasone pretreatment in the rat pup liver, and activity towards 5-hydroxytryptamine was increased in the native microsomal preparations only; this activity was not significantly increased above control values in the maximally activated microsomal preparations.

Table 12.2 Effect of dexamethasone on microsomal UDP-glucuronyltransferase activity in neonatal rat liver

Substrate (activation)		*UDP-glucuronyltransferase activities* Control (4)	Dexamethasone (4)	% Control
Bilirubin	(native)	0.21±0.02	0.44±0.03	211
	(max. act.)	1.34±0.03	2.61±0.10	195
Oestradiol	(native)	0.24±0.03	0.42±0.07	176
	(max. act.)	1.31±0.10	2.04±0.12	156
Oestrone	(native)	0.27±0.01	0.27±0.06	100
	(max. act.)	1.21±0.13	1.00±0.25	83
Testosterone	(native)	0.36±0.08	1.08±0.08	300
	(max. act.)	3.24±0.30	6.14±0.53	190
2-Aminophenol	(native)	0.36±0.05	0.58±0.03	161
	(max. act.)	4.17±0.22	6.91±0.45	166
5-Hydroxytryptamine	(native)	4.08±0.50	7.91±1.20	194
	(max. act.)	13.78±1.47	15.88±0.65	115

Effect of dexamethasone pretreatment on microsomal UDP-glucuronyltransferase activity in liver from rhesus monkey fetuses

Our preliminary results (Leakey, Althaus, Bailey and Slikker, unpublished) indicated that in the rhesus monkey, hepatic UDP-glucuronyltransferase activities from both developmental clusters are increased by dexamethasone *in utero*. Table 12.3 shows that in late gestation, hepatic UDP-glucuronyltransferase activity towards 5-hydroxytryptamine has already developed to near-adult values, but that dexamethasone pretreatment increases it still further. UDP-

Table 12.3 The effect of dexamethasone pretreatment on maximally activated UDP-glucuronyltransferase activities in liver from rhesus monkey fetuses during late gestation

Substrate	*UDP-glucuronyltransferase activity* (% of adult value) *Control*	*Dexamethasone*	*Increase (dex/cont)*
5-Hydroxytryptamine	89	163	1.8
Bilirubin	0.15	13	25.3
Oestradiol	3	13	4.0
Testosterone	3	14	4.3

glucuronyltransferase activities towards bilirubin, oestradiol and testosterone are very low in the fetal liver microsomal suspensions from the control monkeys, but all three activities are markedly increased by dexamethasone pretreatment (25-fold for bilirubin) so that they approach 14–15% of adult values in the treated samples.

DISCUSSION

As expected from earlier work using liver homogenates[3], dexamethasone pretreatment evokes precocious development of microsomal UDP-glucuronyltransferase activities towards 2-aminophenol and 5-hydroxytryptamine in liver from rat fetuses at 17 days gestation, but no stimulation of the activities towards bilirubin, oestradiol or testosterone occurs. Furthermore, at 20 days gestation these Cluster 2 UDP-glucuronyltransferase activities still do not respond to dexamethasone pretreatment. After birth, however, UDP-glucuronyltransferase activities towards bilirubin, oestradiol and testosterone become competent to respond to glucocorticoid, but activity towards oestrone does not. It would appear, therefore, that the forms of UDP-glucuronyltransferase responsible for glucuronidating bilirubin[8] and oestradiol/testosterone[10] are responsive to glucocorticoid stimulation in neonatal rat liver but the form responsible for glucuronidating oestrone[9] is not responsive to glucocorticoid stimulation.

If UDP-glucuronyltransferase activity towards 5-hydroxytryptamine reflects the existence of a single 'late fetal' form of UDP-glucuronyltransferase responsible for all the Cluster 1 activities of the enzyme, then it is probable that this form is induced by glucocorticoids prenatally but not postnatally. The increases in UDP-glucuronyltransferase activity towards 2-aminophenol produced by dexamethasone pretreatment in the neonate, would, therefore, reflect increases in the testosterone/oestradiol form of the transferase rather than the 'late fetal' form, because the testosterone/oestradiol form is known to be active in glucuronidating 2-aminophenol[7].

Although analogous developmental clusters of UDP-glucuronyltransferase exist in the rat and rhesus monkey[11] it appears that the two species differ in the responses of their Cluster 2 UDP-glucuronyltransferase activities to dexamethasone pretreatment. Hepatic UDP-glucuronyltransferase activities towards bilirubin, oestradiol and testosterone all appear at least partially competent to respond to dexamethasone in the rhesus monkey fetuses. It is probable, however, that some form of repression of these activities remains *in utero* as these activities reach less than 15% of adult values.

The premature rhesus monkey has been shown to be susceptible to postnatal jaundice due to low UDP-glucuronyltransferase activity at birth[17]. The large increases (relative to controls) in the transferase activity towards bilirubin we have produced here with dexamethasone implies, therefore, that glucocorticoid therapy may be useful in preventing postnatal jaundice in premature rhesus monkey neonates.

ACKNOWLEDGEMENTS

I thank my collaborators, Dr W. Slikker *et al.* at the National Centre for Toxicological Research, Jefferson, Arkansas, for useful discussion and their contributions to the rhesus monkey data. I also thank Mr R. Forrest for performing some of the oestrone UDP-glucuronyltransferase assays, Mr D. Gardiner and Mrs P. Fotheringham for their skilled technical assistance and the Medical Research Council (UK) and Food and Drug Administration (USA) for financial support.

References

1. Dutton, G. J. and Leakey, J. E. A. (1981). The perinatal development of drug metabolizing enzymes: What factors trigger their onset? *Prog. Drug Res.*, **25**, 189–273
2. Wishart, G. J. (1978). Functional heterogeneity of UDP-glucuronyltransferase as indicated by its differential development and inducibility by glucocorticoids. *Biochem. J.*, **174**, 485–9
3. Wishart, G. J. and Dutton, G. J. (1977). Regulation of onset of development of UDP-glucuronyltransferase activity towards *o*-aminophenol by glucocorticoids in late-foetal rat liver *in utero*. *Biochem. J.*, **168**, 507–11
4. Martin, C. E., Cake, M. H., Hartmann, P. E. and Cook, I. F. (1977). Relationship between fetal corticosteroids, maternal progesterone and parturition in the rat. *Acta Endocrinol.*, **84**, 167–76
5. Leakey, J. E. A., Dutton, G. J. and Wishart, G. J. (1979). Differential stimulation of hepatic mono-oxygenase and glucuronidating systems in chick embryo and neonatal rat by glucocorticoids. *Med. Biol.*, **57**, 756–61
6. Leakey, J. E. A. (1983). Ontogenesis. In Caldwell, J. and Jakoby, W. B. (eds.). *Biological Basis of Detoxication*. pp. 77–103. (New York: Academic Press)
7. Burchell, B. (1981). Identification and purification of multiple forms of UDP-glucuronyltransferase. *Rev. Biochem. Toxicol.*, **3**, 1–32
8. Burchell, B. (1980). Isolation and purification of bilirubin UDP-glucuronyltransferase from rat liver. *FEBS Lett.*, **111**, 131–5
9. Weatherill, P. J. and Burchell, B. (1980). The separation and purification of rat liver UDP-glucuronyltransferase activities towards testosterone and oestrone. *Biochem. J.*, **189**, 377–80
10. Falany, C. N. and Tephly, T. R. (1983). Separation, purification and characterization of three isoenzymes of UDP-glucuronyltransferase from rat liver microsomes. *Arch. Biochem. Biophys.*, **227**, 248–58
11. Leaky, J. E. A., Althaus, Z. R., Bailey, J. R. and Slikker, W. Jr. (1983). UDP-glucuronyltransferase activity exhibits two developmental groups in liver from foetal rhesus monkeys. *Biochem. J.*, **214**, 1007–9
12. Lowry, O. H., Rosebrough, N. J., Farr, A. L. and Randall, R. J. (1951). Protein measurement with the Folin phenol reagent. *J. Biol. Chem.*, **193**, 265–75
13. Dutton, G. J., Leakey, J. E. A. and Pollard, M. R. (1981). Assays for UDP-glucuronyltransferase activities. *Methods Enzymol.*, **77**, 383–91
14. Van Roy, F. P. and Heirwegh, K. P. M. (1968). Determination of bilirubin glucuronide and assay of glucuronyltransferase with bilirubin as acceptor. *Biochem. J.*, **107**, 507–18
15. Leakey, J. E. A. (1978). An improved assay technique for uridine diphosphate glucuronosyltransferase activity towards 5-hydroxytryptamine and some properties of the enzyme. *Biochem. J.*, **175**, 1119–24
16. Rao, G. S., Haueter, G., Rao, M. L. and Breuer, H. (1976). An improved assay for steroid glucuronyltransferase in rat liver microsomes. *Anal. Biochem.*, **74**, 35–40
17. Gartner, L. M., Lee, K.-S., Vaisman, S., Lane, D. and Zarafu, I. (1977). Development of bilirubin transport and metabolism in the newborn rhesus monkey. *J. Paediat.*, **90**, 513–31

13
The isolation of cloned cDNAs coding for liver UDP-glucuronyl-transferases (UDPGT)

B. BURCHELL, M. R. JACKSON, L. McCARTHY AND G. C. BARR

ABSTRACT

We report the isolation of cDNA clones for UDP-glucuronyltransferase (UDPGT) from a rat liver library prepared in the expression vector, λgt11. Four different recombinant phages containing cDNA coding for UDPGT were identified using radioiodinated anti-UDPGT IgG. The hybrid β-galactosidase/UDPGT proteins produced in lysogens in response to the gratuitous inducer, isopropyl-β-D-thiogalactopyranoside, were identified by SDS-polyacrylamide gel electrophoresis and immunoblotting to have molecular weights up to approximately 148 000. The size of cDNA inserts coding for UDPGT range from 1.3 to 2.0 kilobases.

INTRODUCTION

The isolation of genes coding for UDP-glucuronyltransferase will be a major step towards the investigation of the construction, differential induction and genetic deficiencies of these enzymes.

Over the past 2 years we have struggled with the laborious procedures involved in the isolation of transferase genes of plasmid cDNA libraries by screening with enriched preparations of GT mRNA.

The recent construction of the expression vector λgt11[1,2] and its modified form[3] has introduced a general and sensitive technique for the primary purposes of identification of clones cDNAs by using antibodies as probes and isolation of unknown proteins by cloned DNA. In this system foreign DNA was inserted into the β-galactosidase gene *lacZ* to promote synthesis of hybrid proteins. The production of hybrid proteins in response to the β-galactosidase inducer, isopropyl-β-D-thiogalactopyranoside (IPTG), permits screening of the cDNA library using specific antibody. The nature of this bacteriophage also permits the insertion of DNA fragments up to 10 kb sufficient to code for the largest protein subunits[2]. One of the major advantages of using these phage expression vectors is the ability to rapidly obtain the reading frame of the cDNA and hence the amino acid sequence.

We have used this expression vector to facilitate the isolation of UDPGT cDNAs from a rat liver cDNA library using anti-UDPGT antibodies.

MATERIALS AND METHODS

Materials

Escherichia coli strains Y1004, Y1088, Y1089 and Y1090[1,2] were kindly provided by R. Craig and R. Hynes.

Preparation of a rat liver cDNA library in λgt11

The preparation of the rat liver cDNA library used in this work is described by Schwarzbauer *et al.*[4], and we are particularly grateful to R. Hynes who kindly made this library available to us.

Antibodies

Sheep anti-rat UDPGT antiserum was prepared using purified 4-nitrophenol UDPGT[5] by methods previously described[6]. Further characterization of the antiserum will be described elsewhere (S. Kennedy and B. Burchell, unpublished work). Affinity-purified antibodies were prepared to obtain lower backgrounds and facilitate radioiodination of the IgG to high specific activity. Specifically purified IgGs were obtained by binding to 4-nitrophenol UDPGT[5] or bilirubin UDPGT[7] to Sepharose and eluting with 0.1 mol/l glycine-HCl, pH 3.0. Affinity purified antibodies were labelled with ^{125}I as previously described[8]. The specific radioactivity of the anti-UDPGT IgG was 2.5×10^6 cpm/μg protein.

Antibody screening of recombinant phage

100 000 Recombinant phage were screened with anti-UDPGT antibodies. Phage were absorbed to *E. coli* Y1090, plated at a density of 11 000 plaque forming units/9 cm LB-ampicillin plate and grown at 42°C for 5 h. Nitrocellulose filters (Schleicher and Schuell, 0.2 μm) were soaked in 10 mmol/l IPTG for 1 h followed by air drying at room temperature for 1 h. Filters were overlaid on the plaques and β-galactosidase fusion protein synthesis was induced for 2 h at 42°C. Filters were keyed to plaques using a hypodermic needle, removed and washed with 1% bovine serum albumin (Sigma Chemical Co.), 0.05 mol/l Tris-HCl, 0.15 mol/l NaCl, pH 7.5 (BSA/TBS) at room temperature. The filters were then incubated with ^{125}I-labelled affinity purified sheep anti-rat UDPGT antibodies diluted to 1 μg/ml in BSA/TBS by gentle shaking at room temperature for 1 h. Filters were washed three times with BSA/TBS for 15 min each at

room temperature, and finally with TBS for 15 min at room temperature, air-dried and autoradiographed for 16 h at −70°C with intensifying screens.

For immunochemical analysis of proteins after electrophoresis in SDS-polyacrylamide gels[9], proteins were electrophoretically transferred to nitrocellulose for 4 h at pH 8.3[10]. Transferred proteins were reacted with anti-UDPGT antibodies as described above.

Isolation of phage DNA

Candidate positive signals obtained in the first high density screen were taken through four successive rounds of phage purification by antibody screening at progressively lower plaque densities. The resulting repeatedly positive and well-isolated phage plaques were picked and amplified to yield high titre plate stocks[11]. Lysogens were prepared for each clone by infection of *E. coli* strain Y1089 at a multiplicity of infection of 5. Recombinant phage DNA was isolated from induced lysogens as previously described[10].

RESULTS

Isolation of UDP-glucuronyltransferase cDNA clones

Initial plaque screening of 100 000 independent recombinant with affinity purified anti-UDPGT antibodies (*see* Materials and Methods section) identified four putative UDP-glucuronyltransferase clones (Figure 13.1). The clones were

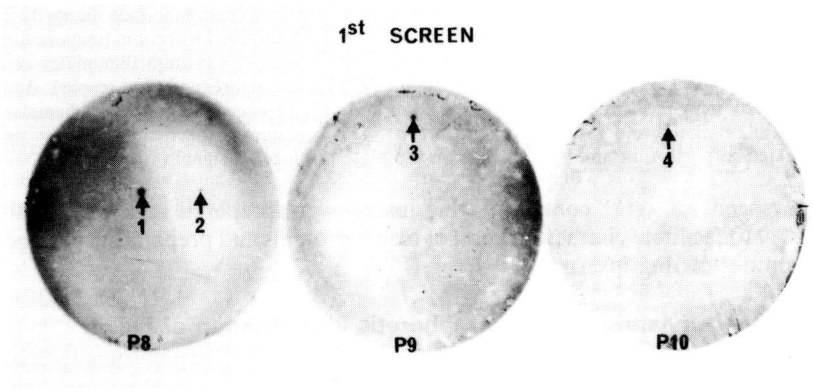

Figure 13.1 Screening a rat liver cDNA library of recombinants with λgtII for UDPGT subunit clones. Plaques (10^5) on nine 90 mm plates formed on a lawn of *E. coli* Y1090 were screened with ^{125}I-labelled anti-UDPGT antibodies (*see* Materials and Methods). The three plates exhibiting positive signals are shown

taken through three rounds of purification and rescreening with antibodies until all plaques gave a positive signal. For examples see rat liver UDP-glucuronyltransferase cDNA clone 3 (λrlug3; Figure 13.2) and the 4th round of purification of λrlug1 and λrlug2 (Figure 13.3).

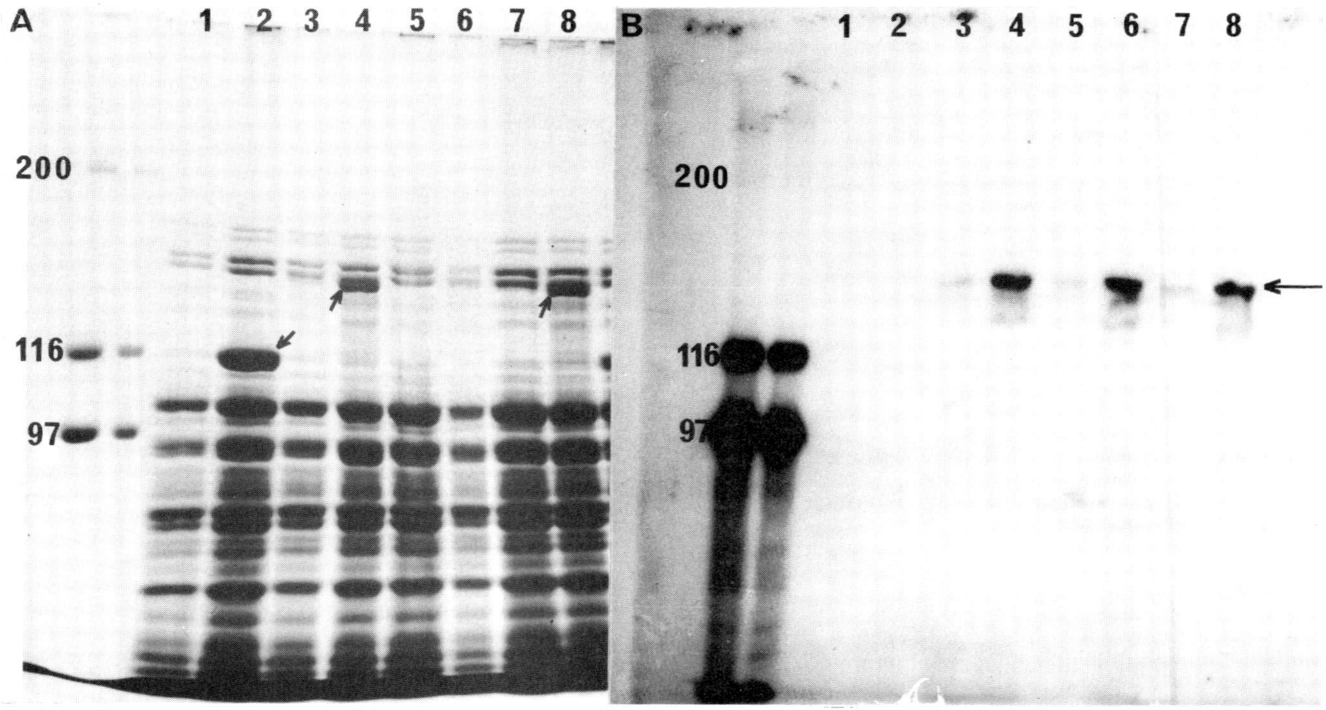

Figure 13.4 Characterization of β-galactosidase/UDPGT fusion proteins. Bacterial ysates were prepared from lysogens of Y1089/λgt11 tracks (1 and 3) and Y1089/rlug 1–4 (tracks 3–8) after inactivation of the temperature sensitive repressor at 42°C, and subsequent induction of fusion proteins in the absence (tracks 1,3,5,7) and presence (tracks 2,4,6,8) of 5 mmol/l IPTG. Reduced samples (100 μg protein) were applied to 6% SDS-polyacrylamide gel. (**A**) Coomassie-blue stained gel. Note IPTG-dependent production of both β-galactosidase (Track 2) and fusion proteins (Tracks 4 and 8). Molecular weights × 10^3 are indicated on the left. (**B**) Western blot of a duplicate gel transferred to nitrocellulose and visualized with affinity purified anti-UDPGT antibodies. Note the labelling of IPTG-dependent fusion protein in lanes 4, 6 and 8 indicated by the arrow

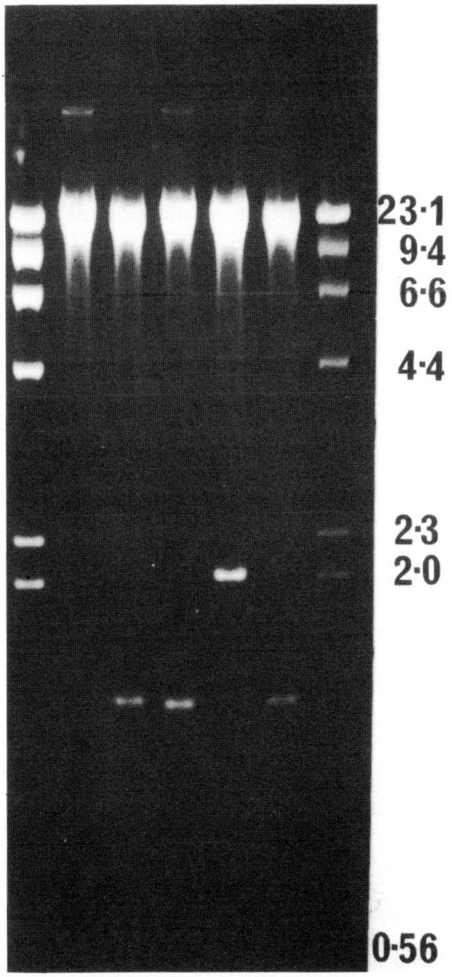

Figure 13.5 Sizing of cDNA inserts in λrlug 1–4. DNA was prepared from recombinant phage and digested with EcoRI restriction endonuclease, fractionated by electrophoresis on a 0.8% agarose gel, and stained with ethidium bromide[10]. Tracks 1 and 7 HindIII digested λDNA fragments used as size markers; track 2, λgt11; track 3, λrlug4; track 4, λrlug3; track 5, λrlug2; track 6, λrlug1

At this stage we have not yet determined which of the UDP-glucuronyltransferases are coded for by these cloned cDNAs, and further confirmation of the presence of individual GTs by radioimmunoassay[2] is restricted by the polyclonal nature of even affinity purified anti-UDPGT antibodies. Recently, we have prepared a number of monoclonal antibodies against UDP-glucuronyltransferases (S. Kennedy and B.Burchell, unpublished work) and these 'monoclonals' which are currently being characterized may help with the identification of individual cloned cDNAs coding for a single isoenzyme.

However, there is no doubt that the ultimate confirmation of the identity of cloned cDNAs with individual UDPGT isoenzymes will result from comparison of DNA and protein sequences. A useful interim strategy will be the comparison of peptide maps of fusion proteins obtained in *E. coli* lysogens and electrophoretically homogeneous preparations of UDPGT isoenzymes obtained from rat liver.

Finally, it should be noted that the fusion proteins obtained in *E. coli* lysogens can be purified and used as 'monoclonal antigens' for raising alternative antisera against fragments of UDPGTs for epitope mapping of unique sites on each isoenzyme. The isolation of these cloned cDNAs for UDP-glucuronyltransferase is a very significant step forward in our goals of investigation of (1) genomic organization of UDPGT structural genes, (2) the genetic regulation of UDPGTs by drugs, hormones and during development and (3) genetic deficiencies of UDPGT. Further, sequencing of cDNA will rapidly provide information about protein structures, protein heterogeneity and structure/activity relationships.

ACKNOWLEDGEMENTS

We are especially grateful to R. Hynes for supplying the rat liver cDNA library in λgt11. We thank I. Duffy for preparation of purified UDP-glucuronyltransferases from rat liver and J. Taylor and R. Craig for their help and encouragement. We also thank the Wellcome Trust for a grant supporting this work. B. B. is a Wellcome Trust Senior Lecturer.

References

1. Young, R. A. and Davis, R. W. (1983). Efficient isolation of genes by using antibody probes. *Proc. Natl. Acad. Sci., USA*, **80,** 1194–8
2. Young, R. A. and Davis, R. W. (1983). Yeast RNA polymerase II genes: Isolation of genes by using antibody probes. *Science*, **222,** 778–82
3. Kemp, D. J., Coppel, R. L., Cowman, A. F., Saint, R. B., Brown, G. V. and Anders, R. F. (1983). Expression of *Plasmodium falciparum* blood-stage antigens in *Escherichia coli*: Detection with antibodies from immune humans. *Proc. Natl. Acad. Sci., USA*, **80,** 3787–91
4. Schwarzbauer, J. E., Tamkum, J. W., Lemischka, I. R. and Hynes, R. O. (1983). Three different fibronectin mRNAs arise by alternative splicing within the coding region. *Cell*, **35,** 421–31
5. Burchell, B. and Weatherill, P. (1981). 4-Nitrophenol UDP-glucuronyltransferase (Rat liver). In Jakoby, W. B. (ed.). *Methods in Enzymology*. Vol. 77, pp. 169–77. (New York: Academic Press)
6. Burchell, G., Kennedy, S. M. E., Jackson, M. R. and McCarthy, L. (1984). The biosynthesis and induction of microsomal UDP-glucuronyltransferase in avian liver. *Biochem. Soc. Trans.*, **12,** 50–3
7. Burchell, B. (1981). Bilirubin UDP-glucuronyltransferase. In Jakoby, W. B. (ed.). *Methods in Enzymology*. Vol. 77, pp. 188–92. (New York: Academic Press)
8. Broome, S. and Gilbert, W. (1978). Immunological screening method to detect specific translation products. *Proc. Natl. Acad. Sci. USA*, **75,** 2746–9
9. Laemmli, U. K. (1970). Cleavage of structural proteins during the assembly of the head of bacteriophage T4. *Nature*, **227,** 680–5
10. Towbin, H., Staehelin, T. and Gordon, J. (1979). Electrophoretic transfer of proteins for polyacrylamide gels to nitrocellulose sheets: Procedure and some applications. *Proc. Natl. Acad. Sci. USA*, **76,** 4350–4
11. Maniatis, T., Fritsch, E. F. and Sambrook, J. (1982). *Molecular Cloning: a Laboratory Manual.* (Cold Spring Harbor Laboratory)

14
Effect of sex and sex steroid hormones on bilirubin conjugation and secretion

J. FEVERY, M. MURACA AND N. BLANCKAERT

INTRODUCTION

Total serum bilirubin levels are higher in healthy adult men than in females; this has been observed by several investigators[1–4]. This difference is not present before puberty and decreases at later ages (Table 14.1), suggesting that sex steroid hormones interact with bilirubin metabolism. Bilirubin production rate is similar in both sexes, but women have a more efficient hepatic bilirubin clearance when expressed per kg of body weight[5].

Table 14.1

Age (years)	*Total serum bilirubin* (mg/dl)	
	Male	*Female*
0–12	0.39	0.43
13–19	0.69	0.61
20–29	0.72*	0.51
30–39	0.65*	0.46
40–49	0.62*	0.47
50–59	0.61*	0.46
60–69	0.55†	0.48
70–79	0.67†	0.48

From Werner *et al.*[3]
* $p<0.001$ † $p<0.01$

Since a close relationship has been suggested between the calculated hepatic

Abbreviations used, UCB: unconjugated bilirubin IX-α; BMC: bilirubin mono-ester conjugates; BDC: bilirubin di-ester conjugates; GTA: glucuronyltransferase activity clearance of injected radiobilirubin and hepatic bilirubin UDP-glucuronyltransferase activity[6], one might expect an influence of sex hormones on the conjugating enzyme system. Results from previous investigations in laboratory animals refer mainly to exogenous substrates[7-13] and cannot be extrapolated to bilirubin conjugation.

Development of a highly sensitive and specific assay of the individual serum bilirubins (UCB, BMC, BDC) by alkaline methanolysis combined with HPLC[14] has permitted detection and measurement of the bilirubin conjugates in serum of healthy humans and rats. As in man, a sex difference was observed

Table 14.2 Concentrations (μmol/l) of bilirubin and its conjugates in serum of healthy adult man and Wistar rat

	Humans		*Wistar rat*	
	Male *(n = 29)*	*Female* *(n = 14)*	*Male* *(n = 8)*	*Female* *(n = 8)*
UCB	6.79 ± 2.62	5.21 ± 2.95	0.96 ± 0.05	0.72 ± 0.05†
BMC	0.10 ± 0.04	0.09 ± 0.06	0.06 ± 0.02	0.05 ± 0.01
BDC	0.12 ± 0.06	0.10 ± 0.07	0.04 ± 0.02	0.02 ± 0.01*
Conjugates as % of total bilirubin	3.5 ± 1.9	3.7 ± 2.1	9.3 ± 2.1	8.6 ± 2.2
BDC as % of total conjugation	55 ± 10	53 ± 12	39 ± 8	32 ± 7

* $p < 0.05$ † $p < 0.001$

in the rat (Table 14.2) allowing the use of this species as an animal model for further investigation of the sex differences.

In the present work, the effects of sex and steroids on bilirubin conjugation in rat liver have been studied both *in vitro* and *in vivo*. The modifications occurring during pregnancy, a condition associated with a high production of female sex steroids, have also been evaluated[15].

HEPATIC UDP-GLUCURONYLTRANSFERASE: DEVELOPMENT OF SEX DIFFERENCE

Bilirubin UDP-glucuronyltransferase was assayed in untreated and/or digitonin-activated liver homogenates or microsomal preparations[16]. Enzyme activity was approximately 2-fold higher in liver preparations from adult females than from adult males (Figure 14.1). However, no difference was observed with livers from rats of 2 and 4 weeks of age (Table 14.3). Puberty occurs in the rat at 7–8 weeks, and this coincided with a decrease of the transferase activity in the male animals and an increase in the females. Three weeks after gonadectomy, enzyme levels were lower in the ovariectomized female and enhanced in the castrated males.

For most substrates previously investigated, conjugation rates were higher in male than in female rats[7,13,17]. However, bilirubin and oestrone, oestradiol and testosterone conjugation[18] is more pronounced in female livers. It is tempting to speculate that the latter transferase activities belong to a different

Table 14.3 Development of rat hepatic bilirubin UDP-glucuronyltransferase

	Activities (nmolh^{-1}mg of protein^{-1})	
Age in weeks	*Male* *(n = 7)*	*Female* *(n = 7)*
2	10.5 ± 1.6	12.1 ± 2.1
4	19.6 ± 1.1	20.3 ± 1.0
6	17.1 ± 3.2	21.6 ± 3.1
8	15.8 ± 1.1	28.4 ± 4.3*
10	14.8 ± 1.1	26.4 ± 1.1*

* $p < 0.001$ difference with males

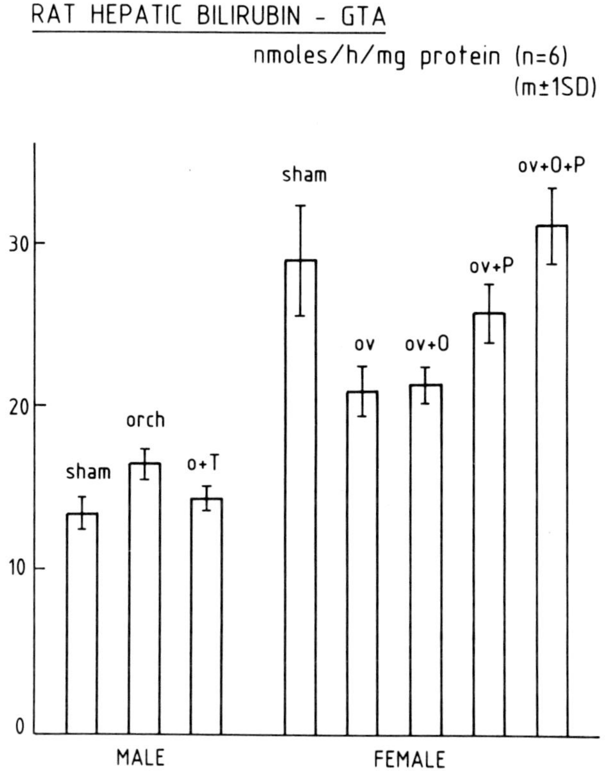

Figure 14.1 Bilirubin UDP-glucuronyltransferase activities in male and female rat liver in controls (sham-operated), and in animals 3 weeks after orchiectomy (orch) or ovariectomy (ov) without or with replacement therapy with testosterone (T), oestradiol (O), progesterone (P) or both (O+P)

enzyme family, e.g. as operationally defined by Wishart *et al.*[19] as the early-neonatal group in contrast to *o*-aminophenol, *p*-nitrophenol and others who are included in the late-fetal group. The latter seems more active in male animals.

EFFECTS OF PHYSIOLOGICAL CONCENTRATIONS OF SEX STEROID HORMONES ON BILIRUBIN UDP-GLUCURONYLTRANSFERASE

At puberty bilirubin GTA decreased in male rats but increased in females. To further investigate the hormones possibly involved, gonadectomy was performed after puberty in male and female rats. Thereafter, the animals were treated for 3 weeks with testosterone, oestradiol and/or progesterone, respectively, in dosages restoring plasma steroid concentrations to the levels observed in healthy adult rats. Treatment with testosterone decreased bilirubin GTA to values found in normal male rats (Figure 14.1). Oestradiol alone had no effect on bilirubin GTA, but progesterone produced a dose-dependent increase. Treatment of ovariectomized females with oestradiol combined with progesterone brought the transferase levels up to values of healthy females (Figure 14.1). Sexual differentiation at puberty of hepatic bilirubin glucuronidation seems thus mediated both by an inhibitory effect of testosterone and a stimulatory action of oestro–progestogens. As prepubertal gondadectomy exerted a decrease but not an abolishment, the sex difference in conjugation seems not exclusively determined by postpubertal gonadal secretion. Neonatal imprinting might thus exist also for bilirubin conjugation.

This phenomenon has been demonstrated for hepatic cortisol-metabolizing enzymes[20,21]: enzymes of animals of both sexes will develop into a feminine pattern except when androgens, presumably secreted by the testicles during the neonatal period, would programme some areas of the brain into a male type of metabolism[21].

RELATIONSHIP BETWEEN BILIRUBIN CONJUGATION AND MAXIMAL SECRETORY RATE (Tm)

To investigate whether these alterations in bilirubin UDP-glucuronyltransferase are meaningful for the *in vivo* handling of bilirubin, a constant i.v. infusion of unconjugated bilirubin saturating the overall hepatic transport was given to male, female and gonadectomized rats having recovered for 3 h from anaesthesia. With this load a constant and maximal biliary secretory rate of bilirubin conjugates (so-called transport maximum, Tm), is obtained[22-24]. After 1 h of bilirubin infusion with monitoring of biliary bile pigment excretion, animals were killed and the serum levels of bilirubins and bilirubin GTA were determined.

The concentration of bilirubin conjugates in bile and the maximal biliary output reached was significantly higher in female than in male animals (Tm values of 73 ± 5 vs. 42 ± 2 nmoles min^{-1} g^{-1} of liver, respectively). Values in gonadectomized animals were intermediate. A highly significant linear correlation was observed between the biliary secretory rate obtained *in vivo* and the hepatic glucuronyltransferase activities, whereby the former levels were approximately 70% of the latter[24]. A similar relationship had been obtained previously in rats treated with phenobarbital or glutethimide[25] and in pregnant, non-lactating and lactating mother rats[15]. This strongly suggests that conjugation, which is a near-absolute requirement for biliary secretion of bilirubin[26], is the major determinant of the maximal biliary output of bilirubins.

This conclusion is reinforced by the observation that plasma levels of bilirubin conjugates at the end of the 60 min bilirubin infusion are low. Indeed only 0.5–1.4% (mean 0.8%) of the serum bilirubins were present in the glucuronidated form, as compared to 6–12% (mean 9%) in unloaded rats (2.5–7.8 μmol/l at the end of Tm vs. 0.06–0.15 μmol/l in control animals, respectively). If the secretory mechanism were rate-limiting, bilirubin conjugates would pile up in the liver, and a more pronounced reflux to plasma would be expected.

CONCLUSIONS

Our findings in male and female rats show that sex differentiation and possibly neonatal sex imprinting lead to higher rates of hepatic bilirubin glucuronidation in mature females compared to males. Testosterone exerts a depressing, and progesterone a stimulatory action on the *in vivo* and *in vitro* glucuronidation of bilirubin. This results in a more efficient handling of a bilirubin load and in lower plasma levels of unconjugated bilirubin.

The results obtained by correlating *in vitro* and *in vivo* findings have an important bearing regarding the theories on the hepatic handling of the pigment. They suggest that conjugation is the determinant factor in the transport of bilirubin from plasma to bile. Hitherto, biliary secretion has commonly been considered the rate-limiting step[27], but this conclusion is probably the result of methodological limitations in the assessment of conjugates in liver and plasma.

As human females also have lower serum values of unconjugated bilirubin and higher hepatic clearance rates[5], it is suggested that their glucuronidation rate is also greater than that of males. Furthermore, as Gilbert's syndrome, characterized by increased unconjugated plasma bilirubin, decreased hepatic clearance rate[6] and decreased hepatic UDP-glucuronyltransferase activity[28], is more prominent in young males, we feel that the upsurge of testosterone secretion at puberty depresses the GTA further in these boys and makes the syndrome clinically evident.

References

1. Schiff, L. (1927). Serum bilirubin in health and in disease. *Arch. Intern. Med.*, **40,** 800–17
2. Brodersen, R., Sparre, H. L. and Vind, I. (1963). Normal bilirubin concentration and the occurrence of other bile pigments in human blood sera. *Scand. Clin. Lab. Invest.*, **15,** 523–8
3. Werner, M., Tolls, R. E., Hultin, J. V. and Mellecker, J. (1970). Influence of sex and age on the normal range of eleven serum constituents. *Zeitschrift. Klin. Chem. Klin. Biochem.*, **8,** 105–15
4. Owens, D. and Evans, J. (1975). Populations studies in Gilbert's syndrome. *J. Med. Genet.*, **12,** 152–6

5. Berk, P. D., Howe, R. B., Bloomer, J. R. and Berlin, N. I. (1969). Studies of bilirubin kinetics in normal adults. *J. Clin. Invest.*, **48,** 2176–90
6. Berk, P. D., Martin, J. F., Blaschke, T. F., Scharschmidt, B. F. and Plotz, P. H. (1975). Unconjugated hyperbilirubinemia. *Ann. Int. Med.*, **82,** 552–70
7. Inscoe, J. K. and Axelrod, J. (1980). Some factors affecting glucuronide formation *in vitro*. *J. Pharmacol. Exp. Ther.*, **129,** 128–31
8. Hartiali, K. J. W. and Pulkkinnen, M. O. (1964). Studies on the possible role of sex hormones on the change in conjugation capacity at various ages in rat. *Ann. Acad. Sci. Fenn.*, **106,** Suppl. 12, 1–8
9. Künzel, B. and Müller-Oerlinghausen, B. (1969). Wirkung von Testosteron und einem Anti-Androgen (Cyproteronacetat) auf die Glukuronidbildung in der Rattenleber. *Pharmak. Exp. Path.*, **262,** 112–23
10. Halac, E. and Sicignano, C. (1969). Re-evaluation of the influence of sex, age, pregnancy and phenobarbital on the activity of UDP-glucuronyltransferase in rat liver. *J. Lab. Clin. Med.*, **73,** 677–85
11. Winsnes, A. (1971). Age and sex dependent variability of the activation characteristics of UDP-glucuronyltransferase *in vitro*. *Biochem. Pharmacol.*, **20,** 1249–58
12. Hietanen, E. (1974). Effect of sex and castration on hepatic and intestinal activity of drug-metabolizing enzymes. *Pharmacology*, **12,** 84–9
13. Chabra, R. S. and Fouts, R. (1974). Sex differences in the metabolism of xenobiotics by extrahepatic tissue in rats. *Drug. Metabol. Disp.*, **2,** 375–9
14. Muraca, M. and Blanckaert, N. (1983). Liquid chromatographic assay and identification of mono- and diester conjugates of bilirubin in normal serum. *Clin. Chem.*, **29,** 1767–71
15. Muraca, M., Leyten, R. and Fevery, J. (1984). Conjugation and maximal biliary excretion of bilirubin in the rat during pregnancy, lactation and during estro–progestogen treatment. *Hepatology*, **4,** 633–8
16. Heirwegh, K. P. M., Van de Vijver, M. and Fevery, J. (1972). Assay and properties of digitonin-activated bilirubin uridine diphosphate glucuronosyl-transferase from rat liver. *Biochem. J.*, **129,** 605–18
17. Lamartiniere, C. A., Dieringer, C. S., Kita, E. and Lucier, G. W. (1979). Altered sexual differentiation of hepatic uridine diphosphate glucuronyltransferase by neonatal hormone treatment in rat. *Biochem. J.*, **180,** 313–8
18. Rao, G. S., Haueter, G., Rao, M. L. and Breuer, H. (1977). Steroid glucuronyltransferases of rat liver. *Biochem. J.*, **162,** 545–56
19. Wishart, G. J., Campbell, M. T. and Dutton, G. J. (1978). Functional heterogeneity of UDP-glucuronyltransferase. In Aitio, A. (ed.). *Conjugation Reactions in Drug Biotransformation*, pp. 179–88. (New York: Elsevier/North Holland)
20. De Moor, P. and Denef, C. (1968). The 'puberty' of rat liver. Feminine pattern of cortisol metabolism in male rats castrated at birth. *Endocrinology*, **83,** 791–8
21. Gustafson, J. A. and Skett, P. (1979). Pituitary control of hepatic steroid metabolism. *Acta Biol. Med. Germ.*, **38,** 307–20
22. Weinbren, K. and Billing, B. H. (1956). Hepatic clearance of bilirubin as an index of cellular function in the regenerating rat liver. *Br. J. Exp. Pathol.*, **37,** 199–204
23. Klaassen, C. D., Roberts, R. J. and Plaa, G. L. (1969). Maximal biliary excretion of bilirubin and sulfobromophthalein during various rates of infusion in rats of different weights and strains. *Toxicol. Appl. Pharmacol.*, **15,** 143-51
24. Muraca, M., De Groote, J. and Fevery, J. (1983). Sex differences of hepatic conjugation of bilirubin determine its maximal biliary excretion in non-anaesthetized male and female rats. *Clin. Sci.*, **64,** 85–90
25. Van Steenbergen, W. and Fevery, J. (1982). Maximal biliary secretion of bilirubin in the anaesthetized rat: dependence on UDP-glucuronyltransferase activity. *Clin. Sci.*, **62,** 521–8
26. Blanckaert, N., Heirwegh, K. P. M. and Zaman, Z. (1977). Comparison of the biliary excretion of the four isomers of bilirubin-IX in Wistar and homozygous Gunn rats. *Biochem. J.*, **164,** 229–36
27. Arias, I. M., Johnson, L. and Wolfson, S. (1961). Biliary excretion of injected conjugated and unconjugated bilirubin by normal and Gunn rats. *Am. J. Physiol.*, **200,** 1091–4
28. Black, M. and Billing, B. H. (1969). Hepatic bilirubin UDP-glucuronyltransferase activity in liver disease and Gilbert's syndrome. *N. Engl. J. Med.*, **280,** 1266–71

15 UDP-glucuronosyltransferase specificity and subcellular localization

B. ANTOINE, G. SIEST AND J. MAGDALOU

INTRODUCTION

The endoplasmic reticulum (ER) of the hepatocyte is known as the major site for drug metabolism. However, the membrane-bound enzymes involved in this process are also associated to other membranes[1,2]. This is particularly the case of UDP-glucuronosyltransferase (UDPGT, E.C. 2.4.1.17) whose activity is also detectable in nuclear membranes[3–7], in Golgi membranes[1,8,9] and in plasma membranes[1,2,8]. Moreover, as in the endoplasmic reticulum, phenobarbital is able to increase UDPGT activity in the plasma membranes[2].

Glucuronidation of structurally different molecules suggests the existence of several enzymes presenting different specificities. In the endoplasmic reticulum, two groups of activities have already been characterized. The late fetal activity[10], which is enhanced by 3-methylcholanthrene[11], is able to conjugate planar molecules or group 1 substrates (GT1)[12]. The neonatal activity[10], inducible by phenobarbital[11], shows a specificity towards bulky aglycones or group 2 substrates (GT2)[12]. Indeed, group 2 substrates could be divided into two subpopulations of aglycones[37]: (1) GT2a which includes monoterpenoid alcohols (borneol) whose conjugation is increased by phenobarbital only in guinea-pig and less deficient in the Gunn rat, and (2) GT2b including bulky aglycones such as morphine.

Finally, conjugation of bilirubin would represent a third group of activities increased by pregnenolone-16α-carbonitrile[13] and clofibrate[14]. We have previously observed that the activity towards group 1 substrates was at least two times higher in microsomes than that measured with group 2 aglycones. This was true for the eight mammalian species studied[37].

In order to establish if the enzyme heterogeneity according to the type of substrates used was also observed in the different subcellular membranes, we have measured the UDPGT activity towards ten aglycones in plasma membranes (PM), Golgi apparatus (Golgi), nuclear envelope (NE) and rough or smooth endoplasmic reticulum (RER, SER) of rat liver. This work was undertaken in order to better understand the functional meaning of the plurilocalization of UDPGT, and to determine if a specialization of a type of membrane towards conjugation of aglycones could exist. We have also determined the true V_{max} and the affinity constants for UDP-glucuronic acid and for one representative substrate of each group of activities.

Finally, the results were discussed in relation to the different phospholipid environments of the UDPGT, according to the type of membrane. Indeed lipid moiety could modulate both substrate accessibility and enzyme conformation[15,16].

MATERIALS AND METHODS

Male Sprague Dawley rats (180–220 g) were purchased from Iffa Credo (St Germain-sur-l'Arbresle, France). After 15 h fasting, the animals, in groups of three, were sacrificed, the livers perfused with ice-cold 0.15 mol/l NaCl, cut into small pieces and homogenized in two parts in the following buffer systems:

(1) 1 mmol/l $NaHCO_3$, pH 7.4 for the preparation of PM according to Neville's technique[17]. The corresponding pellet obtained after centrifugation on the sucrose gradient was used as the NE fraction.
(2) 0.5 mol/l sucrose, 50 mmol/l Tris, 5 mmol/l $MgCl_2$, pH 7.0 for both preparations of SER and RER[18] and Golgi[19].

Protein content was measured by the method of Lowry *et al.*[20] with bovine serum albumin as standard. NADPH cytochrome c reductase activity was determined by the method of Mazel[21]. Alkaline phosphatase and glutamate dehydrogenase activities were estimated on a fast centrifugal analyser (Cobas, Roche Bioelectronique, France) with a BioMerieux kit (Reference 61 371) and a Boehringer kit (Reference 124 320), respectively. γ-Glutamyltransferase activity was measured according to Szasz's method[22] with γ-glutamylparanitroanilide (Sigma Chemical Co., St Louis, USA) as the substrate. UDP-galactose *N*-acetylglucosamine galactosyltransferase (E.C. 2.4.1.38) activity was determined as described by Morré[19]. Glucuronidation rates were estimated at 37°C from Mulder and Van Doorn's assay[23] adapted in our laboratory, on a centrifuge analyser[24]. Bilirubin UDP-glucuronosyltransferase was measured according to Heirwegh *et al.*[25].

RESULTS

Evaluation of the fraction purity

Table 15.1 indicates the enzyme activity or amount of known markers of subcellular fractions in rat liver. RNA was preferentially associated with the RER fraction and was found to be present in similar amounts to those reported in the literature[1,26]. There is currently no good marker for the ER fraction[27].

We measured the NADPH cytochrome c reductase activity which is present to a great extent in the SER fraction[1,8]. In the other endomembranes, its amount was negligible except in the Golgi. As proposed by Ito and Palade[28], this activity could be due mainly to an endogeneous reductase which represents about 30% of the amount found in the microsomal fraction[27]. UDP-galactose *N*-acetylglucosamine galactosyltransferase is a preferentially dictyosomal marker enzyme[29] with which our Golgi fraction was greatly enriched (Table 15.1). Alkaline phosphatase is mainly a marker of liver bile canalicular PM but its intrinsic presence in the Golgi cannot be excluded, as explained by Bergeron *et al.*[30] for AMPase. γ-Glutamyltransferase activity was detectable in all subcellular fractions. This glycoprotein, which can be measured in microsomes, is preferentially located in PM, especially after drug induction[31]. Whatever the fraction studied, we found there was no contamination by mitochondria as estimated by measurement of glutamate dehydrogenase activity.

Finally, the quality of subcellular fractions was also checked by electron microscopy.

Detergent activation pattern of UDPGT in the different types of membrane

The detergent requirement for optimal enzyme activation expressed by Triton X-100 – protein ratio (w/w) has been determined for each subcellular fraction; it was 0.4 for ER and PM and 0.3 for Golgi apparatus and the NE (results not shown). In these conditions, the activities were enhanced 6.0-, 3.0- and 1.3-fold respectively. Surprisingly, in NE, only the activities towards group 1 substrates were increased 3-fold.

Glucuronidation of various substrates in the different subcellular fractions

We compared the UDPGT activity among the different membranes towards ten substrates, after maximal activation with Triton X-100. These were three of the late fetal group or group 1, 4-methylumbelliferone, 4-nitrophenol, eugenol, and five of the neonatal group or group 2, 4-hydroxybiphenyl, 2-aminophenol, borneol, morphine, chloramphenicol, and two endogeneous substrates, testosterone and bilirubin (Figure 15.1). In ER, our results confirm that group 1 (*p*-nitrophenol) presented a conjugation rate at least two times faster than that of group 2 substrates (morphine). Moreover, there was no significant difference between SER and RER. NE possessed the same pattern of UDPGT activity according to the substrate as that found in the ER, but to a smaller extent as the activities in NE represented 22±6% the values found in the ER. The situation in Golgi and PM was very different, as these membranes presented approximately the same glucuronidation rate whatever the substrate used. For group 1 substrates, the activities were between 18–31% those measured in ER. For group 2 substrates, the extent of conjugation by these fractions reached that found with ER, and it was even identical for the bulkiest substrates used such as morphine, chloramphenicol and testosterone.

Table 15.1 Purity of the subcellular membranes of rat liver cells as determined by the measurement of known marker parameters

	RNA (mg/mg prot)	*NADPH cytochrome c* reductase (nmol min^{-1} mg $prot^{-1}$)	*Galactosyl transferase* (*specific activity ratio fraction/homogenate*)	*Alkaline phosphatase* (*specific activity ratio fraction/homogenate*)	*γ-Glutamyltransferase* (nmol min^{-1} mg $prot^{-1}$)	*Glutamate dehydrogenase* (nmol min^{-1} mg $prot^{-1}$)
RER	0.17±0.03	82.74±9.98	0.63±0.41	0.85±0.30	1.86±0.39	18.1±10.1
SER	0.09±0.02	120.47±8.98	2.04±1.08	1.46±0.27	2.24±0.93	18.9± 7.5
Golgi	0.04±0.01	50.05±6.35	51.12±9.94	2.24±0.46	2.73±0.45	ND
Plasma membranes	0.02±0.00	12.51±2.50	1.52±0.61	17.32±1.96	12.53±2.20	43.3± 6.1
Mitochondria	ND	ND	ND	ND	ND	449.0±118

The results are the mean ± SD (n = 4)
ND = not determined

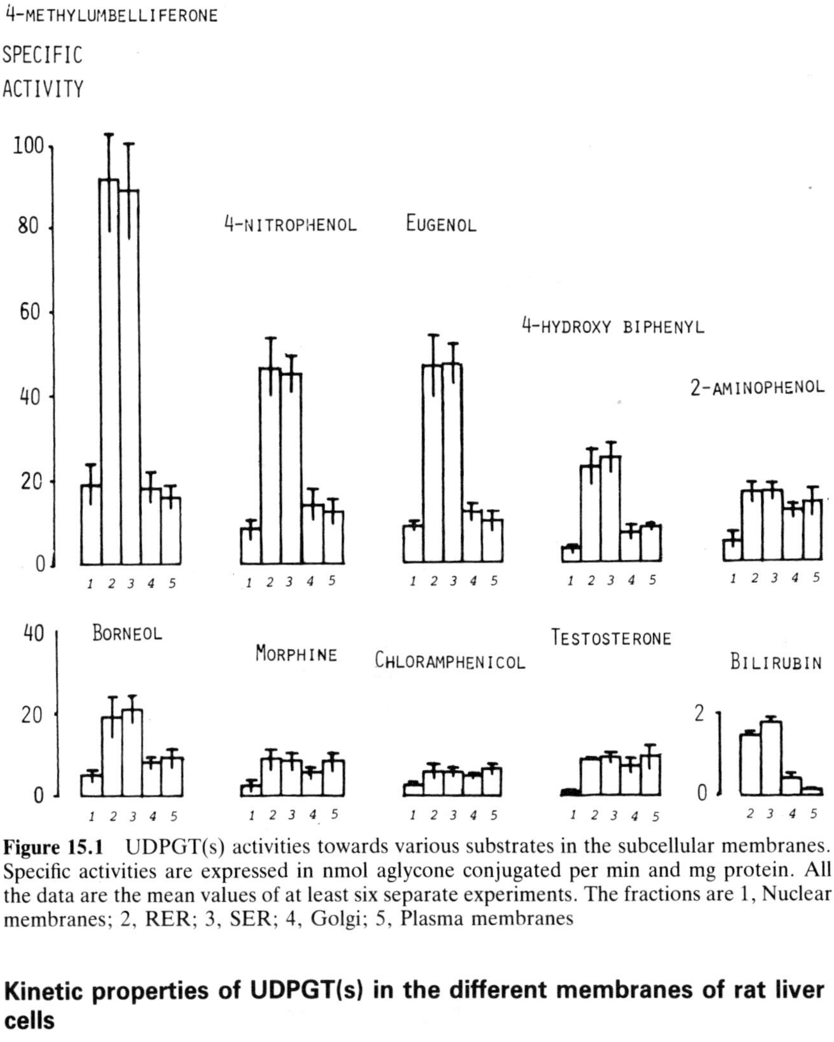

Figure 15.1 UDPGT(s) activities towards various substrates in the subcellular membranes. Specific activities are expressed in nmol aglycone conjugated per min and mg protein. All the data are the mean values of at least six separate experiments. The fractions are 1, Nuclear membranes; 2, RER; 3, SER; 4, Golgi; 5, Plasma membranes

Kinetic properties of UDPGT(s) in the different membranes of rat liver cells

We determined the true V_{max} and also the affinity constants for UDP-glucuronic acid and for one representative substrate of each group of activities: *p*-nitrophenol for GT1, borneol for GT2a and morphine for GT2b groups. The kinetic mechanism of UDPGT is a rapid equilibrium, random bireactant system[32]. Thus, there are two binding constants for each substrate, one for binding of substrate to the free enzyme (K-UDPGA and K-aglycone) and the other for binding to enzyme already saturated with the first substrate (K′-UDPGA and K′-aglycone)[33].

V_{max}

The true V_{max} values are presented in Figure 15.2. The highest V_{max} values were obtained for the glucuronidation of *p*-nitrophenol. V_{max} was 5 and 12 times higher in RER and SER, respectively, than in Golgi and PM. For group 2a (borneol) and group 2b (morphine) substrates, the V_{max} values were markedly depressed in each type of membranes. Interestingly, glucuronidation of morphine occurred at the same low level whatever the membrane considered.

K-UDPGA and K′-UDPGA (Table 15.2)

These terms quantify the enzyme affinity for UDP-glucuronic acid in the presence or absence of aglycone. For a given substrate, K-UDPGA was of the same magnitude in all the membranes except in Golgi for conjugation of *p*-nitrophenol or morphine, where the affinity of the free enzyme was very low.

In the endoplasmic reticulum, the enzyme involved in conjugation of morphine and *p*-nitrophenol presented a K-UDPGA ranging from 0.4 to 0.9; instead of 1.7 and 5.8 for the enzyme which metabolized borneol.

K′-UDPGA was generally lower than the corresponding K-UDPGA value, thus indicating that the fixation of the aglycone also enhanced the enzyme affinity for UDP-glucuronic acid. This was particularly true for enzyme associated with Golgi.

K- and K′-aglycone

The affinity of UDPGT for the substrates used (K-aglycone) was high in all the subcellular membranes. The lowest affinity was observed for *p*-nitrophenol in the endoplasmic reticulum.

Prior fixation of UDP-glucuronic acid increased the enzyme affinity for the aglycone, as the K′-aglycone was rather low. Only in the endoplasmic reticulum the K′ *p*-nitrophenol values remained at a high level, while Golgi and PM presented in that respect high enzyme affinity for *p*-nitrophenol.

DISCUSSION

These results show that ER and NE are the main membrane sites for glucuronidation of group 1 substrates (planar molecules). Indeed specific activities and V_{max} in Golgi and PM only represent from 20 to 30% of the corresponding values in ER. Moreover, surprisingly only GT1 activities were increased three times by Triton X-100 in NE (results not shown).

In the NE, the presence of UDPGT could provide a protective role against damage to genetic material by critical aglycones. Interestingly ER, Golgi and PM present the same conjugation capacities for the bulkiest aglycones such as morphine, chloramphenicol and testosterone: this situation was confirmed by the V_{max} determination in the case of morphine. Borneol which is representative of group 2a substrates exhibited an intermediate behaviour: middle range in specific activities or V_{max} in ER.

It appears that NE, RER and SER are more involved for the conjugation of group 1 substrates, whereas Golgi and PM possess the same potential capacity to conjugate the bulkiest substrates than the ER. This could suggest that, if a

Table 15.2 Kinetic properties of UDP-glucuronosyltransferases in the subcellular membranes

Kinetic constants (mmol/l)	*4-Nitrophenol*				*Borneol*				*Morphine*			
	SER	*RER*	*Golgi*	*PM*	*SER*	*RER*	*Golgi*	*PM*	*SER*	*RER*	*Golgi*	*PM*
K-UDPGA	0.39	0.70	16.61	0.32	5.81	1.71	2.93	4.88	0.71	0.91	4.88	1.58
K′-UDPGA	0.27	0.42	1.67	0.22	1.20	1.91	1.54	2.25	1.63	0.41	2.25	0.48
K-Aglycone	0.34	0.31	0.13	0.054	0.120	0.088	0.054	0.067	0.006	0.079	0.067	0.034
K′-Aglycone	0.23	0.19	0.017	0.037	0.025	0.079	0.029	0.031	0.014	0.041	0.031	0.010

The value of the kinetic constants was determined from the experimental data by linear regression (r better than 0.9)

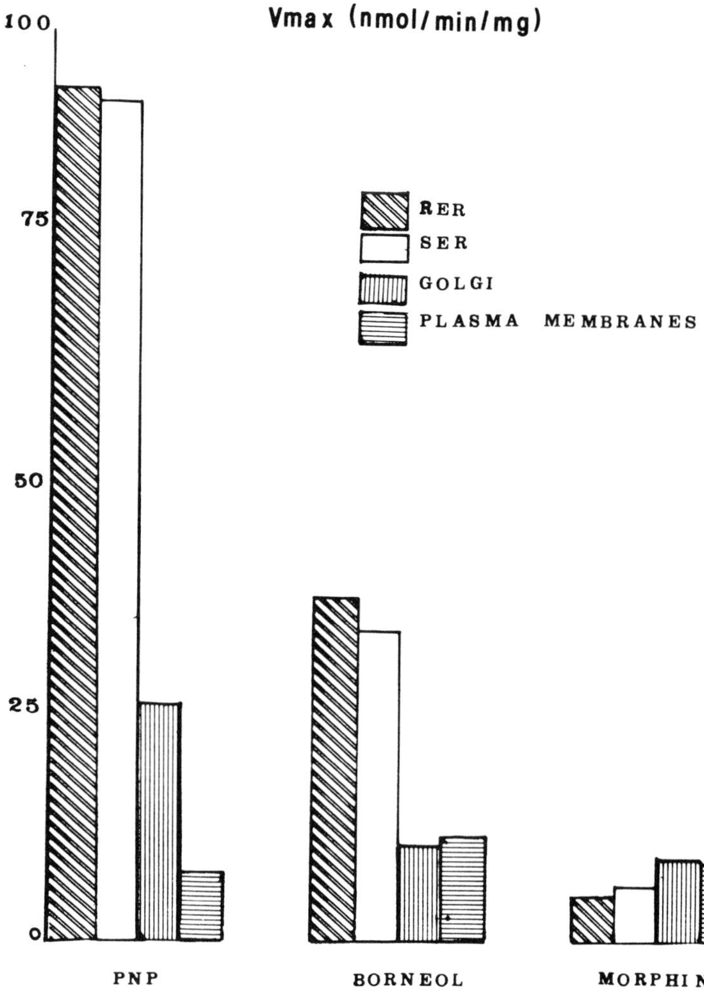

Figure 15.2 V_{max} of glucuronidation of three substrates in the different membranes of rat liver cells

GT1 form is preferentially located in the ER, on the contrary a GT2 form is equally distributed in each type of subcellular membrane.

Comparison of the enzyme affinity for its co-substrate (K-UDPGA), inside a single type of membrane, but according to the group of substrate, can bring information about the number of UDPGT molecular forms. Our results show that in endoplasmic reticulum, the enzyme involved in glucuronidation of morphine and *p*-nitrophenol presents a K-UDPGA ranging from 0.4 to 0.9, whilst 1.7–5.8 for the enzyme which metabolized borneol. These results could suggest the existence of, at least, two populations of binding sites for UDP-glucuronic acid. The same conclusions have been drawn by Hochman *et al.*[34] with the purified enzyme reconstituted in liposomes. Thus, our data suggest the presence in the ER of two distinct forms of UDPGT: the first one which conjugates *p*-nitrophenol has a high affinity for UDPGA as well as high V_{max}; the second one which is involved in borneol transformation presents a much lower affinity and V_{max}.

Interestingly, the affinity for UDP-glucuronic acid in the case of morphine conjugation was the same as that found with *p*-nitrophenol. It was, therefore, attractive to suggest that the enzyme involved in conjugation of *p*-nitrophenol and morphine could possess the same subunit or the same binding site for UDP-glucuronic acid. Weatherill *et al.*[35] indicated that the same antibody precipitated enzyme protein, which supported both glucuronidation of *p*-nitrophenol and morphine.

The main problem with UDP-glucuronosyltransferase activity is to discern what is relevant from the existence of different molecular forms from what is relevant from enzyme activation by phospholipids. Comparison of enzyme affinity for *one* given substrate (K-aglycone) among different membrane phospholipid environments (i.e. among the different subcellular membranes) gives information about the nature of the phospholipid-dependence of UDPGT. Indeed, the phospholipid composition of ER, Golgi and PM varies qualitatively. While in NE, RER and SER the lipid composition is quite similar, the PM fraction exhibits the most different composition when compared to ER, and Golgi presents an intermediate pattern between ER and PM lipid composition. Such a situation suggests affiliation between the different subcellular membranes from ER to PM, via the Golgi.

Table 15.2 shows that K *p*-nitrophenol and K′ *p*-nitrophenol are and remain much higher in ER than in Golgi and PM. This suggests that the enzyme which conjugates group 1 substrates presents a lesser affinity towards these planar substrates in ER than in Golgi or PM. The high level in lysophosphatidylcholine found in Golgi could affect the dissociation constants, as they are known to enhance UDPGT affinity for group 1 substrate (naphthol)[36]. Such a phenomenon is only observed in the case of affinity of group 1 substrates. As group 1 substrates are the most planar molecules, we think that bulkiness and, therefore, the substrate accessibility to the binding site cannot be incriminated.

In conclusion, these results suggest that more than one UDP-glucuronosyltransferase may exist in the different membranes which possess different catalytic properties. We can distinguish namely:

(1) A GT1 form involved in conjugation of planar molecules which presents the following characteristics:
   (a) It is preferentially located in ER where it presents the maximum glucuronidation capacity (high V_{max} and high affinity for UDP-glucuronic acid).
   (b) It is the only one activable by Triton X-100 in NE.

(2) A GT2 form which conjugates the bulkiest molecules. By contrast with GT1, GT2 is rather equally distributed in all the subcellular membranes and presents a low V_{max}.

If the GT2 form corresponds to two distinct molecular forms (GT2a and GT2b), we find that GT2a which conjugates monoterpenoid alcohols presents a low affinity for UDP-glucuronic acid in the ER. In contrast, GT2b which conjugates the bulkiest molecules (morphine) has a high affinity for UDP-glucuronic acid in the ER.

ACKNOWLEDEGMENT

We thank Miss S. Fournel for her helpful assistance in measuring bilirubin conjugation.

References

1. Stasiecki, P., Oesch, F., Bruder, G., Jarasch, E. D. and Franke, W. W. (1980). Distribution of enzymes involved in metabolism of polycyclic aromatic hydrocarbons among rat liver endomembranes and plasma membranes. *Eur. J. Cell Biol.*, **21,** 79–92
2. Magdalou, J., Antoine, B., Ratanasavanh, D. and Siest, G. (1982). Phenobarbital-induction of cytochrome P-450 and UDPGT in rabbit liver plasma membranes. *Enzyme*, **28,** 41–7
3. Wishart, G. J. and Fry, D. J. (1977). UDP-glucuronosyltransferase activity in nuclei and nuclear envelopes of rat liver and its apparent induction by phenobarbital. *Biochem. Soc. Trans.*, **5,** 705–6
4. Wishart, G. J. and Fry, D. J. (1980). Evidence from rat liver nuclear preparations that latency of microsomal UDP-glucuronosyltransferase is associated with vesiculation. *Biochem. J.*, **186,** 687–91
5. Bansal, S. K., Zaleski, J. and Gessner, T. (1981). Glucuronidation of oxygenated benzo(a)pyrene derivatives by UDP-glucuronosyltransferase of nuclear envelope. *Biochem. Biophys. Res. Com.*, **98,** 131–9
6. Elmamlouk, T. H., Mukhtar, H. and Bend, J. R. (1981). The nuclear envelope as a site of glucuronyltransferase in rat liver: properties and effect of inducers on enzyme activity. *J. Pharm. Exp. Ther.*, **219,** 27–34
7. Gonzalez, F. J. and Kasper, C. B. (1982). Differential inducibility of nuclear envelope epoxide hydrolase by trans-stilbene oxide and phenobarbital. *Mol. Pharmacol.*, **21,** 511–6
8. Von Bahr, C., Hietanen, E. and Glaumann, H. (1972). Oxidation and glucuronidation of certain drugs in various subcellular fractions of rat liver. *Acta Pharmacol. Toxicol.*, **31,** 107–20
9. Nyquist, S. E. and Morré, D. J. (1971). Distribution of UDP-glucuronyltransferase among cell fractions of rat liver. *J. Cell. Phys.*, **78,** 9–12
10. Wishart, G. J. (1978). Demonstration of functional heterogeneity of hepatic UDP-glucuronosyltransferase activities after administration of 3-methylcholanthrene and phenobarbital to rats. *Biochem. J.*, **174,** 485–9
11. Bock, K. W., Fröhling, W., Remmer, H. and Rexer, B. (1973). Effects of phenobarbital and 3-methylcholanthrene on substrate specificity of rat liver microsomal UDP-glucuronyltransferase. *Biochim. Biophys. Acta*, **327,** 46–56
12. Okulicz-Kozaryn, I., Schaefer, M., Batt, A. M., Siest, G. and Loppinet, V. (1981). Stereochemical heterogeneity of hepatic UDP-glucuronyltransferase activity in rat liver microsomes. *Biochem. Pharmacol.*, **30,** 1457–61
13. Watkins, J. B., Gregus, Z., Thompson, T. N. and Klaassen, C. D. (1982). Induction studies on the functional heterogeneity of rat liver UDP-glucuronosyltransferases. *Toxicol. Appl. Pharmacol.*, **64,** 439–46
14. Mallet, J., Foliot, A., Amat, D., Petite, J. P., Housset, E. and Camillieri, J. P. (1980). Cytochrome P-450 et bilirubine glucuronosyltransferase hépatiques dans la cirrhose du rat au tetrachlorure de carbone: démonstration d'une induction par le clofibrate. *Gastroenterol. Clin. Biol.*, **4,** 425–31
15. Singh, O. M. P., Graham, A. B. and Wood, G. C. (1981). The phospholipido-dependence of UDP-glucuronosyltransferase. *Eur. J. Biochem.*, **116,** 311–6

16. Magdalou, J., Hochman, Y. and Zakim, D. (1982). Factors modulating the catalytic specificity of a pure form of UDP-glucuronosyltransferase. *J. Biol. Chem.*, **257**, 13624–9
17. Neville, D. M. Jr. (1975). Isolation of cell surface membrane fractions from mammalian cells and organs. *Meth. Membr. Biol.*, **3**, 1–49
18. Blyth, C. A., Freedman, R. B. and Rabin, B. R. (1971). The effects of aflatoxin B1 on the sex-specific binding of steroid hormones to microsomal membranes of rat liver. *Eur. J. Biochem.*, **20**, 580–6
19. Morré, D. J., Cheetham, R. D. and Nyquist, S. E. (1972). A simplified procedure for isolation of Golgi apparatus from rat liver. *Prepar. Biochem.*, **2**, 61–9
20. Lowry, O. H., Rosebrough, N. J., Farr, A. L. and Randall, R. J. (1951). Protein measurement with the Folin phenol reagent. *J. Biol. Chem.*, **193**, 265–75
21. Mazel, P. (1971). In La Du, B. N., Maudel, H. G. and Way, E. L. (eds.). *Fundamentals of Drug Metabolism and Drug Disposition*. pp. 575–7 (Baltimore: Williams and Wilkins)
22. Szasz, G. (1969). A kinetic photometric method for serum gamma-glutamyltransferase peptidase. *Clin. Chem.*, **15**, 124–36
23. Mulder, G. J. and Van Doorn, A. B. D. (1975). A rapid NAD^+ linked for microsomal UDP-glucuronosyltransferase of rat liver and some observations on substrate specificity of the enzyme. *Biochem. J.*, **151**, 131–40
24. Colin-Neiger, A., Kaufmann, I., Boutin, J. A., Fournel, S., Siest, G., Batt, A. M. and Magdalou, J. (1984). Rapid centrifugal analysis of UDP-glucuronosyltransferase activities. Assessment of the Mulder and Van Doorn kinetic procedure. *J. Biomed. Biophys. Meth.*, **9**, 69–79
25. Heirwegh, K. P. M., Van de Vijver, M. amd Fevery, J. (1972). Assay and properties of digitonin-activated bilirubin uridine diphosphate glucuronyltransferase from rat liver. *Biochem. J.*, **129**, 605–18
26. Craft, J. A., Cooper, M. B., Estall, M. R., Rees, D. E. and Rabin, B. R. (1979). The role of components of the ER in the biosynthesis of cytochrome P-450. *Eur. J. Biochem.*, **96**, 379–91
27. Howell, K. E., Ito, A. and Palade, G. E. (1978). Endoplasmic reticulum marker enzymes in Golgi fraction. What does this mean? *J. Cell. Biol.*, **79**, 581–9
28. Ito, A. and Palade, G. E. (1978). Presence of NADPH cytochrome P-450 reductase in rat liver Golgi membranes. *J. Cell. Biol.*, **79**, 590–7
29. Leelavathi, D. E., Estes, L. W., Feingold, D. and Lombardi, B. (1970). Isolation of a Golgi fraction from rat liver. *Biochim. Biophys. Acta*, **211**, 124–38
30. Bergeron, J. J. M., Ehrenreich, J. H., Siekevitz, P. and Palade, G. E. (1973). Golgi fractions prepared from rat liver homogenates. II. Biochemical characterization. *J. Cell. Biol.*, **59**, 73–88
31. Ratanasavanh, D., Tazi, A., Galteau, M. M. and Siest, G. (1979). Localization of gamma-glutamyltransferase in subcellular fractions of rat and rabbit liver: effect of phenobarbital. *Biochem. Pharmacol.*, **28**, 1363–5
32. Vessey, D. A. and Zakim, D. (1972). Regulation of microsomal enzyme by phospholipids. V. Kinetic studies of hepatic UDP-glucuronosyltransferase. *J. Biol. Chem.*, **247**, 3023–8
33. Segel, I. H. (1975). Behaviour and analysis of rapid equilibrium and steady-state enzyme systems. *Enzyme Kinetics*. pp. 273–345. (New York: Wiley Interscience Publ.)
34. Hochman, Y., Kelley, M. and Zakim, D. (1983). Modulation of the number of ligand binding sites of UDP-glucuronosyltransferase by the gel to liquid crystal phase transition of phosphatidylcholines. *J. Biol. Chem.*, **258**, 6509–16
35. Weatherill, P. J., Kennedy, S. M. E. and Burchell, B. (1980). Immunochemical comparison of UDP-glucuronosyltransferase from Gunn and Wistar rats' liver. *Biochem. J.*, **191**, 155–63
36. Hochman, Y., Zakim, D. and Vessey, D. A. (1981). A kinetic mechanism for modulation of the activity of microsomal UDP-glucuronosyltransferase by phospholipids. Effect of lysophosphatidylcholines. *J. Biol. Chem.*, **256**, 4783–8
37. Boutin, J. A., Antoine, B., Batt, A. M. and Siest, G. (1985). Heterogeneity of hepatic microsomal UDP-glucuronosyltransferase(s) activities. Comparison between human and mammalian species activities. *Chem. Biol. Interact.* (In press)

16
Dose related effects of phenobarbital on rat liver microsomal UDP-glucuronyltransferase

P. D. BERK, N. TAVOLONI, H. OKUDA, M. J. T. JONES AND C.-L. KIANG

Administration of phenobarbital to rats at doses of 50–125 mg kg^{-1} day^{-1} accelerates plasma bilirubin clearance while increasing the ratio of bilirubin diglucuronide to monoglucuronide excreted in bile, and augmenting hepatic bilirubin UDP-glucuronyltransferase activity and formation of early labelled bilirubin[1-4]. The increase in bilirubin clearance has been attributed primarily to the increase in glucuronyltransferase. Administration of phenobarbital to man, at doses of 0.5–7.5 mg kg^{-1} day^{-1} also accelerates bilirubin clearance[5,6]. While an increase in the ratio of bilirubin diglucuronide to bilirubin monogluronide has been observed[7], most studies in man have failed to document an increase in bilirubin glucuronyltransferase activity[8,9] or in early labelled bilirubin formation[10] during phenobarbital therapy.

To determine whether reported variations in the effects of phenobarbital in rat and man represent significant species differences in drug-response or are merely dose-related, the activities of cytochrome P-450, glucose-6-phosphatase and both bilirubin- and p-nitrophenol-glucuronyltransferases were measured in hepatic microsomal preparations from control rats and rats treated for 6 days with phenobarbital at doses ranging from 1 to 125 mg kg^{-1} day^{-1} intraperitoneally.

METHODS

Studies were performed in male Sprague-Dawley rats weighing 290 ± (SD) 10 g. All animals were housed in a 22°C temperature controlled room with alternating 12 hour light/dark cycles for at least 1 week prior to study. They were fed Purina Lab Chow *ad libitum* with free access to water, and were not fasted prior to sacrifice. Animals were killed by stunning followed by exsanguination. Livers were excised, homogenized and microsomal suspensions prepared in 250 mmol/l sucrose/1 mmol/l EDTA as previously described[11].

Microsomal cytochrome P-450 activity was determined by its dithionite difference spectrum as described by Omura and Sato[12]. Glucose-6-phosphatase activity in native or deoxycholate-activated microsomes was determined by the method of Nordlie and Arion[13].

For the measurement of glucuronyltransferase activity, extensive preliminary studies reported in detail elsewhere[11] indicated that, in addition to such conventional variables as enzyme, substrate and magnesium concentration, pH and temperature, observed enzyme activity was markedly influenced by several additional variables, standardization of which is often neglected. These included whether the microsomes were prepared in sucrose/EDTA or KCl; frequency of freezing and thawing prior to assay; choice of activator; and species and concentration of albumin employed to solubilize bilirubin[14].

Accordingly, glucuronyltransferase activity was assayed using the standardized conditions shown in Table 16.1. When assaying bilirubin UDP-glucuronyltransferase activity, conjugated bilirubin formation was determined by extraction into the polar layer of a modified Weber–Schalm partition system[15] prior to coupling with diazotized sulphanilic acid, as described by Strebel and Odell[16]. When all other conditions are standardized, the use of this endpoint has been shown[11] to yield results identical to those obtained by the method of Heirwegh and colleagues[17–19], involving selective coupling of conjugated bilirubin by diazotized ethyl anthranilate at pH 2.7. P-nitrophenol-UDP-glucuronyltransferase was assayed as previously described[20].

Table 16.1 Conditions for assay of UDP-glucuronyltransferase

Variable	*Acceptor* *Bilirubin (BR)*	 *P-nitrophenol (PNP)*
Buffer: 250 mmol/l Tris	pH 7.9	pH 7.4
$MgCl_2$ (mmol/l)	10	10
UDPGA (mmol/l)	5.17	5.17
Substrate	0.214 mmol/l BR	0.75 mmol/l PNP
Carrier	6.25 mg/ml BSA	None
Microsomal protein	0.3–0.5 mg	0.3–0.5 mg
Total incubation volume	1 ml	1 ml
Incubation time (min at 37°C)	30	10
Microsome activation studies	'Native', UDPNAG, digitonin, deoxycholate	'Native', UPDNAG, deoxycholate

Microsome preparation: 250 mmol/l sucrose/1 mmol/l EDTA
Microsome storage: −20°C for up to 7 days; use immediately after initial thawing

RESULTS

Validation of methods

Using the standard incubation mixture described above, conjugated bilirubin formation (bilirubin–UDP–glucuronyltransferase activity) in 'native' microsomes was 3.85 ± 0.48 nmol 10 min^{-1} mg microsomal $protein^{-1}$ as assayed by the sulphanilic acid endpoint (SA) of Strebel and Odell[16], and 3.72 ± 0.44 nmol/ 10 min^{-1} mg^{-1} by the ethyl anthranilate endpoint (EA) of Heirwegh and colleagues[17–19]. Equivalent results were also obtained by the two endpoint techniques with UDPNAG (SA: 6.46 ± 0.69; EA: 6.08 ± 0.79) or digitonin activated microsomes (SA: 13.70 ± 2.16; EA: 14.78 ± 1.59)[11]. When bile pigments were extracted from the incubation mixtures by affinity chromatography over albumin–agarose gel and examined by thin layer chromatography[21], both bilirubin diglucuronide (BDG) and bilirubin monoglucuronide (BMG) were always identified as reaction products in addition to the unconjugated bilirubin –IXα substrate, irrespective of whether the incubated enzyme was 'native', or UDPNAG- or digitonin activated[21]. Of the conventional 1-*O*-acyl glucuronide conjugates detected, BDG accounted for 38–60%, the remainder being BMG. Occasionally, bands believed to represent 2,3- or 4-*O*-acyl conjugates were observed. There was no consistent difference in the relative proportions of BDG and BMG as a function of the activation status of the microsomal preparation employed.

Cytochrome P-450

Cytochrome P-450 activity in control rats was 0.76 ± 0.11 nmol/mg microsomal protein, and at 0.79 ± 0.09 nmol/mg was not enhanced significantly following treatment with phenobarbital at 1 mg kg^{-1} day^{-1}. A statistically significant induction to 0.98 ± 0.07 nmol/mg was observed at 3 mg kg^{-1} day^{-1} of phenobarbital, beyond which a dose-related induction was observed at all doses up to a maximum of 75 mg kg^{-1} day^{-1} (Figure 16.1). The lesser degree of induction observed at 125 mg/kg may be secondary to reduced food intake in turn resulting from excessive somnolence. Both weight gain and the increase in the liver weight/body weight ratio were lower at this phenobarbital dose than in any of the next three lower doses.

UDP-glucuronyltransferase

To determine whether the induction of UDP-glucuronyltransferase by phenobarbital was influenced by the activation status of the enzyme, drug effects were measured in native microsomes, in microsomes activated allosterically with UDPNAG and in detergent activated preparations. In untreated animals, UDPNAG produced an increase in measured enzyme activity to 165% of that in native microsomes, whereas digitonin and deoxycholate produced much greater mean increases of 370 and 430%, respectively (Table 16.2). Irrespective of the activation status of the microsomes, a statistically significant and dose-related induction of bilirubin UDP-glucuronyltransferase activity was observed at all phenobarbital doses equal to or greater than 3 mg kg^{-1} day^{-1}. Maximal induction was observed with the highest dose of phenobarbital employed. The degree of maximal induction at 125 mg kg^{-1} day^{-1} was similar in native and in each of the activated enzyme preparations, ranging from 218 to 260% of control values (Table 16.2)[22].

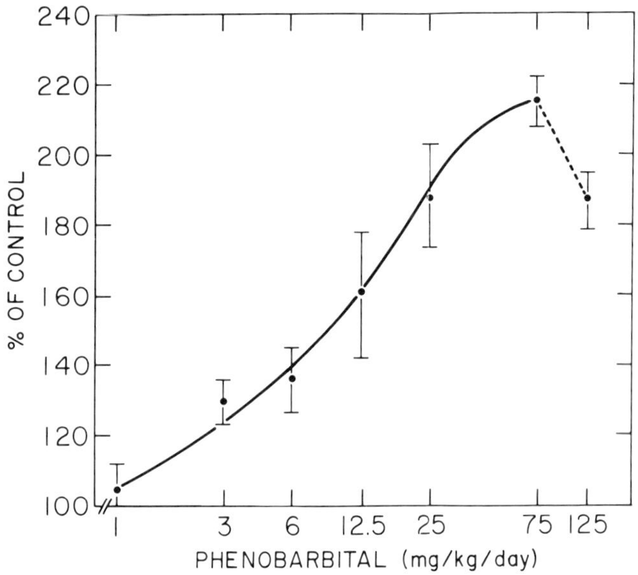

Figure 16.1 Effect of phenobarbital treatment on hepatic cytochrome P-450 activity of rat liver microsomes. Doses of the drug are in a log scale. Values are means ± SD and represent the percentage increase over the control activity (nmol/mg microsomal protein). Reproduced from [22] with permission

Table 16.2 Effect of phenobarbital treatment (PB, mg kg^{-1} day^{-1}) on bilirubin UDP-glucuronyltransferase activity of rat liver microsomes[a]

Treatment		*'Native'*	*UDPNAG*	*Digitonin*	*Deoxycholate*
Controls	(*n* = 8)[b]	3.64 ± 0.48	5.96 ± 0.75	13.33 ± 1.71	15.68 ± 2.39
PB 1	(*n* = 7)	3.85 ± 0.59	6.19 ± 0.64	14.94 ± 2.82	16.38 ± 3.00
PB 3	(*n* = 7)	4.50 ± 0.55*	6.90 ± 1.06*	16.51 ± 1.35*	18.33 ± 2.37*
PB 6	(*n* = 6)	4.75 ± 0.80	7.56 ± 1.28*	18.72 ± 2.53*	19.92 ± 3.02*
PB 12.5	(*n* = 6)	6.22 ± 0.54	9.50 ± 0.68*	22.75 ± 2.46*	26.35 ± 2.39*
PB 25	(*n* = 6)	6.71 ± 1.36	9.95 ± 1.75*	23.99 ± 1.34*	27.45 ± 3.57*
PB 75	(*n* = 7)	7.87 ± 1.38	11.03 ± 1.40*	26.81 ± 2.90*	31.10 ± 2.74*
PB 125	(*n* = 6)	9.32 ± 0.71	12.98 ± 1.64*	32.78 ± 3.55*	40.86 ± 5.47*

[a] Values are means ± SD and represent μmol 10 min^{-1} mg microsome $protein^{-1}$
[b] number of animals
* Regardless of the enzyme activation status, all activities from rats treated with a dose of PB of 3 mg/kg or greater are significantly greater than controls ($p < 0.05$–0.001)
Reproduced from [22] with permission

As with bilirubin UDP-glucuronyltransferase, detergent activation of *p*-nitrophenol glucuronyltransferase was greater than that observed with UDPNAG (Table 16.3). For all three microsomal preparations studied, a statistically significant induction of enzyme activity was observed at phenobarbital doses as low as 3 mg kg^{-1} day^{-1}. The degree of induction at this dose,

Table 16.3 Effect of phenobarbital (PB) treatment on *p*-nitrophenol UDPGT activity in rat liver microsomes*

Treatment		*'Native'*	*Enzyme activation†* *UDPNAG*	*Deoxycholate*
Controls	(n = 6)	3.54 ± 0.74	12.94 ± 2.65	39.31 ± 9.83
PB 1 mg/kg	(n = 5)	3.97 ± 0.81	14.52 ± 2.71	47.61 ± 8.07
PB 3 mg/kg	(n = 7)	5.33 ± 1.25‡	21.46 ± 3.32‡	58.65 ± 7.93‡

* Values (means ± SD) are nmol min^{-1} mg microsomal $protein^{-1}$ (number of animals in parenthesis)
† UDPNAG was added to the incubation mixture at 3.07 mmol/l; deoxycholate (0.125/100 ml) was added to the microsome suspension (12.5/100 ml) 30 min before use
‡ Student's *t*-test: $p < 0.05$–0.001 compared to corresponding control group
Reproduced from [20] with permission

approximately 150–165%, was similar in each type of microsomal preparation[20].

Glucose-6-phosphatase

In contrast to the other enzymes studied, glucose-6-phosphatase activity was decreased by phenobarbital in a dose-related fashion (Figure 16.2), significant depression being observed with doses as low as 3 mg kg^{-1} day^{-1}. This depression

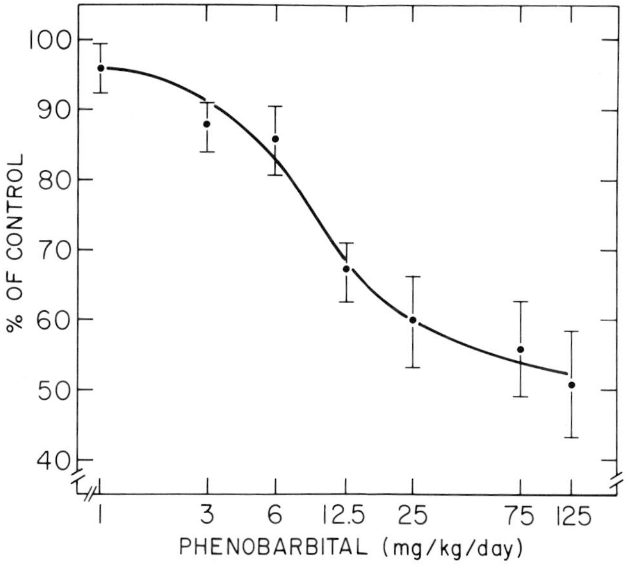

Figure 16.2 Effect of phenobarbital treatment on glucose-6-phosphatase activity of rat liver microsomes. Doses of the drug are in a log scale. Values are means ± SD and represent the percentage decrease of the deoxycholate-activated enzyme specific activity (nmol mg^{-1} mg^{-1} microsomal protein) from controls. Reproduced from [22] with permission

was observed equally with native or deoxycholate activated enzyme, and irrespective of whether the results were expressed as enzyme specific activity (nmol min^{-1} mg microsomal $protein^{-1}$) or total hepatic activity (μmol min^{-1} 100 gm body $weight^{-1}$)[22].

DISCUSSION

Although other investigators have examined the dose response effects of phenobarbital on microsomal enzyme activity[23-26], no study has previously examined systematically the dose response curve for bilirubin conjugation. Our results indicate that phenobarbital produces a dose-related induction of rat liver cytochrome P-450 and both bilirubin- and *p*-nitrophenol UDP-glucuronyltransferases, which is statistically significant at doses of 3 mg kg^{-1} day^{-1} or more. For the glucuronyltransferases, in contrast to prior reports[27], the degree of induction by phenobarbital is equivalent for native, UDPNAG and detergent activated enzyme, although absolute values depend on the activation status of the microsomes. Moreover, the inducing effect is enzyme specific since, in contrast to P-450 and glucuronyltransferase, phenobarbital at 3 mg/kg or more produces a dose-related depression of glucose-6-phosphatase activity.

The lowest absolute dose of phenobarbital producing these inducing effects on *in vitro* bilirubin conjugation in rat liver is similar to doses employed clinically, and even lower if corrected for species differences in the rate of drug metabolism between man and rat[28-31]. Accordingly, we conclude that the failure to detect measurable induction of bilirubin UDP-glucuronyltransferase by phenobarbital in man is not merely dose-related. The same presumably holds true for the failure of phenobarbital to increase incorporation of 4-^{14}C-δ-aminolaevulinic acid into early labelled bilirubin in man[10], as it does in the rat[4]. Either methodologic artefacts or an appreciable species difference in response to the drug must underlie the reported differences between man and rat in its effect on bilirubin conjugation *in vitro* and early labelled bilirubin formation *in vivo*.

ACKNOWLEDGEMENTS

The authors are indebted to Ms Mary Barrett for rapid and accurate preparation of the manuscript. This work was supported in part by Grant AM-26438 from the National Institute of Arthritis, Diabetes, Digestive and Kidney Disease; and by generous gifts from the Jack Martin Fund and the Polly Annenberg Levee Charitable Trust.

References

1. Berk, P. D., Blaschke, T. F. and Gisselbrecht, C. (1977). Discrepancy between drug effects on early labeling and bilirubin production. In Berk, P. D. and Berlin, N. I. (eds.). *The Chemistry and Physiology of Bile Pigments*, DHEW Publication No. NIH 77-1100, pp. 254–62. (Washington: US Government Printing Office)

2. Schmid, R., Marver, H. S. and Hammaker, L. (1966). Enhanced formation of rapidly labeled bilirubin by phenobarbital: hepatic microsomal cytochromes as a possible source. *Biochem. Biophys. Res. Commun.*, **24,** 319–28
3. Robinson, S. H., Yannoni, C. and Nagasawa, S. (1971). Bilirubin excretion in rats with normal and impaired bilirubin conjugation. Effect of phenobarbital. *J. Clin. Invest.*, **50,** 2606–13
4. Levitt, M., Schachter, B. A., Zipursky, A. and Israels, L. G. (1968). The nonerythropoietic component of early bilirubin. *J. Clin. Invest.*, **47,** 1281–94
5. Blaschke, T. F., Berk, P. D., Rodkey, F. L., Scharschmidt, B. F., Collison, H. A. and Waggoner, J. G. (1974). Drugs and the liver. 1. Effects of glutethimide and phenobarbital on hepatic bilirubin clearance, plasma bilirubin turnover, and carbon monoxide production in man. *Biochem. Pharmacol.*, **23,** 2795–2806
6. Black, M., Fevery, J., Parker, D., Jacobson, J., Billing, B. H. and Carson, E. R. (1974). Effect of phenobarbitone on plasma (^{14}C) bilirubin clearance in patients with unconjugated hyperbilirubinaemia. *Clin. Sci. Mol. Med.*, **46,** 1–17
7. Fevery, J., Blanckaert, N., Heirwegh, K. P. M., Preaux, A.-M. and Berthelot, P. (1977). Unconjugated bilirubin and an increased proportion of bilirubin monoconjugates in the bile of patients with Gilbert's syndrome and Crigler–Najjar syndrome. *J. Clin. Invest.*, **60,** 970–9
8. Felsher, B. F., Craig, J. R. and Carpio, N. (1973). Hepatic bilirubin glucuronidation in Gilbert's syndrome. *J. Lab. Clin. Med.*, **81,** 829–37
9. Black, M. and Sherlock, S. (1970). Treatment of Gilbert's syndrome with phenobarbitone. *Lancet*, **1,** 1359–62
10. Berk, P. D., Blaschke, T. F., Waggoner, J. G. and Shrager, R. I. (1980). Phenobarbital does not increase hepatic heme turnover in man. *Gastroenterology*, **79,** 1004 (Abstr)
11. Tavoloni, N., Jones, M. J. T., Wittman, R., Kiang, C.-L. and Berk, P. D. (1983). Comparison of different activators and diazotization procedures in the assay of bilirubin-UDP-glucuronyltransferase activity in rat liver. *Clin. Chim. Act.*, **128,** 209–21
12. Omura, T. and Sato, R. (1964). The carbon monoxide-binding pigment of liver microsomes. Evidence for its hemoprotein nature. *J. Biol. Chem.*, **239,** 2370–8
13. Nordlie, R. C. and Arion, W. J. (1966). Glucose-6-phosphatase. In Woods, W. A. (ed.). *Methods in Enzymology*, Vol. 9, p. 619. (New York: Academic Press)
14. Tavoloni, N., Jones, M. J. T., Isola, L. M. J. and Berk, P. D. (1984). Effect of albumin on the *in vitro* conjugation of bilirubin by rat liver microsomes. *Proc. Soc. Exp. Biol. Med.*, **176,** 356–65
15. Weber, A. P. and Schalm, L. (1962). Quantitative separation and determination of bilirubin and conjugated bilirubin human serum. *Clin. Chim. Acta*, **7,** 805–10
16. Strebel, L. and Odell, G. B. (1971). Bilirubin uridine diphospho-glucuronyltransferase in rat liver microsomes: genetic variation and maturation. *Pediatr. Res.*, **5,** 548–59
17. Van Roy, F. P. and Heirwegh, K. P. M. (1968). Determination of bilirubin glucuronide and assay of glucuronyltransferase with bilirubin as acceptor. *Biochem. J.*, **107,** 507–18
18. Heirwegh, K. P. M., Van De Vijver, M. and Fevery, J. (1972). Assay and properties of digitonin-activated bilirubin uridine diphosphate glucuronyltransferase from rat liver. *Biochem. J.*, **129,** 605–18
19. Black, M., Billing, B. H. and Heirwegh, K. P. M. (1970). Determination of bilirubin UDP-glucuronyltransferase activity in needle-biopsy specimens of human liver. *Clin. Chim. Acta*, **29,** 27–35
20. Tavoloni, N., Wittman, R., Jones, M. J. T. and Berk, P. D. (1983). Effect of low-dose phenobarbital on hepatic microsomal UDP-glucuronyltransferase activity. *Biochem. Pharmacol.*, **32,** 2143–7
21. Okuda, H., Tavoloni, N., Kiang, C.-L., Jones, M. J. T. and Berk, P. D. (1983). Bilirubin diglucuronide formation by rat liver microsomes: demonstration by affinity and thin layer chromatography of bile pigment tetrapyrroles. *Biochem. Biophys. Res. Commun.*, **117,** 406–12
22. Tavoloni, N., Jones, M. J. T. and Berk, P. D. (1983). Dose-related effects of phenobarbital on hepatic microsomal enzymes. *Proc. Soc. Exp. Biol. Med.*, **174,** 20–7
23. Breckenridge, A., Orme, M. L. E., Davies, L., Thorgeirsson, S. S. and Davies, S. S. (1973). Dose-dependent enzyme induction. *Clin. Pharmacol. Ther.*, **14,** 514–20
24. Valerino, D. M., Vesell, E. S., Johnson, A. O. and Aurori, K. C. (1973). Effects of

various centrally active drugs on hepatic microsomal enzymes: a comparative study. *Drug Metab. Dispos.*, **1,** 669–78

25. Valerino, D. M., Vesell, E. S., Aurori, K. C. and Johnson, A. O. (1974). Effects of various barbiturates on hepatic microsomal enzymes. *Drug. Metab. Dispos.*, **2,** 448–57
26. Heath, E. C. and Dingell, J. V. (1974). The interaction of foreign chemical compounds with the glucuronidation of estrogens *in vitro*. *Drug Metab. Dispos.*, **2,** 556–65
27. Wisnes, A. (1971). Variable effect of phenobarbital treatment of mice on hepatic UDP-glucuronyltransferase activity when judged by slightly different enzyme-assay techniques. *Biochem. Pharmacol.*, **20,** 1853–7
28. Conomy, J. P. (1978). Long-term use of the major anticonvulsant drugs. *Am. Fam. Phys.*, **18,** 107–18
29. Hvidberg, E. F. and Dam, M. (1976). Clinical pharmacokinetics of anticonvulsants. *Clin. Pharmacokinet.*, **1,** 161–88
30. Cooper, D. Y., Schleyer, H., Levin, S. S., Touchstone, J. C., Eisenhardt, R. H., Vars, H. M., Rosenthal, O., Rastigar, H. and Harken, A. (1978). Biliary and urinary excretion of phenobarbital and parahydroxyphenobarbital in rats with bile fistula. In Estabrook, R. W. and Lindenlaub, E. (eds.). *The Induction of Drug Metabolism*, p. 252. (Stuttgart: Schattaner)
31. Croft, J. E., Caldwell, J. and Smith, R. L. (1978). Phenobarbitone disposition in relation to tolerance. *Biochem. Soc. Trans.*, **6,** 246–8

Section 5
Cellular Control of Glucuronide Formation

Chairman: C. D. Klaassen

17
Changes in hepatic UDP-glucuronate contents induced by pyrimidine precursors and uridylate-trapping sugar analogues

D. KEPPLER, C. SCHIESSEL AND C. FORSTHOVE

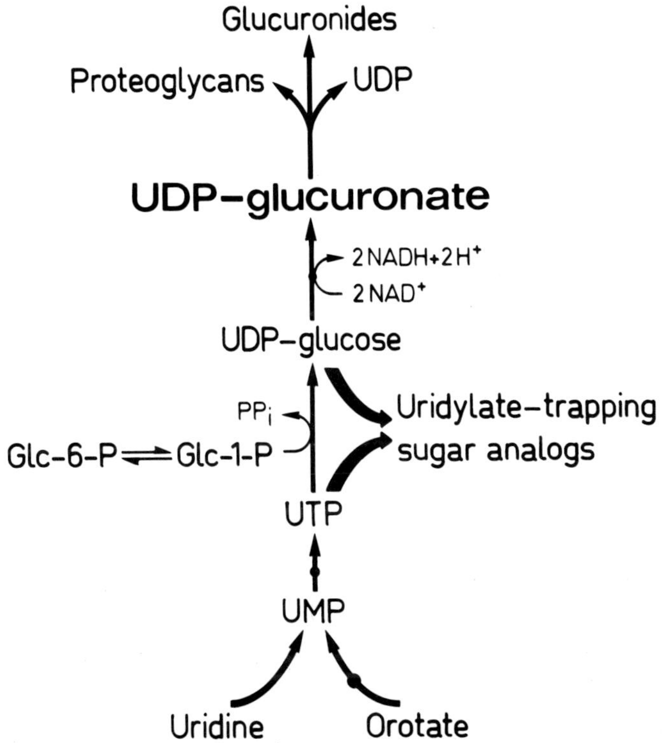

Figure 17.1 Biosynthesis and metabolism of UDP-glucuronate. The diversion of uridylate from UTP- or UDP-glucose by uridylate-trapping sugar analogues is indicated

Cellular levels of UDP-glucuronate (UDP-GlcA) are controlled by its biosynthesis from UDP-glucose as well as by its utilization in the reactions of glucuronide synthesis and proteoglycan formation. Interference of this balance between utilization and biosynthesis may result – on the side of biosynthesis – from an inhibition of UDP-glucose dehydrogenase by a rise in the NADH/NAD ratio[1], from a diversion of uridylate by uridylate-trapping sugar analogues yielding UDP-sugar analogues[2,3], or from inadequate rates of uridylate synthesis from orotate or uridine (Figure 17.1). It is not clear whether nucleotide pyrophosphatase (EC 3.6.1.9) can contribute to an *intracellular* breakdown of UDP-glucuronate yielding UMP and glucuronate 1-pyrophosphate.

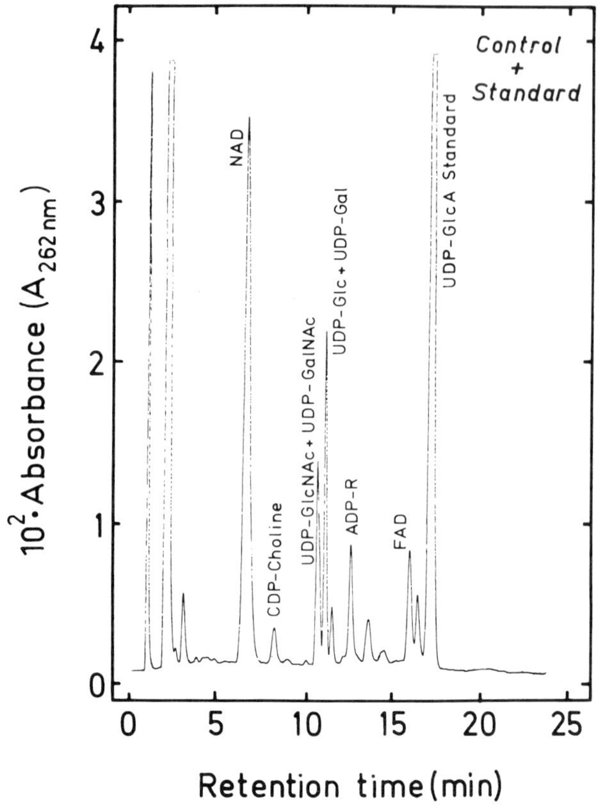

Figure 17.2 Separation of an internal UDP-glucuronate standard from rat liver nucleotides by anion-exchange HPLC. Rat liver was freeze-clamped *in situ* and homogenized in cold perchloric acid (0.6 mol/l)[2,3]. The supernatant, after centrifugation, was separated from the pellet and neutralized with KOH. Treatment with alkaline phosphatase (15 units/ml)[10] was performed at 30°C for 30 min. After the addition of UDP-glucuronate (100 nmol) as a standard, the nucleotides corresponding to 2 mg of liver wet weight were separated by anion-exchange HPLC[13]. As a result of the phosphatase treatment, NAD includes NADP; moreover, ADP-ribose (ADP-R) includes ADP-ribose phosphate. The latter are produced during acidic deproteinization from NADH and NADPH, respectively. The UDP-glucuronate (UDP-GlcA) standard is eluted as the last nucleotide on the chromatogram

METHODS FOR DETERMINATION OF UDP-GLUCURONATE

The analysis of UDP-glucuronate has mostly employed the UDP-glucuronosyl-transferase-catalysed formation of conjugates which can be chromogenic[4], fluorescent[5,6], or radioactive[7,8]. Another method has employed the specific enzymatic analysis of the UMP moiety of UDP-glucuronate after its chromatographic separation[2]. More recently, high-performance liquid chromatography (HPLC) with detection of the uracil absorbance has become available for rapid analysis, in which separation of the nucleotides can be achieved both by anion-

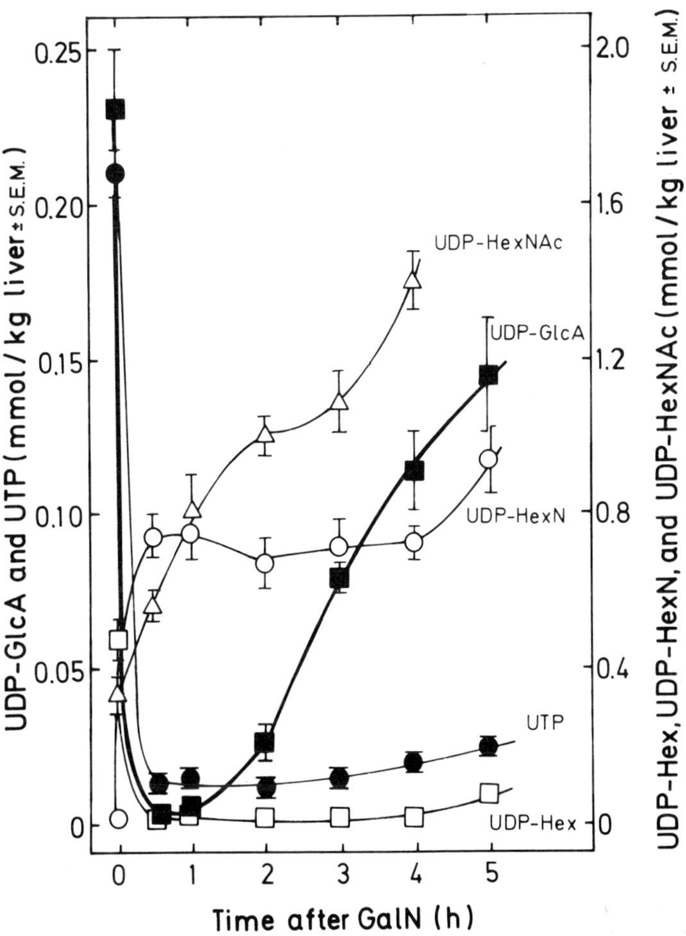

Figure 17.3 Depletion of rat liver UDP-glucuronate and associated changes in uracil nucleotide contents induced by D-galactosamine. Female rats of the Wistar strain were injected i.p. with D-galactosamine (GalN; 3 mmol/kg). Freeze-clamped livers were analysed by HPLC[3,10,12,13]. UDP-HexNAc designates the sum of UDP-*N*-acetylglucosamine and UDP-*N*-acetylgalactosamine, UDP-HexN the sum of UDP-glucosamine and UDP-galactosamine, UDP-Hex the sum of UDP-glucose and UDP-galactose

exchange[3,9,10] or ion-pair reversed-phase[11] chromatography. Separation of UDP-glucuronate by anion-exchange HPLC can be improved by treatment of the extract with alkaline phosphatase, which hydrolyses all nucleoside phosphates but leaves the UDP-sugars intact[10]. The HPLC determination of UDP-glucuronate should be initiated by freezing or freeze-clamping of cells or tissues prior to deproteinization with cold perchloric acid[2,3,10]. An advantage of this HPLC analysis is the simultaneous detection of other nucleotides, such as UDP-glucose, NAD, NADH, and UDP-*N*-acetylglucosamine[10,12], which function as precursor or as regulators in UDP-glucuronate metabolism (Figure 17.2).

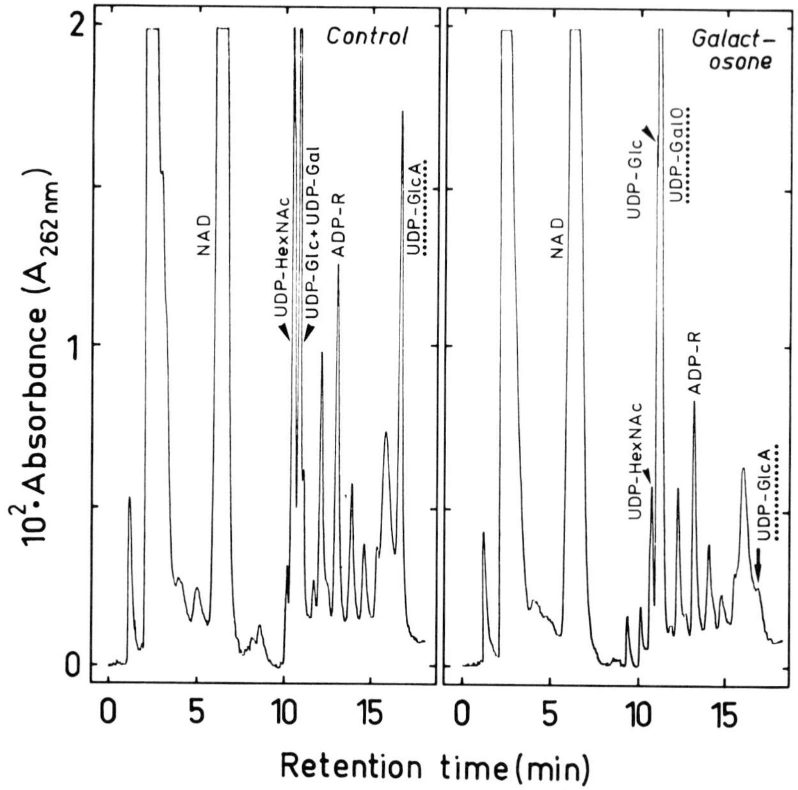

Figure 17.4 UDP-sugars in cultured hepatocytes exposed to D-galactosone. Cultured rat hepatocytes[18], kindly provided by Dr T.-A. Tran-Thi, were frozen in liquid nitrogen[10] after an exposure for 2 h to D-galactosone (2 mmol/l). Perchloric acid extracts were treated for 30 min at pH 8.5 with alkaline phosphatase[10] (30 units/ml) for hydrolysis of nucleoside phosphates and partial degradation of alkali-labile UDP-derivatives of D-galactosone[3]. Note the accumulation of UDP-galactosone (UDP-GalO), and the decrease in UDP-*N*-acetylhexosamines (UDP-HexNAc) and in UDP-glucuronate from 0.24 to 0.07 and from 0.22 to < 0.02 mmol/kg wet hepatocytes, respectively. The extract injected for HPLC corresponded to about 2 mg of cultured hepatocytes

MODIFICATION OF UDP-GLUCURONATE CONTENTS BY PYRIMIDINE PRECURSORS AND SUGAR ANALOGUES

An expansion of the UDP-glucuronate pool is observed after administration of pyrimidine precursors such as orotate or uridine. Uridine (4 mmol/kg, i.p.) increased the content of UDP-glucuronate in rat liver two-fold within 2 h, simultaneous with an expansion of UDP-glucose and UDP-*N*-acetylglucosamine pools. Glucosamine, however, markedly increased UDP-glucuronate and UDP-*N*-acetylglucosamine while decreasing UDP-glucose both in liver[2] and in colon carcinoma cells[10].

A depletion of UDP-glucuronate can be induced by uridylate-trapping sugar analogues[2,3]. As a consequence, glucuronidation of several substrates is impaired in liver slices[14], in isolated hepatocytes[15], in perfused liver[16] and in the rat *in vivo*[17]. A single dose of D-galactosamine decreased hepatic UDP-glucuronate to 5% of control within 30 min (Figure 17.3). The early recovery of the UDP-glucuronate level follows the galactosamine-induced rise in UDP-*N*-acetylglucosamine and UDP-*N*-acetylgalactosamine.

D-Galactosone has been identified recently as another uridylate-trapping galactose analogue[3]. D-Galactosone is metabolized by enzymes of the galactose pathway yielding the alkali-labile derivative UDP-galactosone[3]. Furthermore, UDP-glucosone is oxidized by UDP-glucose dehydrogenase[13]. D-Galactosone depletes UDP-glucuronate in rat liver *in vivo*[3] and in cultured hepatocytes (Figure 17.4). In contrast to the effect of D-galactosamine, D-galactosone also reduces the cellular content of UDP-*N*-acetylhexosamines.

The sugar analogues, particularly the galactose analogues, can be employed for a depletion of the cellular UDP-glucuronate pool which causes a reduced rate of glucuronide conjugation. The choice of the sugar analogue modifies the associated changes in the concentration of other UDP-sugars such as UDP-glucose and UDP-*N*-acetylglucosamine (Figure 17.5). Uridine, as a rapidly phosphorylated pyrimidine nucleotide precursor, can be used to replenish depleted UDP-glucuronate pools.

	GalN	GalO	GlcN	Oro	Urd
UDP-GlcA	↓	↓	↑	↑	↑
UDP-glucose	↓	↓	↓	↑	↑
UDP-N-acetyl-hexosamines	↑	↓	↑	↑	↑
UDP-sugar analogs	↑	↑	–	–	–

Figure 17.5 Changes in hepatic UDP-glucuronate and UDP-sugar levels induced by sugar analogues or pyrimidine precursors. GalN, D-galactosamine; GalO, D-galactosone; GlcN, D-glucosamine; Oro, orotate; Urd, uridine. The increase in UDP-sugar analogues induced by D-galactosamine refers to UDP-galactosamine and UDP-glucosamine; the increase after D-galactosone refers to UDP-galactosone and its UDP-derivatives

ACKNOWLEDGEMENTS

Thanks are due to Dr T.-A. Tran-Thi for providing us with cultured rat hepatocytes. This work has been supported by the Deutsche Forschungsgemeinschaft through Sonderforschungsbereich 154 'Hepatologie', Freiburg.

References

1. Zalitis, J. and Feingold, D. S. (1968). The mechanism of action of UDPG dehydrogenase. *Biochem. Biophys. Res. Commun.*, **31**, 693–8
2. Keppler, D., Rudigier, J., Bischoff, E. and Decker, K. (1970). The trapping of uridine phosphates by D-galactosamine, D-glucosamine, and 2-deoxy-D-galactose. A study on the mechanism of galactosamine hepatitis. *Eur. J. Biochem.*, **17**, 246–53
3. Keppler, D., Schulz-Holstege, C., Fauler, J., Reiffen, K. A. and Schneider, F. (1982). Uridylate trapping, induction of UTP deficiency, and stimulation of pyrimidine synthesis *de novo* by D-galactosone. *Biochem. J.*, **206**, 139–46
4. Dutton, G. J. and Storey, I. D. E. (1962). Glucuronide-forming enzymes. *Meth. Enzymol.*, **5**, 159–64
5. Wong, K. P. and Sourkes, T. L. (1967). Determination of UDPG and UDPGA in tissues. *Anal. Biochem.*, **21**, 444–53
6. Singh, J., Schwarz, L. R. and Wiebel, F. J. (1980). A rapid enzymic procedure for the determination of picomole amounts of UDP-glucuronic acid. *Biochem. J.*, **189**, 369–72
7. Lehnert, W., Wagner, T. O. F., Fürst, M. W. and Künzer, W. (1979). Eine radioenzymatische Mikromethode zur Bestimmung der UDP-Glucuronsäure. *J. Clin. Chem. Clin. Biochem.*, **17**, 363–7
8. Schiller, C. M., Dieringer, C. S., Twine, M. E. and Jeffcoat, A. R. (1982). Determination of tissue UDP-glucuronic acid levels by high-pressure liquid chromatograhy. *Anal. Biochem.*, **127**, 68–72
9. Patterson, D., Vannais, D. B. and Laas, W. (1983). Isolation and characterization of a Chinese hamster ovary cell mutant which accumulates UDP-glucuronic acid and requires uridine for growth. *J. Cell. Physiol.*, **116**, 257–64
10. Krug, E., Zweibaum, A., Schulz-Holstege, C. and Keppler, D. (1984). D-Glucosamine-induced changes in nucleotide metabolism and growth of colon-carcinoma cells in culture. *Biochem. J.*, **217**, 701–8
11. Aw, T. Y. and Jones, D. P. (1982). Direct determination of UDP-glucuronic acid in cell extracts by high-performance liquid chromatography. *Anal. Biochem.*, **127**, 32–6
12. Weckbecker, G. and Keppler, D. (1983). Separation and analysis of 4-epimeric UDP-sugars by borate high-performance liquid chromatography. *Anal. Biochem.*, **132**, 405–12
13. Holstege, A., Schulz-Holstege, C., Henninger, H., Reiffen, K. A., Schneider, F. and Keppler, D. (1982). Uridylate trapping induced by the C-2-modified D-glucose analogs glucosone, fluoroglucose, and glucosamine. *Eur. J. Biochem.*, **121**, 469–74
14. Hänninen, O. and Marniemi, J. (1970). Inhibition of glucuronide synthesis by physiological metabolites in liver slices. *FEBS Lett.*, **6**, 177–81
15. Greim, H., Summer, K.-H. and Schwarz, L. R. (1984). Metabolic inactivation of toxins. In Keppler, D., Popper, H., Bianchi, L. and Reutter, W. (eds.). *Mechanisms of Hepatocyte Injury and Death*. pp. 369–77. (Lancaster: MTP Press)
16. Otani, G., Abou-El-Makarem, M. M. and Bock, K. W. (1976). UDP-glucuronyltransferase in perfused rat liver and in microsomes – III. Effects of galactosamine and carbon tetrachloride on the glucuronidation of 1-naphthol and bilirubin. *Biochem. Pharmacol.*, **25**, 1293–7
17. Watkins, J. B., Gregus, Z., Thompson, T. N. and Klassen, C. D. (1982). Depletion of hepatic UDP-glucuronic acid (UDPGA) decreases the biliary excretion of drugs. *Hepatology*, **2**, 702
18. Gross, V., Andus, T., Tran-Thi, T.-A., Bauer, J., Decker, K. and Heinrich, P. C. (1984). Induction of acute phase proteins by dexamethasone in rat hepatocyte primary cultures. *Exp. Cell Res.*, **151**, 46–54

18
Chemical influences on UDP-glucuronic acid concentration

C. D. KLAASSEN, R. L. DILLS, Z. GREGUS, G. A. HAZELTON, J. J. HJELLE, C.-P. SIEGERS AND J. B. WATKINS

Glucuronidation is an important conjugation reaction involved in metabolic conversion of endogenous and exogenous substances to more aqueous soluble compounds that can be excreted into urine or bile. Glucuronidation is dependent upon the enzymatic activity of UDP-glucuronosyltransferase and the intracellular concentration of UDP-glucuronic acid.

The effect of chemicals on hepatic UDP-glucuronosyltransferase activity has been extensively studied, but less is known regarding xenobiotic-induced changes in UDP-glucuronic acid concentrations. Therefore, the purpose of the present study was to determine the effect of chemicals on UDP-glucuronic acid concentration, and whether an alteration of the cosubstrate concentration would affect the glucuronidation and excretion of various xenobiotics.

The effects of the anaesthetic diethyl ether on the concentration of UDP-glucuronic acid in rat liver, duodenum, kidney and lung are shown in Figure 18.1. In this experiment rats were exposed to diethyl ether for 10 min. Diethyl ether markedly decreased UDP-glucuronic acid in liver, kidney, and lung by 95, 38, and 69%, respectively, immediately after the 10 min exposure. Although significantly lower at 15, 30, and 45 min (decreased 88, 80, and 50%, respectively), hepatic UDP-glucuronic acid concentration rapidly returned to control values by 1 h after exposure. In the lung, UDP-glucuronic acid was depressed 60 and 65% at 15 and 30 min, respectively, before recovering to control levels. The concentration of UDP-glucuronic acid in kidney was significantly decreased immediately after exposure and was higher than controls at 2 h after exposure to diethyl ether. UDP-glucuronic acid concentration in the duodenum was not altered by inhalation of this anaesthetic.

The effect of diethyl ether depletion of UDP-glucuronic acid concentration on the biliary excretion of compounds which are glucuronidated before excretion into bile is shown in Table 18.1. Diethyl ether had no effect on the biliary excretion of phenolphthalein. Unlike phenolphthalein, the biliary excretion of iopanoic acid glucuronide was markedly reduced by diethyl ether anaesthesia.

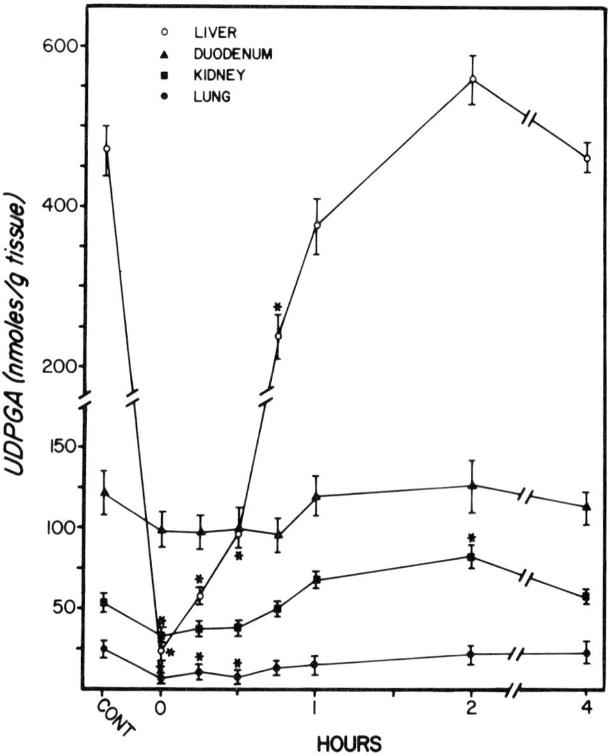

Figure 18.1 Effect of recovery time after a 10 min exposure to diethyl ether on the concentration of UDP-glucuronic acid in liver, duodenum, kidney, and lung[3]

The biliary excretion of bilirubin, primarily as its diglucuronide conjugate, was diminished by diethyl ether anaesthesia. Biliary excretion of diethylstilboestrol glucuronide, the main form of diethylstilboestrol in bile, was slightly affected by diethyl ether. The biliary excretion of valproic acid glucuronide was also diminished by diethyl ether. Thus, diethyl ether decreases the biliary excretion of compounds requiring glucuronidation before excretion.

Because the studies described above demonstrated that the concentration of UDP-glucuronic acid can affect the excretion of chemicals, it was of interest to determine whether the glucuronidation of acetaminophen, a widely used antipyretic and analgesic, is saturable, and if it was, to determine if it might be due to limited availability of UDP-glucuronic acid. The effect of various dosages of acetaminophen administered intravenously to urethane anaesthetized rats on the biliary excretion of acetaminophen glucuronide is shown in Figure 18.2. The predominant form of acetaminophen in bile was acetaminophen-glucuronide, which reached a biliary excretion rate of 700 μg equivalents of acetaminophen per minute per kilogram after the highest dosage. Peak biliary excretion rates were observed 15–30 min after administration of the three lowest dosages, but were delayed after the two higher dosages of acetaminophen. While the amount of acetaminophen-glucuronide in the bile increased as the dose was increased, there was not a doubling of excretion when the dose

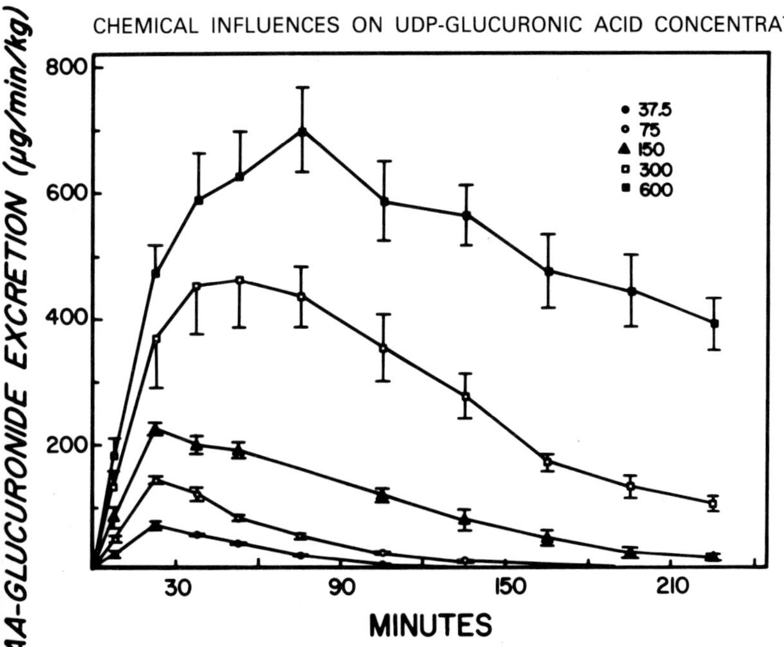

Figure 18.2 Biliary excretion rate of acetaminophen-glucuronide after acetaminophen i.v. These data are expressed as microgram equivalents of acetaminophen. Each point represents the mean ± SE of four to eight rats. From Hjelle and Klaassen[2]

Table 18.1 Biliary excretion of glucuronides of cholephils in control (urethane) and diethyl ether-anaesthetized rats

	Dosage (µmol/kg)	*Biliary excretion* (% of control)
Phenolphthalein	200	95
	15	112
Iopanoic acid	200	37*
	15	24*
Bilirubin	60	73*
	5	59*
Diethylstilboestrol	60	82
	5	71*
Valproic acid	1000	72*

* Significantly different ($p < 0.05$) from control
Based on Gregus *et al.*[1]

was increased from 300 to 600 mg/kg. The apparent first-order formation rate constants for glucuronidation were determined as the product of the plasma elimination rate constant and the fraction of the recovered dose excreted in urine and bile as the glucuronide. Table 18.2 indicates that the rate constant for acetaminophen-glucuronide formation decreased as the dosages increased, and was statistically less at the two higher doses.

It can be calculated from peak biliary excretion data that at least 35% of the hepatic steady-state pool of UDP-glucuronic acid (control values of 325 nmol/g

Table 18.2 Glucuronide formation rate constants (K'_f) after various dosages of acetaminophen

Dosage (mg/kg)	*Acetaminophen-Glucuronide* (mean ± SE) ($K'_f \times 10^3 \times min^{-1}$)
37.5	7.81 ± 0.49
75	7.52 ± 0.60
150	6.66 ± 0.72
300	5.37 ± 1.17*
600	4.40 ± 0.34*

* Significantly different ($p < 0.05$) from the 37.5 mg/kg dose. Based on Hjelle and Klaassen[2]

of liver) is consumed per minute by acetaminophen glucuronidation after the 600 mg/kg dosage. Thus, when glucuronide excretion into urine is also taken into account, the amount of UDP-glucuronic acid consumed per minute may be approximately 45–55% of its steady-state pool. Therefore, it is possible that capacity-limited glucuronidation may be related to lowered cosubstrate availability. In fact, recent studies in our laboratory demonstrate that 600 mg/kg of acetaminophen decreases UDP-glucuronic acid concentration over 90% within 30 min after administration.

In conclusion, these studies demonstrate that various chemicals can alter UDP-glucuronic acid levels, and this appears to markedly influence the glucuronidation and excretion of chemicals. Furthermore , substrate (e.g. acetaminophen) induced-depletion of UDP-glucuronic acid may, in certain instances, account for their capacity-limited glucuronidation. The maximal rate at which chemicals are glucuronidated may be more dependent on UDP-glucuronic acid concentration than UDP-glucuronosyltransferase activity.

ACKNOWLEDGEMENTS

The authors acknowledge permission from the American Society for Pharmacology and Experimental Therapeutics to use information previously published.

This work was supported by USPHS Grants ES-03192 and ES-07079.

References

1. Gregus, Z., Watkins, J. B., Thompson, T. N. and Klaassen, C. D. (1983). Depletion of hepatic UDP-glucuronic acid decreases the biliary excretion of drugs. *J. Pharmacol. Exp. Ther.*, **225,** 256–62
2. Hjelle, J. J. and Klaassen, C. D. (1984). Glucuronidation and biliary excretion of acetaminophen in rats. *J. Pharmacol. Exp. Ther.*, **228,** 407–13
3. Watkins, J. B. and Klaassen, C. D. (1983). Chemically-induced alterations of UDP-glucuronic acid concentration in rat liver. *Drug Metab. Disp.*, **11,** 37–40

19
Glucuronide conjugation in isolated cells from intestine, liver and kidney

M. SCHWENK

INTRODUCTION

The altered pharmacokinetics of drugs in disease can only be correctly interpreted if we know the contribution that extrahepatic organs play in biotransformation. A valid comparison between the drug metabolizing activities of these organs requires the use of identical experimental set-ups. Isolated cells are excellently suitable for such studies. In the case of glucuronidation freshly isolated cells have been employed to study liver[1–7], kidneys[3,8], and small intestine[4,9–11]. However, a wider knowledge of the affinities and activities of glucuronyltransferases in the major drug metabolizing organs is required. In addition, those factors, modulating the contribution of these organs *in vivo*, such as route of administration or transcellular transport are not fully understood, and should be elucidated in animal and human preparations.

Based on these unsolved problems, the present study had three aims. First, to compare the kinetics of 1-naphthol glucuronidation in freshly isolated cells of liver, jejunum, ileum, colon and kidney of guinea-pig. Second, to study the relationship between transcellular transport and conjugation in the rat, and third, to see if human colon cells would conjugate 1-naphthol. 1-Naphthol is a useful substrate for such studies, because it is rapidly taken up by cells[5], and transport, therefore, does not provide a rate-limiting step.

MATERIALS AND METHODS

Chemicals

1[^{14}C]Naphthol (56 mCi/mmol) was obtained from Radiochemical Centre (Amersham, England), collagenase from Boehringer (Mannheim, FRG), minimum essential medium with Earl's salts (MEM) from Serva (Heidelberg, FRG). Silica gel G thin-layer foils were from Merck (Darmstadt, FRG) and silicon oil was obtained from Wacker Chemie (Munich, FRG). All other chemicals were obtained at the highest purity available from Merck (Darmstadt, FRG).

Biological material

Male guinea-pigs (300–400 g) and male rats (250–300 g) were obtained from Ivanovas (Kisslegg, FRG). Human colon material was obtained from surgical specimens.

Cell isolation

Liver cells from rat[12] and guinea-pig[13] were isolated by collagenase perfusion of the liver. Jejunal epithelial cells were prepared from the first quarter, ileal cells from the last quarter of the small intestine and colon cells from the whole length of the colon of guinea-pig. These cells were isolated by treatment of the intestine with medium A (containing citrate) and medium B (containing EDTA and dithiothreitol) as first described by Weiser[14], and modified by Hegazy *et al.*[15]. Human colon crypts were prepared from normal tissue from surgical preparations. Medium A was injected into the submucosa. The mucosa was very carefully cut off the submucosa with a pair of sharp bent scissors. Small mucosal strips were gained, which were incubated for 90 min in medium B. The detached cellular material consisted mainly of intact colonic crypts (besides some single colonocytes); they were collected every 10 min and stored in ice-cold MEM. Kidney tubule fragments ('kidney cells') were isolated from guinea-pig by treatment of the kidney cortex mash with collagenase-containing medium, according to the method of Guder and colleagues[16].

Cell viability

Each cell preparation was examined by light microscopy. In addition, respiration was recorded in the basal state, in the presence of oligomycin (more than 50% inhibition), and after addition of the uncoupler carbonyl-cyanide-*p*-trifluoromethoxy-phenyl-hydrazone[15]. Electron micrographs were also made as described[15]. Figure 19.1 shows the electron micrograph of an isolated intestinal epithelial cell, which has preserved its typical brush border. Figure 19.2 depicts the light-microscopic appearance of a cluster of isolated human colon crypts. The small tips represent the crypt bases, and the wide ends represent the transition to the mucosal surface.

Organ preparations

The isolated perfused rat liver with cannulated bile duct was prepared according to Miller[17]. The isolated intestinal loop was prepared as described[18]. The intestinal lumen was connected with a tube, which allowed sampling of luminal contents at the desired times.

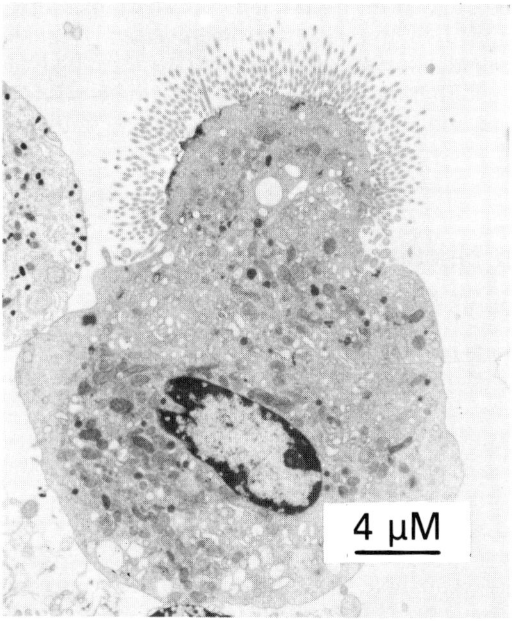

Figure 19.1 Electron micrograph of an isolated jejunal epithelial cell of guinea-pig

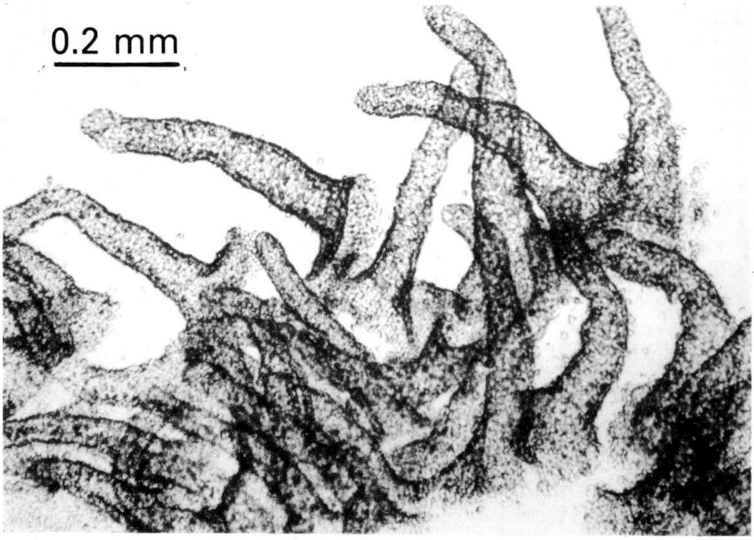

Figure 19.2 Light micrograph of isolated human colon crypts

Analysis of 1-naphthol conjugates

The biological samples were brought up to an aqueous volume of 200 μl. They were then denatured in 400 μl of a mixture of methanol and chloroform (1 : 3);

after shaking, 600 μl chloroform were added. Twenty microlitres of the aqueous phases were applied to thin-layer chromatography foils (silica gel G). 1-Naphthol glucuronide was separated from 1-naphthol sulphate in a solvent system, consisting of n-butanol : 0.01 mol/l Tris : proprionic acid (75 : 14 : 1.1)[5]. The foils were cut into 20 fractions and the strips were placed in scintillation vials.

RESULTS AND DISCUSSION

Glucuronidation in cells from different organs

Since it was the aim to compare the apparent K_m- and V_{max}-values in cells from different organs of the guinea-pig, various 1-naphthol concentrations were employed. Figure 19.3 shows, as an example, the results which were gained with jejunal cells. The left panel depicts the time course of glucuronidation, and the right panel shows the respective Lineweaver–Burk plot, which was derived from initial rates. In all five cell types, the Lineweaver–Burk plots were linear; the results are summarized in Figure 19.4. The apparent K_m-values ranged between $17 \pm 4\,\mu$mol/l and $32 \pm 8\,\mu$mol/l. Since they were so close together, they are compatible with the presence of a single, genetically identical 1-napthol-glucuronyltransferase in cells from all tissues. The small differences observed may be due to experimental factors, or to the partial overlapping of multiple enzyme forms[19]. Interestingly, the apparent K_m-values corresponded well with those found in rat intestinal epithelial cells[10] or rat hepatocytes[6].

The bars in Figure 19.4 represent the V_{max} values of each organ. The highest glucuronyltransferase activity was found in jejunum. The activity decreased towards the aboral end of the intestine in accordance with findings on 7-hydroxycoumarin conjugation[20]. Liver cells exhibited an intermediate activity, comparable to that in rat liver cells[6], and kidney cells a very low activity. Unfortunately, these V_{max}-values do not directly reflect the contribution of each organ in 1-naphthol conjugation, because physiologically the extent of glucuronidation depends on the route of administration, as shown in the following section.

Glucuronidation and transcellular transport

If 1-naphthol is added to the lumen of an intestinal loop *in situ*, it is absorbed and appears in the mesenteric vein predominantly in the glucuronidated form, besides some free 1-naphthol[21] (Figure 19.5). Thus, after oral application, the small intestine plays the major role in glucuronidation. Interestingly, 1-napthol glucuronide is released back into the lumen, together with 1-naphthol sulphate. A similar release has been observed with oestrogens in rat preparations[18,22]; it represents a presystemic elimination of the drug, which may then be excreted with the faeces, because its reabsorption is quite slow (not shown). The different movement of glucuronide (preferentially through basal membrane) and sulphate (exclusively through the brush border membrane) might reflect a different distribution of carriers for these two conjugates.

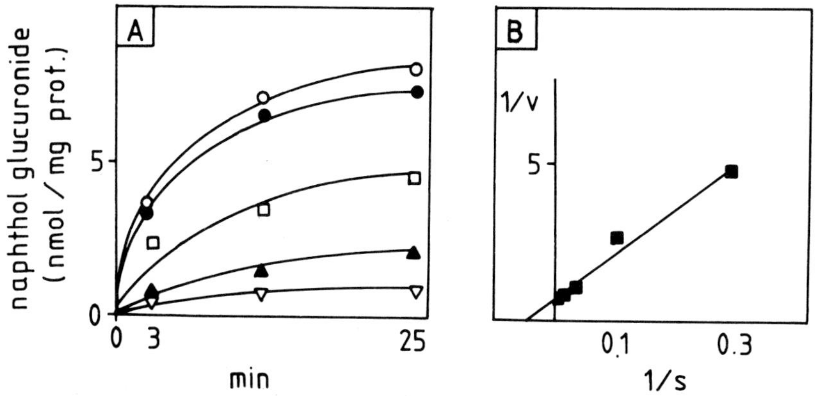

Figure 19.3 1-Naphthol-glucuronidation in isolated jejunal cells of guinea-pig. Cells (1.5 mg protein) were incubated in 1.5 ml MEM while stirring at 37°C. After 10 min of preincubation, [^{14}C]naphthol was added to the following final concentrations: 3.5 μmol/l (▽), 10 μmol/l (▲), 30 μmol/l (□), 60 μmol/l (●), 200 μmol/l (○). Panel **A**; Time course of glucuronide conjugation. Panel **B**: Lineweaver–Burk plot; v is expressed as nmol/mg prot^{-1} min^{-1} and s is expressed as μmol/l

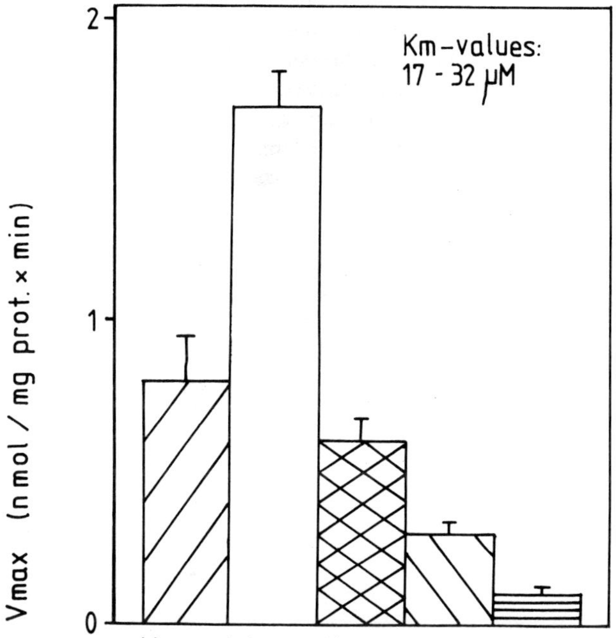

Figure 19.4 Kinetic constants of 1-naphthol glucuronidation in isolated guinea-pig cells. Cells of each organ were incubated as described in Figure 19.3. Apparent K_m- and V_{max}-values were derived from the Lineweaver–Burk plots after duplicate measurements in five preparations

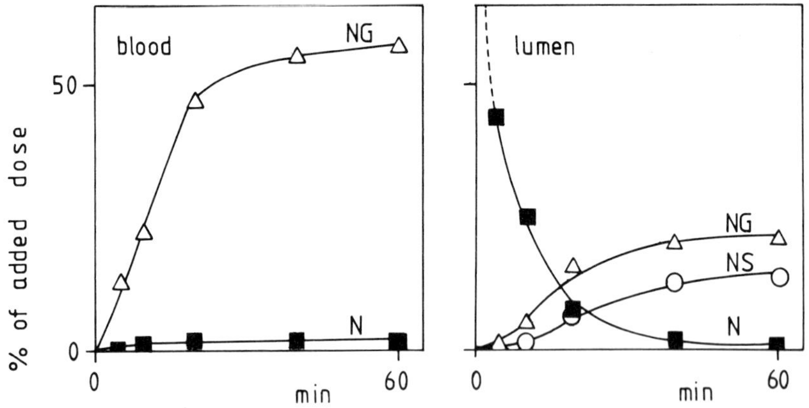

Figure 19.5 1-Naphthol disposition in the isolated intestinal loop of the rat. [^{14}C]Naphthol (final concentration 10 μmol/l), dissolved in 1 ml 0.9% NaCl, was instilled into the intestinal lumen of an isolated jejunal loop *in situ*. Blood from the draining mesenteric vein was quantitatively collected in fractions. Small samples from the lumen were withdrawn at the times indicated. The curves represent the cumulative radioactivities, expressed as % added dose. N = 1-naphthol, NG = 1-naphthol glucuronide, NS = 1-naphthol sulphate

What happens with free 1-naphthol in the liver? If 1-naphthol was added to the perfusion medium of an isolated perfused rat liver, bile contained exclusively conjugates, and no free 1-naphthol[23] (Figure 19.6). Newly formed conjugates were also released into the medium, where they were accumulating. As in the intestine, the sulphates and glucuronides were released at different ratios to the two sides of the polar cells.

The question came up, whether these complicated kinetics might be analysed in isolated cell preparations. Figure 19.7 shows an experiment with isolated rat liver cells, where extracellular (upper panel) and intracellular (lower panel) kinetics were separately analysed. 1-Naphthol was initially absorbed by the cells and was then conjugated with glucuronic acid and sulphate. These conjugates were released into the medium. This experimental set-up may be helpful in studying the carriers involved in glucuronide secretion, since a similar design enables us to characterize the carrier for bromosulphophthalein conjugates[24].

Attempts were also made to see whether 1-naphthol-glucuronide, contained in the portal blood, would be taken up by the liver. So far there was only indirect evidence for its uptake, because it was deconjugated and reconjugated with sulphate in liver cell preparations[25]. We saw now that 1-naphthol-glucuronide is taken up by liver cells. But it is hardly accumulated, presumably because the carrier for its secretion from the cell is very active. The uptake was saturable and energy-dependent in liver cells of guinea-pig, and there was also a specific active uptake by small intestinal cells. But further experiments must be awaited before the involved transport system can be definitively characterized.

Figure 19.7 also shows that glucuronidation and sulphation proceeded at similar rates initially, but later glucuronidation continued, while sulphation stagnated. Similar shifts have previously been seen by others[2]. Here the shift is probably not due to sulphate depletion, because the 1-naphthol concentration was very low. The shift may rather reflect an equilibrium between secretion and reabsorption as well as conjugation and enzymatic cleavage of the conjugates.

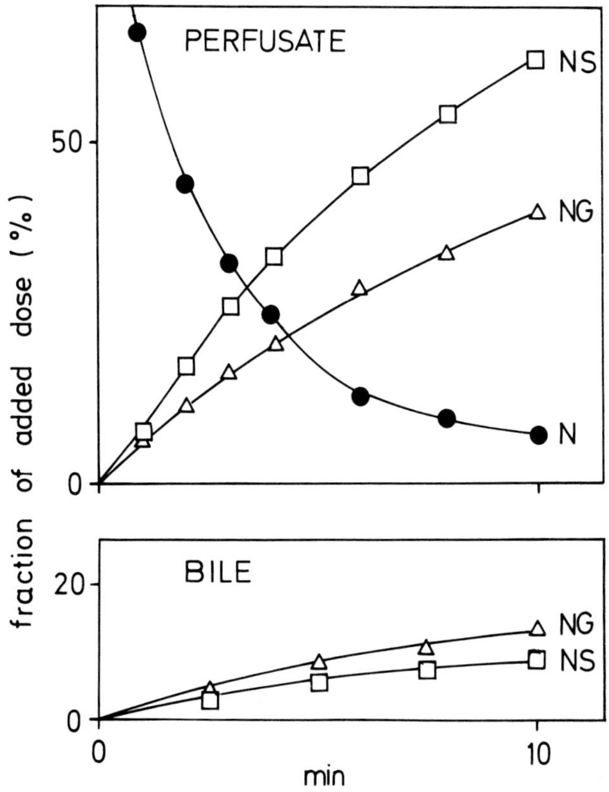

Figure 19.6 Disposition of 1-naphthol in the isolated perfused rat liver. The liver from a male rat (250 g body weight) was perfused in a recirculating system under carbogen at 37°C. [^{14}C]Naphthol was added to the medium at a final concentration of 10 μmol/l. Samples of bile and of the perfusion medium were withdrawn at various times and analysed for metabolites. N = 1-naphthol, NG = 1-naphthol glucuronide, NS = 1-naphthol sulphate

Figure 19.8 schematically summarizes the kinetics of 1-naphthol in intestine and liver. The postulated carriers are identified by circles.

Glucuronidation in human material

We have started a project where the conjugating activities are studied in human cells from different organs. Figure 19.9 shows preliminary results from isolated human colon crypts. In contrast to other organs, there was more sulphation (76%) than glucuronidation (24%), in accordance with findings in human colon tissue cultures[26]. The mean V_{max} for both reactions was tentatively derived from a Lineweaver–Burk plot. It amounted to 0.2 nmol/mg protein × min, and thus was lower than in the guinea-pig.

In conclusion, the 1-naphthol glucuronyltransferases of different organs from guinea-pig might be identical, because they have similar apparent K_m-values. Second, the route of administration determines the contribution that each organ plays in glucuronidation. Finally, human colonic crypts conjugate 1-naphthol in a similar way as do guinea-pig colon cells.

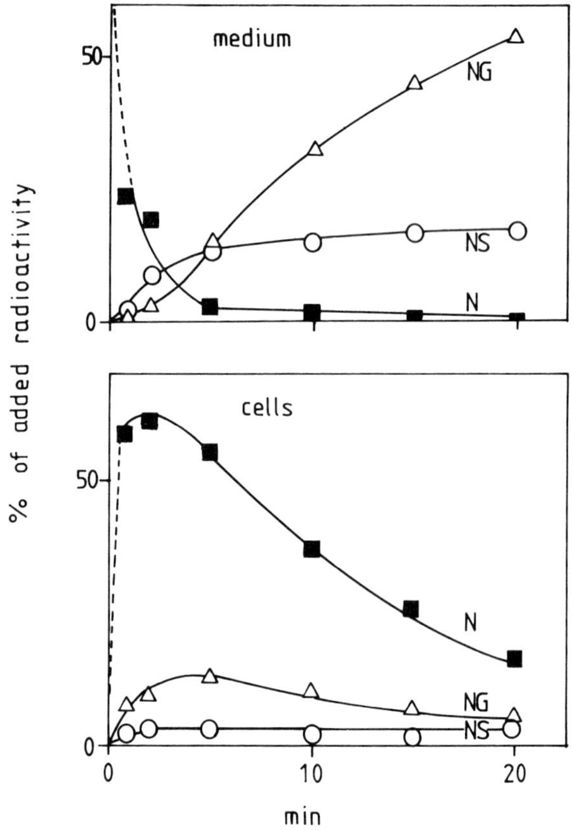

Figure 19.7 Disposition of 1-naphthol in isolated rat liver cells. Liver cells (1.5 mg prot) were incubated in MEM at 37°C while stirring. After 10 min preincubation, [^{14}C]naphthol was added to the final concentration of 30 μmol/l. Samples of 200 μl were withdrawn at various times and cells were separated from the medium by centrifugation[25]. Symbols as in Figure 19.5

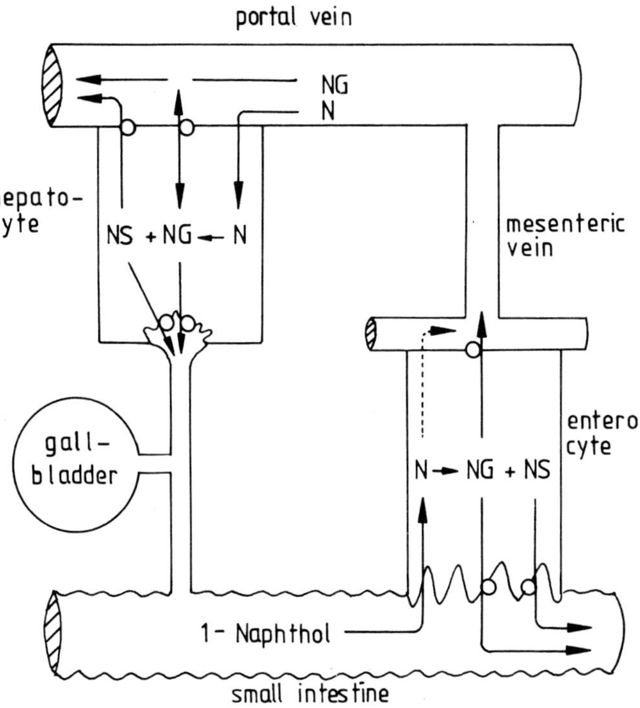

Figure 19.8 Schematic drawing of 1-naphthol kinetics in intestine and liver. 1-Naphthol is transported across the membrane by diffusion. The circles indicate the proposed carriers for 1-naphthol sulphate and 1-naphthol glucuronide

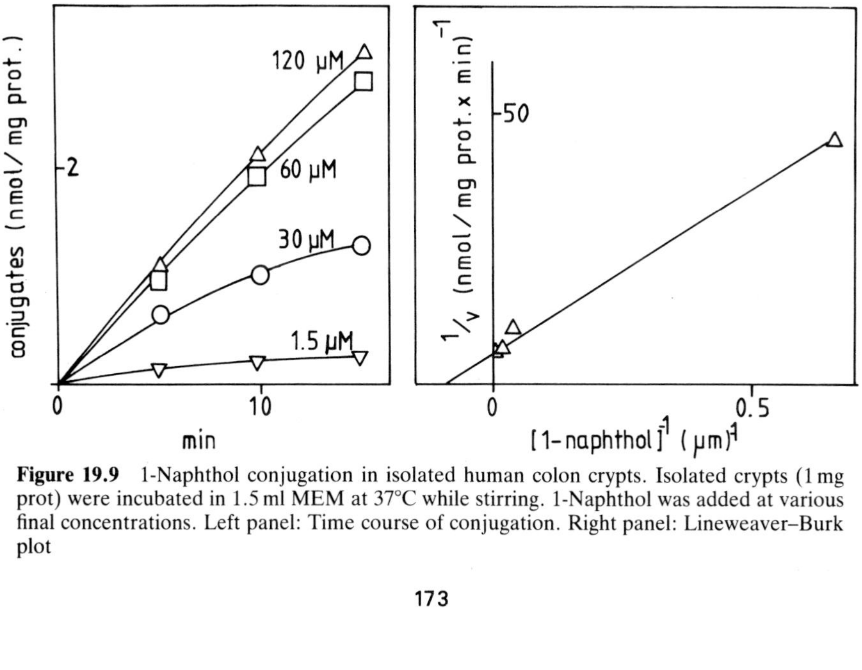

Figure 19.9 1-Naphthol conjugation in isolated human colon crypts. Isolated crypts (1 mg prot) were incubated in 1.5 ml MEM at 37°C while stirring. 1-Naphthol was added at various final concentrations. Left panel: Time course of conjugation. Right panel: Lineweaver–Burk plot

References

1. Moldeus, P., Högberg, J. and Orrenius, S. (1978). Isolation and use of liver cells. *Meth. Enzymol.*, **52,** part C, 60–71
2. Koster, H., Halsema, I., Scholtens, E., Knippers, M. and Mulder, G. J. (1981). Dose-dependent shifts in the sulfation and glucuronidation of phenolic compounds in the rat *in vivo* and in isolated hepatocytes. *Biochem. Pharmacol.*, **30,** 2569–75
3. Fry, J. R., Wiebkin, P., Kao, J., Jones, C. A., Gwynn, J. and Bridges, J. W. (1978). A comparison of drug-metabolizing capability in isolated viable rat hepatocytes and renal tubule fragments. *Xenobiotica*, **8,** 113–20
4. Shirkey, R. J., Kao, J., Fry, J. R. and Bridges, J. W. (1979). A comparison of xenobiotic metabolism in cells isolated from rat liver and small intestinal mucosa. *Biochem. Pharmacol.*, **28,** 1461–6
5. Schwenk, M., Lopez del Pino, V. and Remmer, H. (1979). An experimental model for the study of hepatic transport and metabolism of toxic compounds. *Arch. Toxicol.*, **Suppl. 2,** 339–43
6. Schwarz, L. R. (1980). Modulation of sulfation and glucuronidation of 1-naphthol in isolated rat liver cells. *Arch. Toxicol.*, **44,** 137–45
7. Ullrich, D. and Bock, K. W. (1984). Glucuronide formation of various drugs in liver microsomes and in isolated hepatocytes from phenobarbital- and 3-methylcholanthrene-treated rats. *Biochem. Pharmacol.*, **33,** 97–101
8. Jones, D. P., Sundby, G. B., Ormstad, K. and Orrenius, S. (1979). Use of isolated kidney cells for study of drug metabolism. *Biochem. Pharmacol.*, **28,** 929–35
9. Koster, A. S. and Noordhoek, J. (1983). Glucuronidation in the rat intestinal wall. Comparison of isolated mucosal cells, latent microsomes and activated microsomes. *Biochem. Pharmacol.*, **32,** 895–900
10. Grafstrom, R., Moldeus, P., Andersson, B. and Orrenius, S. (1979). Xenobiotic metabolism by isolated rat small intestinal cells. *Med. Biol.*, **57,** 287–93
11. Dawson, J. R. and Bridges, J. W. (1979). Xenobiotic metabolism by isolated intestinal epithelial cells from guinea-pigs. *Biochem. Pharmacol.*, **28,** 3299–305
12. Berry, M. N. and Friend, D. S. (1969). High yield preparation of isolated rat liver parenchymal cells. *J. Cell Biol.*, **43,** 506–20
13. Hauber, G., Frommberger, R., Remmer, H. and Schwenk, M. (1984). Metabolism of low concentrations of *N*-nitrosodimethylamine in isolated liver cells of the guinea-pig. *Cancer Res.*, **44,** 1343–6
14. Weiser, M. M. (1973). Intestinal cell surface membrane glycoprotein synthesis. *J. Biol. Chem.*, **248,** 2536–41
15. Hegazy, E., Lopez del Pino, V. and Schwenk, M. (1983). Isolated intestinal mucosa cells of high viability from guinea-pig. *Eur. J. Cell Biol.*, **30,** 132–6
16. Guder, W., Wiesner, W., Stukowski, B. and Wieland, O. (1971). Metabolism of isolated kidney tubules. *Hoppe Seyler's Z. Physiol. Chem.*, **352,** 1319–28
17. Miller, L. L., Bly, C. G., Watson, M. L. and Bale, W. F. (1951). The dominant role of the liver in plasma protein synthesis. *J. Exp. Med.*, **94,** 431–53
18. Schwenk, M., Frank, B., Bolt, H. M. and Winne, D. (1981). Intestinal first pass effects of estrone sulfate and estrone in the rat. *Drug Res.*, **31,** 1254–7
19. Bock, K. W., Burchell, B., Dutton, G. J., Hänninen, O., Mulder, G. J., Owens, I. S., Siest, G. and Tephly, T. R. (1983). UDP-Glucuronyltransferase activities. *Biochem. Pharmacol.*, **32,** 953–5
20. Dawson, J. R. and Bridges, J. W. (1979). Conjugation and excretion of metabolites of 7-hydroxycoumarin in the small intestine of rats and guinea pigs. *Biochem. Pharmacol.*, **28,** 3291–7
21. Bock, K. W. and Winne, D. (1975). Glucuronidation of 1-naphthol in the rat intestinal loop. *Biochem. Pharmacol.*, **24,** 859–62
22. Schwenk, M., Schiemenz, C., Lopez del Pino, V. and Remmer, H. (1982). First pass biotransformation of ethinylestradiol in rat small intestine *in situ. Naun. Schmiedeb. Arch. Pharmacol.*, **321,** 223-5
23. Bock, K. W. and White, I. N. H. (1974). UDP-glucuronyltransferase in perfused rat liver and in microsomes: Influence of phenobarbital and 3-methylcholanthrene. *Eur. J. Biochem.*, **46,** 451–9

24. Schwarz, L. R., Summer, K. H. and Schwenk, M. (1979). Transport and metabolism of bromosulfophthalein by isolated rat liver cells. *Eur. J. Biochem.*, **94,** 617–22
25. Schwenk, M. (1980). Transport systems of isolated hepatocytes. *Arch. Toxicol.*, **44,** 113–26
26. Cohen, G. M., Grafstrom, R. C., Gibby, E. M., Smith, L., Autrup, H. and Harris, C. C. (1983). Metabolism of benzo(a)pyrene and 1-naphthol in cultured tumorous and nontumorous colon. *Cancer Res.*, **43,** 1312–5

20
Intestinal glucuronidation. *In vivo* and *in vitro* model systems

A. Sj. KOSTER

INTRODUCTION

It is being increasingly recognized that the intestine has a large capacity for metabolizing xenobiotics[1-3]. Together with the intestinal mucous layer and the gastrointestinal immune system, the biotransformational enzymes can be considered to form an important defence mechanism against possible deleterious environmental influences. Intestinal metabolism is one of the presystemic strategies[4] of animals for coping with the excessive number of xenobiotics, present in their normal diet[5]. This point is nicely illustrated by the presence, in the intestinal wall[6], of UDP-glucuronosyltransferase (UDPGT) which will effectively detoxify the widely occurring phenolic constituents of plant material[5,7].

Since the intestine is an important entry point for xenobiotics it is not surprising that all major biotransformational enzyme activities can be found in the intestinal wall. Various mono-oxygenase activities[2,8,9], mono-amine oxidase[10] and conjugation reactions, such as glucuronidation[6], sulphation[11-13], glutathione conjugation[14,15], glycine conjugation[16], acetylation[17] and epoxide hydrolase activity[18] have been described (*see also* Ref. 1). Systemic availability of orally administered xenobiotics like phenacetin[19], hexamethylmelamine[20], propachlor[15], carbaryl[21], phenol[22], diethylstilboestrol[23], 1-naphthol[24], salicylamide[25] and morphine[26] can be very effectively reduced by intestinal first-pass metabolism in experimental animals and man (*see* Ref. 27). The role of the intestine in eliminating systemically administered xenobiotics is less well understood, although recent evidence suggests that intestinal glucuronidation may play an important role in eliminating intravenously administered L-dopa[28] and 4-methylumbelliferone[29].

It is – often tacitly – assumed that *in vitro* and *in vivo* model systems can be used to predict intestinal metabolism quantitatively or at least qualitatively. Model systems, ranging from microsomes to *in situ* perfused intestinal loops, are undoubtedly useful in the investigation of various aspects of intestinal glucuronidation. *In vitro* models make it possible to study details such as, e.g. enzyme kinetics or polarity of transport of conjugates. *In vitro* models will, therefore, increase our scientific understanding without the need to use large numbers of live animals. However, the ultimate goal of assessing intestinal metabolism and its effects on systemic availability of orally administered xenobiotics can only be investigated by *in vivo* experiments. It is the purpose of this paper to evaluate how different *in vitro* and *in vivo* model systems can be used to assess intestinal glucuronidation. Furthermore, an attempt will be made to review the recent literature and to describe the major points of interest that have to be considered when investigating the intestinal glucuronidation of xenobiotics.

INTESTINAL GLUCURONIDATION

Species distribution

Intestinal glucuronidation of various xenobiotics has been shown to occur in the rat, mouse, guinea-pig and rabbit (Tables 20.1 and 20.2). It has been claimed that in the dog[50,65] and the pig[60] intestinal glucuronidation can occur. Glucuronidation of 1-naphthol[39,41], metabolites of benzo(*a*)pyrene[69], oestrogens[63], morphine[53] and bilirubin[123] has been demonstrated in biopsies of the human intestine.

Table 20.1 Conjugation of xenobiotics in isolated intestinal epithelial cells and intact intestinal segments of several species

Species	*Xenobiotic*	*% Glucuronides*[a]	*References*
Rat	phenol	82–95	22, 30
	1-naphthol	>95	24, 31–33
	7-hydroxycoumarin	80–90	30, 31, 34
	paracetamol	70–85	32, 35
	salicylamide	50	25, 36
	morphine	>80	35, 37
Mouse	1-naphthol	33	38
Guinea pig	1-naphthol	50	39
	7-hydroxycoumarin	20–60	34, 40
	2-hydroxybiphenyl	>95	40
	4-hydroxybiphenyl	50	40
Rabbit	salicylamide	80	25
Human	1-naphthol	10–30	41

[a] expressed as percentage of total conjugates formed. The remainder is conjugated with sulphate and glutathione (in the case of paracetamol) or with sulphate

The typical substrates for intestinal glucuronidation are phenolic xenobiotics (Table 20.2), the resulting products being ethereal glucuronides. There is some evidence to indicate that ester-glucuronides[66] and *N*-glucuronides[67] can be formed in the rat intestinal wall. Since most phenolic substrates can also be

Table 20.2 Xenobiotics glucuronidated in the intestinal wall

Class and xenobiotics	*Level studied*[a]	*Major references*[b]
Group-1 substrates[c]		
Phenol	— C O	22, 30
p-Nitrophenol	S — —	42–44
1-Naphthol	S C O	24, 31, 38[M], 41[H], 45, 46, 47[G], 48[M],
7-Hydroxycoumarin	S C —	31, 49, 34[G], 40[G]
4-Methylumbelliferone	S — —	42, 48[M], 50[D]
2-Naphthol, harmol	— C —	32
3-OH-Benzo(*a*)pyrene, *N*-OH-2-naphthylamine	S — —	51
Group-2 substrates[c]		
4-Hydroxybiphenyl	S C —	51, 40[G], 48[M]
2-Hydroxybiphenyl	— C —	40[G]
Morphine	S C O	37, 51, 52, 48[M], 53[H]
Chloramphenicol, bilirubin	S C —	51, 54, 123, 123[H]
Antipyretics, analgesics		
Paracetamol	— C O	32, 35
Salicylamide	— C O	25, 25[R], 55[R], 56[R]
Etorphine, dihydromorphine, buprenorphine, diprenorphine, naloxone, nalorphine	— — O	52, 57, 58
β-Sympathomimetics		
Orciprenaline, terbutaline, fenoterol, bamethan, salbutamol, ritodrine	S C —	37
Procaterol	S — —	59
Hormones		
(Ethinyl)oestradiol, mestranol, levonorgestrel, oestrone	— C O	60[P], 61, 62, 63[H]
Diethylstilboestrol	— — O	23, 64
Testosterone	— — O	65[D]
Miscellaneous		
Ipodate sodium[d], prontosil[d]	— — O	66, 67
Phenolphthalein, desacetylbisacodyl, oxyphenisatin	— — O	68

[a] Studied at the subcellular (S: microsomes, lysed cells, total intestinal homogenate, postmitochondrial supernate), cellular (C: isolated mucosal cells, intestinal biopsies) or organ level (O: everted sacs, perfused segments, *in situ* perfused loops)
[b] Rat unless otherwise indicated: [D] dog, [G] guinea-pig, [H] human, [M] mouse, [P] pig, [R] rabbit
[c] According to Bock *et al.*[48,51]
[d] The product is an ester-glucuronide (ipodate) or *N*-glucuronide (prontosil). All other xenobiotics mentioned form ethereal glucuronides

conjugated with sulphate[70] it is interesting to establish the relationship between intestinal sulphation and glucuronidation. Most substrates investigated are partly conjugated with sulphate and partly with glucuronic acid (UDPGlcUA; Table 20.1) A direct inter-species comparison between the rabbit and rat[25] confirms that the general pattern for the rat is to form a large percentage of glucuronide conjugates (Table 20.1). Various narcotic analgesics[57,58], hormones[23,61,62,64] and laxatives[68] are almost exclusively conjugated with UDPGlcUA in the rat intestine.

In rat hepatocytes phenols are preferentially conjugated with sulphate at lower substrate concentrations, while at higher concentrations glucuronidation prevails[71–73]. The situation is different in isolated cells of the rat intestine since glucuronidation is dominant already at very low substrate concentrations[31,49]. This may be caused by the presence of an inhibitor of sulphotransferase in the adult rat intestine[74]. It is not known whether the balance between sulphation and glucuronidation can be changed by environmental factors. It is, however, interesting to note that the glucuronidation of 1-naphthol is enhanced in tumourous human colon tissue with respect to adjacent non-tumourous tissue[41].

Intestinal conjugation with UDPGlcUA not only occurs with added phenolic substrates, but also with primary metabolites, formed in the intestinal wall by mono-oxygenase metabolism of naphthalene[75], carbaryl[21], 7-ethoxycoumarin[49,76] (Figure 20.1) and benzo(*a*)pyrene[69,77]. For further details concerning intestinal glucuronidation and sulphation the reader is referred to reviews by Hartiala[1], Aitio and Marniemi[6], Powell and Roy[11] and Dutton[78].

Heterogeneity and induction

In the rat liver at least four different forms of UDPGT occur[79,80] and substrates can be classified into at least two groups, which are glucuronidated by chromatographically separable forms of the enzyme[80,81]. The GT-1 group of substrates consists of relatively flat molecules[82] which are glucuronidated by the 3-methylcholanthrene (3MC) inducible enzyme-form[81] and the GT-2 group of substrates consists of bulky molecules[82], glucuronidated by one (or more) phenobarbital inducible form(s) of the enzyme[79,80]. Recent studies suggest that functional heterogeneity towards the same two groups of substrates can be found in the rat[51] and mouse[48] intestinal wall (Table 20.2). However, no purification of the intestinal UDPGT forms has been reported. Evidence obtained with intestinal microsomes suggests that 1-naphthol and morphine are glucuronidated by different enzyme forms and that fenoterol and ritodrine are glucuronidated by the form that also glucuronidates morphine[37] (and unpublished observations). With regard to all other xenobiotics mentioned in Table 20.2 it is uncertain by which enzyme form they are conjugated.

The intestinal UDPGT can be induced by 2,3,7,8-tetrachlorodibenzo-*p*-dioxin[83,84], 3MC[43,85,86] and benzo(*a*)pyrene[85,87], but relatively high doses are required (100 mg/kg for 3MC[85,86]). Lower doses, which are effective in inducing hepatic UDPGT, do not induce the intestinal enzyme in intact epithelial cells[30,32,49] and microsomes[88]. Oral administration of 3MC is more effective than intraperitoneal administration[86]. UDPGT activity towards bilirubin is induced by spironolactone[54].

The effect of a large number of dietary modifications on the glucuronidation of *p*-nitrophenol in intestinal homogenate has been studied by Hietanen and co-workers[43,85,89–95] and by others[83,96–99]. UDPGT activity is increased by a high-cholesterol diet[43,89–91] or by a low-protein diet[43,93] and is decreased by a cholesterol-free diet[43,91], an olive-oil enriched diet[89], by CCl_4-treatment[43,94], by aflatoxin-treatment[99] or by vitamin-A deficiency[99]. Intestinal glucuronidation is not affected by a high-protein diet[43,93], by an ethanol-containing diet[95], by riboflavin deficiency[93] or by inclusion in the diet of large amounts of cabbage or Brussels sprouts[98]. There is no difference in intestinal glucuronidation between germ-free and SPF-animals[92]. The effect of a fat-free diet[90,96] and of starvation[43,97] are ambiguous. Unfortunately, similar studies have not been done with intact epithelial cells, everted sacs or intestinal loops. The *in vivo* significance of these modifications can, therefore, not be properly assessed (*see* below).

Longitudinal and crypt–villus distribution

It has been often stated that the activity of intestinal UDPGT varies along the length of the intestine, the highest activity being found in the duodenum. A gradual decrease in specific activity is observed further down the intestinal tract[6]. Unfortunately, most of these studies were done with intestinal homogenates, supplied with high UDPGlcUA concentrations, and therefore the *in vivo* significance of these observations can not be assessed (*see* below). In more

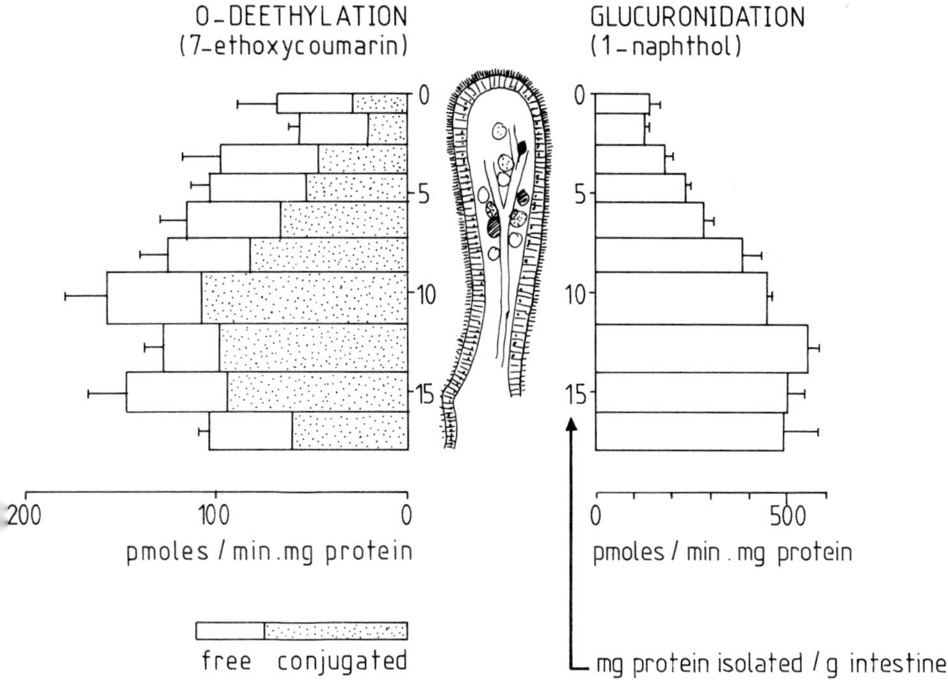

Figure 20.1 Distribution of biotransformational enzymes along the crypt–villus axis of the rat intestine. The data represent the means ±SEM of duplicate determinations with three batches of isolated mucosal cells, each prepared from two rats. Data taken from Ref. 76 with permission

recent studies with perfused segments[46] or *in situ* perfused loops[23] of the rat intestine no significant differences in the total glucuronidation capacity of proximal, distal and intermediate segments of the small intestine (i.e. jejunum and ileum) could be found. In everted sacs of the guinea-pig intestine a gradual decrease of the capacity for glucuronidation was observed from duodenum to distal ileum[34].

A discrepancy between the activity of UDPGT in cell homogenates[84] and the capacity for glucuronidation in intact cells[76] seems to exist for the crypt–villus distribution. Schiller and Lucier[84] found the highest activity of UDPGT in lysed mature tip cells supplied with 0.8 mmol/l UDPGlcUA. More recently we established that the glucuronidation capacity was highest in intact cells isolated from the lower villous region[76]. In mature tip cells the glucuronidation capacity is much smaller (Figure 20.1).

IN VITRO MODEL SYSTEMS

Homogenates and microsomes

A number of different subcellular systems have been used to obtain evidence for the glucuronidation of xenobiotics by the intestinal UDPGT, including lysed cells[84], total intestinal homogenate[50,53] and postmitochondrial supernates[43,83,85,86,89–100]. More detailed studies have been done with microsomes prepared from total intestinal homogenates[44,101,102], scraped-off mucosa[35,42,48,51,54] or isolated epithelial cells[31,45,47,88,103]. When subcellular organelles are isolated, incomplete recovery has to be taken into consideration

Table 20.3 Main factors to be considered in choosing model systems to study intestinal glucuronidation

Model system	*Main considerations*
Subcellular preparations (e.g. microsomes)	– loss of mucosal–serosal polarity – loss of cellular diffusion barriers – artefacts, caused by isolation conditions, e.g. incomplete recovery of UDPGT – artefacts, caused by inducation conditions, in particular activation of latent UDPGT-activity and unphysiological UDPGlcUA levels
Isolated cells	– loss of mucosal–serosal polarity – artefacts, caused by isolation conditions, e.g. cellular damage, selection of cell populations
Everted sacs	– unphysiological serosal barrier and serosal volume – inadequate oxygenation of serosal side
Perfused segments	– unphysiological serosal barrier
Vascularly perfused segments	– complex perfusion media (or blood) required – difficult preparation
In situ perfused loops	– relatively large number of animals (incl. blood donor animals) required – complex preparation, anaesthesia needed

(Table 20.3). Microsomal recovery can be measured with arylesterase as a marker and recoveries of approximately 50% have been observed[104,105] when microsomes are prepared from isolated mucosal cells. The presence of intestinal mucus[106] forms a particular problem with the homogenization of intestinal cells, especially when the rat is used as an experimental animal (*see also* Ref.

39). It is, therefore, preferable to isolate intestinal microsomes from isolated mucosal cells, which can be prepared relatively free of mucus (*see* below). Another reason for preparing microsomes from isolated cells is that latent microsomes can be prepared in this way[31,45,103]. When microsomes are prepared from total intestinal homogenate[100] or mucosal scrapings[35,42] activation inevitably occurs.

Latency of intestinal UDPGT has not been investigated systematically until recently[31,103]. Latency in intestinal microsomes appears to be comparable to latency in hepatic microsomes[31,45,78,103]. Maximum activation is obtained with 0.01% Triton X-100 and various concentrations of $MgCl_2$ (10–50 mmol/l, depending on the substrate used[31,37]) when 0.1–0.3 mg microsomal protein per ml incubate is used. Activation affects both the K_m^{app} and V_{max} values for 1-naphthol; the slope function of double reciprocal plots is, however, not altered[31,45]. This suggests that in the absence of activators uncompetitive inhibition occurs, which can be explained by end-product inhibition by UDP[45]. The effect of UDPGlcNAc (UDP-*N*-acetylglucosamine, an activator of hepatic UDPGT[78]) on intestinal UDPGT is complicated. With respect to UDPGlcUA it acts as a fully competitive inhibitor. With regard to 1-naphthol, UDPGlcNAc exhibited a dual effect: both inhibition and activation were observed, depending on the activation conditions used[45,103]. The intestinal microsomal UDPGT may resemble the enzyme in phospholipase-A treated guinea-pig liver microsomes in this respect[107]. In fully activated microsomes the intestinal UDPGT (with 1-naphthol as a substrate) follows an ordered Bi-Bi reaction sequence in which 1-naphthol and UDPGlcUA are the first and second binding substrates, and UDP and 1-naphthol glucuronide the first and second product, respectively[45].

Inhibition and activation by UDP, UDPGlcNAc, $MgCl_2$, and Triton X-100, and the concentration of UDPGlcUA used, profoundly affect the activity measured *in vitro*. These factors will complicate the use of *in vitro* obtained data to predict the *in vivo* significance of intestinal glucuronidation. At best, subcellular systems can be used to measure the potentially present activity of UDPGT and its modification by diverse environmental factors[43,83,85,89–99]. A direct comparison between isolated mucosal cells, latent microsomes and activated microsomes demonstrates that the use of microsomes may lead to a systematic overestimation of the glucuronidation capacity of the intestinal wall, especially at higher substrate concentrations[31] (*see* below). Intestinal microsomes are, nevertheless, suitable for studying biochemical details such as activation phenomena and enzyme kinetic properties[31,45]. Microsomes will probably also serve as good starting material for purifying possible multiple forms of the intestinal UDPGT[39,48,51].

Isolated mucosal cells

Glucuronidation has been studied in mucosal cells isolated from the rat[30–32,37,49,76,108], guinea-pig[39,40] and human intestine[39]. Cells can be isolated by enzymic treatment of intact intestinal segments[30,40,123], or mucosal scrapings[32,49] and by treatment of intestinal segments with Ca^{2+}-chelating agents, such as EDTA[30,37,49,76,108]. The latter method is preferable with respect to cell yield, cellular viability (as assessed by LDH leakage and trypan blue exclusion) and inter-experiment variability[49,109]. When EDTA-chelation is combined with strong longitudinal vibration[106,110] a very rapid release of cell material occurs and a mixed population of villus and crypt cells is obtained[76] (Figure 20.2). The intestinal mucus can be removed efficiently by a preliminary 2 minute vibration in phosphate-buffered saline[106,110]. EDTA-chelation can also be used to sequentially isolate cells from different levels of the crypt–villus axis[111]. The localization of biotransformational enzymes along the intestinal villi has been investigated[76] in this way (Figure 20.1). Artefacts can be introduced by the isolation and incubation conditions (Table 20.3). The use of Tris-buffers during cell isolation has to be avoided, since this affects glucuronidation rates adversely (unpublished observations). Furthermore, it has to be taken into consideration that different cell populations may be isolated by different cell isolation procedures[49], and that pretreatment of the animals with 3MC before cell isolation may affect the metabolism studied negatively, even though this is not measured as a change in cell viability[49]. Various media have been used to incubate intestinal cells[31,32,40,76,112]. There is no distinct advantage of more complex media over the relatively simple Krebs–Ringer bicarbonate buffer[32,112], provided that adequate oxygenation and buffering by CO_2 is maintained. HEPES can be added to control pH when incubations are carried out in closed incubation vessels[32,108]. Linearity of metabolism with time is only maintained for approximately 30 minutes when rat cells are used[32,112] (and Koster, unpublished observations). This may be due to the rapid production of mucus by rat intestinal cells[39,106,112].

Isolated cells offer the advantage that glucuronidation can be investigated in relation to other biotransformation reactions taking place simultaneously, such as sulphation[30,32,39,40,49], glutathione conjugation[32] and mono-oxygenase activities[32,76]. Furthermore, the influence of various environmental factors can be easily investigated in one pool of isolated cells[39,108]. Inter-experiment variation and the need to use large numbers of experimental animals can be largely avoided in this way.

A major determinant of the glucuronidation in mucosal cells appears to be the availability of UDPGlcUA[31], because the addition of D-galactosamine decreases the glucuronidation of 1-naphthol[108]. Furthermore, glucuronidation in intestinal cells is directly dependent on the presence of extracellular carbohydrates (glucose or fructose)[108]. No intracellular carbohydrate reserves appear to be present in intestinal cells since fasting of the experimental animals before cell isolation does not affect glucuronidation in the isolated cells[108]. Glucuronidation in intestinal cells is not significantly changed by incubation with ethanol, diethyl ether or sorbitol[108].

Isolated cells can be used to investigate possible interactions between different xenobiotics that are glucuronidated[37]. It remains to be established whether these interactions also occur in the intact animal[37,108]. In our opinion isolated mucosal cells constitute a highly suitable *in vitro* model system which gives a reasonably accurate prediction of various aspects of intestinal glucuronidation. A major disadvantage is, however, the loss of mucosal–serosal polarity, which is a distinct feature of the intact intestine.

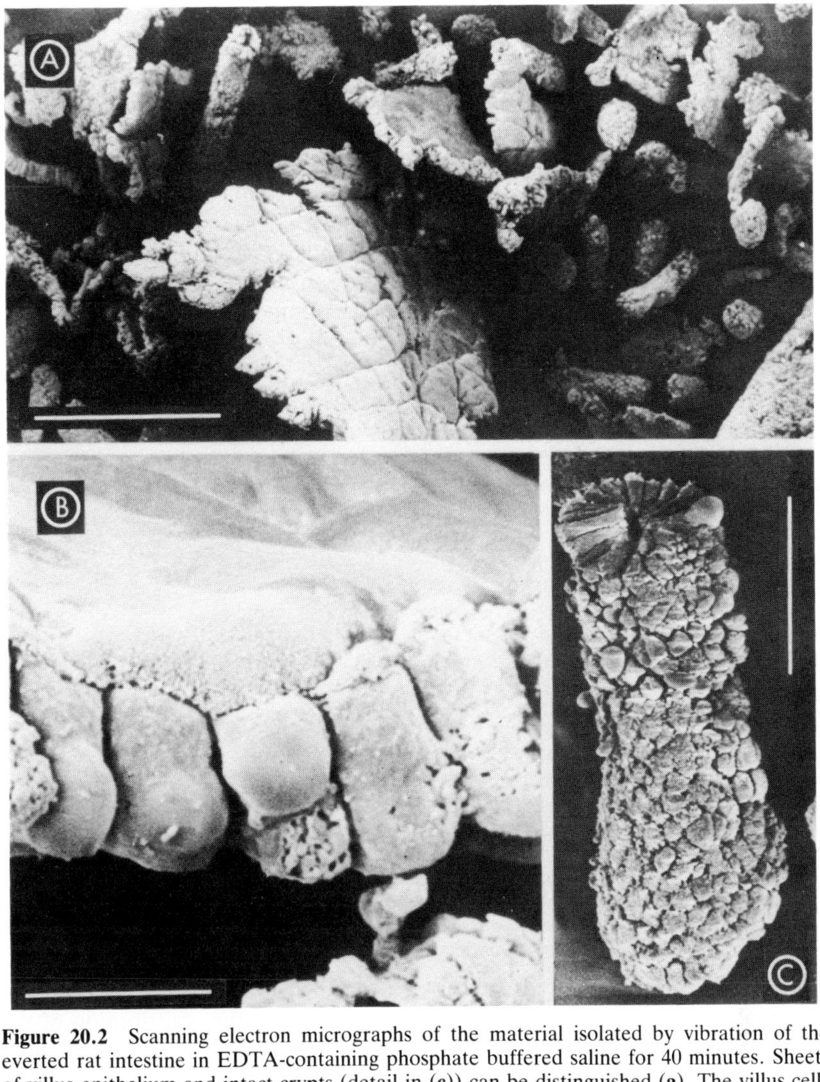

Figure 20.2 Scanning electron micrographs of the material isolated by vibration of the everted rat intestine in EDTA-containing phosphate buffered saline for 40 minutes. Sheets of villus epithelium and intact crypts (detail in (**c**)) can be distinguished (**a**). The villus cells remain attached at their luminal apex (detail in (**b**)). Scale bars: 200 μm (**a**), 10 μm (**b**) and 40 μm (**c**). Figure taken from Ref. 76, with permission

Everted and perfused segments

Intestinal glucuronidation can be studied in everted sacs[33,34,55–58,64,67,68] or in intestinal segments in which the lumen is perfused[22,46,66]. A preparation in which the intestinal vascular bed is perfused as well has been introduced recently[38]. Some potential disadvantages of each system are mentioned in Table 20.3. The maintenance of the mucosal–serosal polarity of the intact intestine makes it possible to investigate the release of conjugates to the intestinal lumen as well as to the serosal side (Table 20.4). An additional advantage of the vascularly perfused intestine is that the vascular perfusate[38] or blood[36] flow can be varied at will. In this way it was shown that the release of conjugates to the vascular bed is flow-dependent in the mouse[38]. In the last-mentioned study no conjugates in the intestinal lumen could be detected. This observation raises the possibility that also in species other than the mouse the appearance of conjugates on the mucosal side in non-vascularly perfused preparations is an artefact, caused by the unphysiological nature of the serosal barrier. This interpretation is, however, contradicted by the observation that mucosal conjugates are found in *in situ* perfused intestinal loops (Table 20.4 and below). It has been suggested that glucuronide-conjugates are actively transported from the metabolizing tissue to both the serosal and mucosal side of the intestine[33,46,66].

Table 20.4 Release of conjugates to the mucosal and serosal side after administration of xenobiotics in the intestinal lumen

Xenobiotic	*Concentration* (μmol/l)	*System*[a]	*% Conjugates on serosal side*[b]	*% Mucosal conjugates*[c]	*Ref.*[d]
1-Naphthol	10–100	P	100	44	46
1-Naphthol	200	IS	75	26	24
7-Hydroxycoumarin	100	E	100	70	34[G]
Salicylamide	100–10 000	IS	~50	25	55[R]
Ethinyloestradiol	3.4	IS	50	50	61
Oestrone	74	IS	28	23	62
Diethylstilboestrol	20	E	94	30	64
Diethylstilboestrol	100–5000	IS	45	30	23
Ipodate sodium	3.2–100	P	57	50	66
Phenolphthalein	20 and 100	E	>95	67	68
Desacetylbisacodyl	20 and 100	E	>95	75	68
Oxyphenisatin	20 and 100	E	>95	75	68

[a] P = Perfused intestinal segment, IS = *in situ* perfused intestinal loops, E = everted sac
[b] Expressed as percentage of total xenobiotic present in serosal fluid or portal blood
[c] Expressed as percentage of total conjugate formed
[d] Rat unless otherwise indicated: [G] guinea-pig, [R] rabbit

Intestinal segments can also be used to investigate the glucuronidation of xenobiotics after serosal administration[46]. In this way the contribution of the intestine to pre-absorptive and post-absorptive metabolism[113] can be estimated independently. Our recent observation that 1-naphthol is glucuronidated when administered to the serosal side of perfused segments[46] suggests that the intestine may play a role in postabsorptive metabolism. The contribution of the intestinal wall to systemic clearance will probably be limited by the mucosal blood flow, but evidence obtained with *in vivo* experiments indicates that intestinal metabolism of systemically administered L-dopa[28] and 4-methylumbelliferone[29] may be quantitatively important.

We recently found that the glucuronidation rate of 1-naphthol in perfused segments, when administered to the serosal side, is 3- to 4-fold higher than after mucosal administration. This suggests that glucuronidation after mucosal administration is limited by the entry of 1-naphthol into the metabolizing tissue[46]. Slow uptake of a substrate will tend to cause a greater presystemic intestinal first-pass effect because saturation of the metabolizing enzyme will not occur.

IN VIVO MODEL SYSTEM

The *in situ* perfused intestinal loop with complete venous collection[114,115] closely resembles the *in vivo* situation. Glucuronidation of phenol[22], 1-naphthol[17,24,35], morphine[35,52], paracetamol[35], salicylamide[25,55,56,116] and various analgesics[58] and hormones[23,61,62] has been studied in this system. The major advantage of this method is that intestinal metabolism and intestinal uptake of the (unmetabolized) xenobiotic can be studied in conjunction. *In vitro* intestinal segments can be used for this purpose, but evidence obtained with 1-naphthol and diethylstilboestrol suggests that uptake of the unmetabolized xenobiotic tends to be underestimated when *in vitro* preparations are used (Table 20.4). The unphysiological nature of the serosal diffusion barrier and the absence of serosal blood flow in *in vitro* intestinal segments may affect the uptake of the unmetabolized xenobiotic and the conjugates differently. When conjugates are actively transported out of the metabolizing tissue (*see* above) the amount appearing in the portal blood of *in situ* perfused intestinal loops can be expected not to be very different from the amount appearing on the serosal side of *in vitro* perfused segments. The available data are too fragmentary to definitely decide whether or not *in vitro* intestinal segments give a reliable indication of the amount of conjugates transported to the serosal side. It seems advisable to use *in situ* perfused intestinal loops when an accurate quantitative estimation of the uptake of a xenobiotic and its conjugates has to be made[23,24,58,61,62]. The potential use of vascularly perfused intestinal loops *in vitro*[38] needs to be investigated.

Anaesthesia is needed for *in vivo* experiments. Since diethyl ether, halothane and enflurane can affect hepatic glucuronidation adversely[117–120] the use of these anaesthetics should be avoided, even though intestinal glucuronidation seems not to be as sensitive in this respect as hepatic glucuronidation[108,120].

AN EXAMPLE, 1-NAPHTHOL

A quantitative comparison between different model systems can be made for 1-naphthol (Table 20.5). It can be concluded that when 1-naphthol is added in the intestinal lumen there is a reasonable correspondence between everted sacs, perfused segments and *in situ* perfused intestinal loops. When 1-naphthol is administered to the serosal side of the perfused intestine a considerably higher glucuronidation rate is observed (*see* above). Because both the mucosal and serosal surface of isolated cells are exposed to the incubation medium, the glucuronidation in isolated mucosal cells must be compared to the glucuronidation in perfused segments after mucosal plus serosal administration (*see* above); the quantitative difference can presumably be explained by loss of cell viability and/or incomplete recovery during the cell isolation procedure. Data obtained with microsomes (whether activated or not) tend to overestimate the intestinal glucuronidation of 1-naphthol (*see* above).

Table 20.5 Glucuronidation of 1-naphthol in the rat intestine

Model system	*Concentration* (μmol/l)	*Max. glucuronidation* (nmol min^{-1} g $intestine^{-1}$)	K_m^{app} [a] (μmol/l)	*Mucosal conjugates*[b]	*Ref.*
Microsomes[c]					
Latent	20–200	70.6±11.5[e]	10.5± 1.4	—	31, 45
Maximally activated[d]	20–200	393 ±58[e]	67 ±11	—	31, 45
Mucosal cells	10–200	14.1± 1.0[f]	10	—	31
Everted sacs					
Mucosal administration	10	2.0 – 2.5[g]	not determined	present	33
Perfused segments					
Mucosal administration	10–100	10.8± 0.9	40	44±3	46
Serosal administration	10–100	30.7± 2.0	25	22±3	46
Mucosal + serosal admin.	10–100	32.7± 1.7	25	16±2	46
In situ *perfused loops*					
Mucosal administration	65	6.7	not determined	26	24

[a] The use of K_m^{app} is only justified with microsomes. In other model systems the concentration at which half-maximal glucuronidation occurs is given
[b] Expressed as percentage of total conjugates formed
[c] Prepared from isolated mucosal cells
[d] 50 mmol/l $MgCl_2$ plus 0.01% Triton X-100
[e] Using a yield of 2.4 mg microsomal protein/g intestine (Ref. 31) and a microsomal recovery of 50% (Refs. 104, 105). Measured in the presence of 3 mmol/l UDPGlcUA
[f] Using a yield of 18.1 mg cell protein/g intestine (Refs. 31, 76). Corrected for cell viability (85%)
[g] Tends to be an underestimate because only the amount of glucuronide produced during a 2 hour incubation period is given in Ref. 33 and because a 10 μmol/l concentration was used

CONCLUSIONS

The intestinal glucuronidation of xenobiotics has not been studied in a systematic way until recently. A large number of widely differing xenobiotics and model systems have been used (Table 20.2). Conclusions regarding the suitability of different model systems can, therefore, be only tentative. In our opinion isolated mucosal cells are a very useful research tool for investigating intestinal glucuronidation. A reasonably reliable prediction can be obtained with isolated cells, and a large number of factors that can influence intestinal glucuronidation can be easily investigated in this way. Intact intestinal segments can be used to gain additional evidence concerning the polarity of transport of conjugates. When intestinal metabolism has to be quantified in conjunction with uptake of the unmetabolized xenobiotic, the *in situ* perfused intestinal loop appears to be the method of choice. Subcellular preparations of the intestinal wall are not very useful to predict intestinal metabolism in a quantitatively reliable way. They can, however, be used to clarify biochemical details.

Even though many details have become available during the last 10 years, our understanding of the intestinal glucuronidation of xenobiotics is still fragmentary. Future research goals should be centred on the following topics:

(1) Modification of intestinal glucuronidation by dietary and other environmental factors should be investigated with intact cellular or supracellular systems.
(2) The possible active transport of conjugates should be studied.
(3) The occurrence of different forms of intestinal UDP-glucuronosyltransferase and the substrate specificities of chromatographically separable isozymes should be determined.
(4) Relationships between the chemical structure and the glucuronidation for a range of (chemically related) xenobiotics should be investigated.

Furthermore, it is recommended that the relationship between intestinal metabolism and intestinal uptake should be more thoroughly investigated. It is necessary to find out how the balance between metabolism and uptake is influenced by the physico–chemical characteristics of a xenobiotic. Only in this way will it be possible to understand why some orally administered xenobiotics are largely metabolized in the intestinal wall, and why some others – even if closely related – are not[20,121,122].

ACKNOWLEDGEMENTS

The author wishes to thank Dr P. J. A. Borm, Dr P. J. M. Klippert and Prof. Dr J. Noordhoek for their continued interest in intestinal drug metabolism; Mrs S. M. McNabb for improving the English and Mrs A. van Putten for typing the manuscript.

References

1. Hartiala, K. (1973). Metabolism of hormones, drugs and other substances by the gut. *Physiol. Rev.*, **53,** 496–534
2. Vianio, H. and Hietanen, E. (1980). Role of extrahepatic metabolism. In Jenner, P. and Testa, B. (eds.). *Concepts in Drug Metabolism*, part A, pp. 251–84. (New York: Marcel Dekker)
3. Gram, Th. E. (ed.) (1980). *Extrahepatic Metabolism of Drugs and other Foreign Compounds*. (Lancaster: MTP Press)
4. Boxenbaum, M. (1983). Evolutionary biology, animal behavior, fourth-dimensional space, and the *raison d'être* of drug metabolism and pharmacokinetics. *Drug Metab. Rev.*, **14,** 1057–97
5. Harborne, J. B. (1977). *Introduction to Ecological Biochemistry*. (London: Academic Press)
6. Aitio, A. and Marniemi, J. (1980). Extrahepatic glucuronide conjugation. In Gram, Th. E. (ed.). *Extrahepatic Metabolism of Drugs and other Foreign Compounds*, pp. 365–87. (Lancaster: MTP Press)
7. Swain, T. (1978). Plant-animal coevolution: A synoptic view of the paleozoic and mesozoic. In Harborne, J. B. (ed.). *Biochemical Aspects of Plant and Animal Coevolution*, pp. 3–19. (New York: Academic Press)

8. Chhabra, R. S. (1979). Intestinal absorption and metabolism of xenobiotics. *Environ. Health Perspect.*, **33,** 61–9
9. Hoensch, H. P. and Hartmann, F. (1981). The intestinal enzymatic biotransformation system – Potential role in protection from colon cancer. *Hepat. Gastroenterol*, **28,** 221–8
10. Strolin Benedetti, M., Boucher, T., Carlsson, A. and Fowler, C. J. (1983). Intestinal metabolism of tyramine by both forms of monoamine oxidase in the rat. *Biochem. Pharmacol.*, **32,** 47–52
11. Powell, G. M. and Roy, A. B. (1980). Sulphate conjugation. In Gram, Th.E. (ed.). *Extrahepatic Metabolism of Drugs and other Foreign Compounds*, pp. 389–425. (Lancaster: MTP Press)
12. Wong, K. P. and Yeo, T. (1982). Importance of extrahepatic sulphate conjugation. *Biochem. Pharmacol.*, **31,** 4001–4
13. Dawson, J. R. and Bridges, J. W. (1981). Guinea pig intestinal sulphotransferases: an investigation using the cytosol fraction. *Biochem. Pharmacol.*, **30,** 2409–13
14. Pinkus, L. M., Ketley, J. N. and Jakoby, W. B. (1977). The glutathione S-transferases as a possible detoxification system of rat intestinal epithelium. *Biochem. Pharmacol.*, **26,** 2359–63
15. Pekas, J. C., Larsen, G. L. and Feil, V. J. (1979). Propachlor detoxication in the small intestine: cysteine conjugation. *J. Toxicol. Environ. Health*, **5,** 653–62
16. Strahl, N. R. and Barr, W. H. (1971). Intestinal drug absorption and metabolism III: Glycine conjugation and accumulation of benzoic acid in rat intestinal tissue. *J. Pharm. Sci.*, **60,** 278–81
17. Turner, J. C., Shanks, V., Kelly, W. J. and Green, R. S. (1980). Studies on the conjugation of 1-naphthol and aniline by small intestinal loops of the rat and guinea-pig *in vivo*. *Gen. Pharmacol.*, **11,** 165–8
18. James, M. O., Fouts, J. R. and Bend, J. R. (1976). Hepatic and extrahepatic metabolism, *in vitro*, of an epoxide (8–^{14}C-styrene oxide) in the rabbit. *Biochem. Pharmacol.*, **25,** 187–93
19. Klippert, P. J. M., Littel, R. J. J. and Noordhoek, J. (1983). *In vivo O*-de-ethylation of phenacetin in 3-methylcholanthrene-pretreated rats: Gut wall and liver first-pass metabolism. *J. Pharmacol. Exp. Therap.*, **225,** 153–7
20. Klippert, P. J. M., Hulshoff, A., Mingels, M.-J. J., Hofman, G. and Noordhoek, J. (1983). Low oral bioavailability of hexamethylmelamine in the rat due to simultaneous hepatic and intestinal metabolism. *Cancer Res.*, **43,** 3160–4
21. Pekas, J. C. (1983). Intestinal metabolism and absorption of carbaryl studied with a portal fistula. *Pestic. Biochem. Physiol.*, **19,** 36–43
22. Powell, G. M., Miller, J. J., Olavesen, A. H. and Curtis, C. G. (1974). Liver as major organ of phenol detoxication? *Nature (Lond.)*, **252,** 234–5
23. Lasker, J. and Rickert, D. E. (1978). Absorption and glucuronylation of diethylstilbestrol by the rat small intestine. *Xenobiotica*, **8,** 665–72
24. Bock, K. W. and Winne, D. (1975). Glucuronidation of 1-naphthol in the rat intestinal loop. *Biochem. Pharmacol.*, **24,** 859–62
25. Shibasaki, J., Konishi, R., Koike, M., Imamura, A. and Sueyasu, M. (1981). Some quantitative evaluation of first-pass metabolism of salicylamide in rabbit and rat. *J. Pharm. Dyn.*, **4,** 91–100
26. Iwamoto, K. and Klaassen, C. D. (1977). First-pass effect of morphine in rats. *J. Pharmacol. Exp. Therap.*, **200,** 236–44
27. George, C. F. (1981). Drug metabolism by the gastrointestinal mucosa. *Clin. Pharmacokin,*, **6,** 259–74
28. Landsberg, L., Berardino, M. B. and Silva, P. (1975). Metabolism of ^{3}H-L-DOPA by the rat gut *in vivo* – Evidence for glucuronide conjugation. *Biochem. Pharmacol.*, **24,** 1167–74
29. Mulder, G. J., Brouwer, S. and Scholtens, E. (1984). High-rate intestinal conjugation of 4-methylumbelliferone during intravenous infusion in the rat *in vivo*. *Biochem. Pharmacol.*, **33**
30. Shirkey, R. J., Kao, J., Frey, J. R. and Bridges, J. W. (1979). A comparison of xenobiotic metabolism in cells isolated from rat liver and small intestinal mucosa. *Biochem. Pharmacol.*, **28,** 1461–6
31. Koster, A. Sj. and Noordhoek, J. (1983). Glucuronidation in the rat intestinal wall.

Comparison of isolated mucosal cells, latent microsomes and activated microsomes. *Biochem. Pharmacol.*, **32,** 895–900

32. Grafström, R., Moldéus, P., Andersson, B. and Orrenius, S. (1979). Xenobiotic metabolism by isolated rat small intestinal cells. *Med. Biol.*, **57,** 287–93
33. Pekas, J. C. (1974). Naphthol metabolism: Glucuronide conjugation and transport by the rat intestine *in vitro*. *Toxicol. Appl. Pharmacol.*, **29,** 404–19
34. Dawson, J. R. and Bridges, J. W. (1979). Conjugation and excretion of metabolites of 7-hydroxycoumarin in the small intestine of rats and guinea-pigs. *Biochem. Pharmacol.*, **28,** 3291–7
35. Josting, D., Winne, D. and Bock, K. W. (1976). Glucuronidation of paracetamol, morphine and 1-naphthol in the rat intestinal loop. *Biochem. Pharmacol.*, **25,** 613–6
36. Sakai, K., Akima, M., Hinohara, Y., Sasaki, M. and Niki, R. (1980). Vascularly perfused rat small intestine: a research model for drug absorption. *Jpn. J. Pharmacol.*, **30,** 231–41
37. Koster, A. Sj., Frankhuijzen-Sierevogel, A. C. and Noordhoek, J. (1984). Glucuronidation of morphine and six β-sympathomimetics in isolated rat intestinal epithelial cells. *Drug. Metab. Disp.* (in press)
38. Wollenberg, P., Ullrich, V. and Rummel, W. (1983). Conjugation of 1-naphthol and transport of 1-naphthol-conjugates in the vascularly perfused small intestine of the mouse. *Biochem. Pharmacol.*, **32,** 2103–7
39. Schwenk, M. (1984). Glucuronide conjugation in isolated cells from intestine, liver and kidney. In Matern, S., Bock, K. W. and Gerok, W. (eds.). *Advances in Glucuronide Conjugation*, pp. 163–73. (Lancaster: MTP Press)
40. Dawson, J. R. and Bridges, J. W. (1979). Xenobiotic metabolism by isolated intestinal epithelial cells from guinea-pigs. *Biochem. Pharmacol.*, **28,** 3299–305
41. Cohen, G. M., Grafström, R. C., Gibby, E. M., Smith, L., Autrup, H. and Harris, C. G. (1983). Metabolism of benzo(*a*)pyrene and 1-naphthol in cultured human tumorous and nontumorous colon. *Cancer Res.*, **43,** 1312–6
42. Aitio, A. (1974). Effect of various membrane perturbating agents on the UDP-glucuronosyltransferase activity in different rat tissues. *Int. J. Biochem.*, **5,** 617–21
43. Hietanen, E. and Lang, M. (1978). Control of glucuronide biosynthesis in the gastrointestinal mucosa. In Aitio, A. (ed.) *Conjugation Reactions in Drug Biotransformation*, pp. 399–408. (Amsterdam: Elsevier/North Holland)
44. Lucier, G. W., Sonawane, B. R. and McDaniel, O. S. (1977). Glucuronidation and deglucuronidation reactions in hepatic and extrahepatic tissues during perinatal development. *Drug Metab. Disp.*, **5,** 279–87
45. Koster, A. Sj. and Noordhoek, J. (1983). Kinetic properties of the rat intestinal microsomal 1-naphthol: UDP-glucuronosyltransferase. Inhibition by UDP and UDP-*N*-acetylglucosamine. *Biochim. Biophys. Acta*, **761,** 76–85
46. Koster, A. Sj. and Noordhoek, J. (1983). Glucuronidation in isolated perfused rat intestinal segments after mucosal and serosal administration of 1-naphthol. *J. Pharmacol. Exp. Therap.*, **226,** 533–8
47. Dawson, J. R. and Bridges, J. W. (1981). Intestinal microsomal drug metabolism. A comparison of rat and guinea-pig enzymes, and of rat crypt and villus tip cell enzymes. *Biochem. Pharmacol.*, **30,** 2415–20
48. Bock, K. W., Lilienblum, W. and Pfeil, H. (1982). Functional heterogeneity of UDP-glucuronosyltransferase activities in C57Bl/6 and DBA/2 mice. *Biochem. Pharmacol.*, **31,** 1273–7
49. Borm, P. J. A., Koster, A. Sj., Frankhuijzen-Sierevogel, A. and Noordhoek, J. (1983). Comparison of two cell isolation procedures to study *in vitro* intestinal wall biotransformation in control and 3-methylcholanthrene pretreated rats. *Cell Biochem. Funct.*, **1,** 161–7
50. Toivonen, L., Hänninen, O. and Hartiala, K. (1973). Drug metabolism in canine duodenum. *Ann. Med. Exp. Biol. Fenn.*, **51,** 8–10
51. Bock, K. W., Clausbruch, U. C. von, Kaufmann, R., Lilienblum, W., Oesch, F., Pfeil, H. and Platt, K. L. (1980). Functional heterogeneity of UDP-glucuronyltransferase in rat tissues. *Biochem. Pharmacol.*, **29,** 495–500
52. Iwamoto, K. and Klaassen, C. D. (1977). First-pass effect of nalorphine in rats. *J. Pharmacol. Exp. Therap.*, **203,** 365–76

53. Pacifici, G. M. and Rane, A. (1982). Distribution of UDP-glucuronyltransferase in different human foetal tissues. *J. Clin. Pharmacol.*, **13,** 732–5
54. Morisoli, L. S., Mottino, A. D., Pellegrino, J. M., Guibert, E. E. and Rodriguez-Garay, E. A. (1982). Effect of spironolactone on bilirubin metabolism in rat liver and small intestinal mucosa. *Biochem. Pharmacol.*, **31,** 1469–74
55. Barr, W. H. and Riegelman, S. (1970). Intestinal drug absorption and metabolism I: Comparison of methods and models to study physiological factors of *in vitro* and *in vivo* intestinal absorption. *J. Pharm. Sci.*, **59,** 154–63
56. Barr, W. H. and Riegelman, S. (1970). Intestinal drug absorption and metabolism II: Kinetic aspects of intestinal glucuronide conjugation. *J. Pharm. Sci*, **59,** 164–8
57. Rance, M. J. and Shillingford, J. S. (1976). The role of the gut in the metabolism of strong analgesics. *Biochem. Pharmacol.*, **25,** 735–41
58. Rance, M. J. and Shillingford, J. S. (1977). The metabolism of phenolic opiates by rat intestine. *Xenobiotica*, **7,** 529–36
59. Shimuzu, T., Mori, H., Tabusa, E., Morita, S., Miyamoto, G., Yasuda, Y. and Nakagawa, K. (1978). The metabolism of a bronchodilater procaterol•HCl in the rat *in vitro* and *in vivo*. *Xenobiotica*, **8,** 349–58
60. Moore, A. B., Bottoms, G. D., Coppoc, G. L., Pohland, R. C. and Roesel, O. F. (1982). Metabolism of estrogens in the gastrointestinal tract of swine•I• instilled estradiol. *J. Anim. Sci.*, **55,** 124–34
61. Schwenk, M., Schiemenz, C., Lopez del Pino, V. and Remmer, H. (1982). First-pass biotransformation of ethinylestradiol in rat small intestine *in situ*. *Naun. Schmied. Arch. Pharmacol.*, **321,** 223–5
62. Schwenk, M., Frank, B., Bolt, H. M. and Winne, D. (1981). Intestinal first-pass effects of estrone sulfate and estrone in the rat. *Arzneim. Forsch. Drug Res.*, **31,** 1254–7
63. Back, D. J., Bates, M., Breckenridge, A. M., Ellis, A., Hall, J. M., MacIver, M., Orme, M. L.'E. and Rowe, P. M. (1981). The *in vitro* metabolism of ethinylestradiol, mestranol and levonorgestrel by human jejunal mucosa. *Br. J. Clin. Pharmacol.*, **11,** 275–8
64. Fischer, L. J. and Millburn, P. (1970). Stilbestrol transport and glucuronide formation in everted sacs of rat intestine. *J. Pharmacol. Exp. Therap.*, **175,** 267–75
65. Harri, M. P. and Nienstedt, W. (1981). Intestinal absorption and metabolism of dihydrotestosterone in the dog. *Int. J. Biochem.*, **13,** 761–4
66. Komp, B. and Forth, W. (1980). Transfer across mucosal epithelium, tissue content and metabolic fate of ^{125}I-(ipodate sodium) on isolated everted segments of rat small intestine. *Naun. Schmied. Arch. Pharmacol.*, **311,** 273–84
67. Gingell, R. and Bridges, J. W. (1973). Intestinal azo-reduction and glucuronide conjugation of Prontosil. *Xenobiotica*, **3,** 599–604
68. Sund, R. B. and Hillestad, B. (1982). Uptake, conjugation and transport of laxative diphenols by everted sacs of the rat jejunum and stripped colon. *Acta Pharmacol. Toxicol.*, **51,** 377–87
69. Autrup, H., Harris, C. C., Trump, B. F. and Jeffrey, A. M. (1978). Metabolism of benzo(*a*)pyrene and identification of the major benzo(*a*)pyrene adducts in cultured human colon. *Cancer Res.*, **38,** 3689–96
70. Mulder, G. J. (1982). Conjugation of phenols. In Jakoby, W. B., Bend, J. R. and Caldwell, J. (eds.). *Metabolic Basis of Detoxication. Metabolism of Functional Groups*, pp. 247–70. (New York: Academic Press)
71. Wiebkin, P., Fry, J. R., Jones, C. A., Lowing, R. K. and Bridges, J. W. (1978). Biphenyl metabolism in isolated rat hepatocytes: Effect of induction and nature of the conjugates. *Biochem. Pharmacol.*, **27,** 1899–1907
72. Koster, H., Halsema, I., Scholtens, E., Knippers, M. and Mulder, G. J. (1981). Dose-dependent shifts in the sulfation and glucuronidation of phenolic compounds in the rat *in vivo* and in isolated hepatocytes. The role of saturation of phenolsulfotransferase. *Biochem. Pharmacol.*, **30,** 2569–75
73. Sundheimer, D. W. and Brendel, K. (1983). Metabolism of harmol and transport of harmol conjugates in isolated rat hepatocytes. *Drug Metab. Disp.*, **11,** 433–40
74. Powell, G. M. and Curtis, C. G. (1978). Sites of sulphation and the fates of sulphate esters. In Aitio, A. (ed.). *Conjugation Reactions in Drug Biotransformation*, pp. 409–16. (Amsterdam: Elsevier/North Holland Biomedical Press)

75. Bock, K. W., Clausbruch, U. C. von, and Winne, D. (1979). Absorption and metabolism of naphthalene and benzo(*a*)pyrene in the rat jejunum *in situ*. *Med. Biol.*, **57**, 262–4
76. Koster, A. Sj., Borm, P. J. A., Dohmen, M. R. and Noordhoek, J. (1984). Localization of biotransformational enzymes along the crypt–villus axis of the rat intestine. Evaluation of two cell isolation precedures. *Cell Biochem. Funct.*, **2**, 95–101
77. Hietanen, E. (1980). Oxidation and subsequent glucuronidation of 3,4-benzopyrene in everted intestinal sacs in control and 3-methylcholanthrene-pretreated rats. *Pharmacology*, **21**, 233–43
78. Dutton, G. J. (1980). *Glucuronidation of Drugs and Other Compounds*. (Boca Raton: CRC Press)
79. Burchell, B. (1981). Identification and purification of multiple forms of UDP-glucuronosyltransferase. *Rev. Biochem. Toxicol.*, **3**, 1–32
80. Falany, C. N. and Tephly, T. R. (1983). Separation, purification and characterization of three isozymes of UDP-glucuronyltransferase from rat liver microsomes. *Arch. Biochem. Biophys.*, **227**, 248–58
81. Bock, K. W., Josting, D., Lilienblum, W. and Pfeil, H. (1979). Purification of rat-liver microsomal UDP-glucuronyltransferase. Separation of two enzyme forms inducible by 3-methylcholanthrene and phenobarbital. *Eur. J. Biochem.*, **98**, 19–26
82. Okulicz-Kozaryn, I., Schaefer, M., Batt, A-M., Siest, G. and Loppinet, V. (1981). Stereochemical heterogeneity of hepatic UDP-glucuronosyltransferase activity in rat liver microsomes. *Biochem. Pharmacol.*, **30**, 1457–61
83. Marselos, M., Törrönen, R. and Aitio, A. (1978). Responses of the D-glucuronic acid pathway in rat tissues to treatment with tetrachlorodibenzodioxin. *Xenobiotica*, **8**, 397–402
84. Schiller, C. M. and Lucier, G. W. (1978). The differential response of isolated intestinal crypt and tip cells to the inductive actions of 2,3,7,8-tetrachlorodibenzo-*p*-dioxin. *Chem. Biol. Interact.*, **22**, 199–209
85. Aitio, A., Vainio, H. and Hänninen, O. (1972). Enhancement of drug oxidation and conjugation by carcinogens in different rat tissues. *FEBS Lett.*, **24**, 237–40
86. Hietanen, E., Laitinen, M. and Koivusaari, U. (1980). Effect of administration route of 3-methylcholanthrene on the inducibility of intestinal drug-metabolizing enzymes. *Enzyme*, **25**, 153–7
87. Turner, J. C., Shanks, V., Kelly, W. J. and Green, R. S. (1977). The effect of sodium phenobarbital and 3,4-benzpyrene on the glucuronidation of 1-naphthol in rat small intestinal loops *in vivo*. *Gen. Pharmacol.*, **8**, 51–3
88. Shirkey, R. S., Chakraborty, J. and Bridges, J. W. (1979). Comparison of the drug metabolizing ability of rat intestinal mucosal microsomes with that of liver. *Biochem. Pharmacol.*, **28**, 2835–9
89. Hietanen, E., Laitinen, M., Vainio, H. and Hänninen, O. (1975). Dietary fats and properties of endoplasmic reticulum II: dietary lipid induces changes in activities of drug metabolizing enzymes in liver and duodenum of rat. *Lipids*, **10**, 467–72
90. Hietanen, E. and Laitinen, M. (1977). Regulation of intestinal UDP-glucuronosyltransferase activity by fatty acids in the rat. *Enzyme*, **22**, 316–21
91. Hietanen, E. and Laitinen, M. (1978). Dependence of intestinal biotransformation on dietary cholesterol. *Biochem. Pharmacol.*, **27**, 1095–7
92. Hietanen, E. and Pelkonen, K. (1979). Hepatic and extrahepatic induction of drug-metabolizing enzymes in specific pathogen free and germ-free rats. *Gen. Pharmacol.*, **10**, 239–47
93. Hietanen, E. (1981). Adaption of intestinal biotransformation to nutritional variation. *Adv. Physiol. Sci.*, **29**, 373–84
94. Koivusaari, U., Lang, M. and Hietanen, E. (1980). Differences in the response of hepatic and intestinal drug metabolizing enzymes in rats following carbon tetrachloride and/or phenobarbital treatment. *Acta Pharmacol. Toxicol.*, **46**, 37–42
95. Koivusaari, U., Norling, A., Lang, M. and Hietanen, E. (1981). Structural and biotransformational membrane changes in the liver and intestine during chronic ethanol administration. *Toxicology*, **20**, 173–83
96. Laitinen, M. (1976). Hepatic and duodenal drug metabolism in the rat during fat deficiency. *Gen. Pharmacol.*, **7**, 263–6
97. Marselos, M. and Laitinen, M. (1975). Starvation and phenobarbital treatment effects

on drug hydroxylation and glucuronidation in the rat liver and small intestinal mucosa. *Biochem. Pharmacol.*, **24,** 1529–35

98. Uotila, P. and Aitio, A. (1979). The effect of dietary vegetables on rat intestinal and hepatic metabolism of xenobiotics. *Res. Comm. Chem. Pathol. Pharmacol.*, **26,** 425–8
99. Nair, C. R., Chauhan, D. P., Gupta, P. H. and Mehta, S. K. (1982). Intestinal drug metabolizing systems (phase I and phase II) in rats fed vitamin-A deficient diet and aflatoxin B1. *Digestion*, **24,** 190–4
100. Aitio, A. (1974). UDP-glucuronyltransferase activity in various rat tissues. *Int. J. Biochem.*, **5,** 325–30
101. Del Villar, E., Sanchez, E. and Tephly, T. R. (1974). Morphine metabolism II. Studies on morphine glucuronyltransferase activity in intestinal microsomes of rats. *Drug Metab. Disp.*, **2,** 370–4
102. Hook, G. E. R., Haseman, J. K. and Lucier, G. W. (1975). Induction and suppression of hepatic and extrahepatic microsomal foreign-compound-metabolizing enzyme systems by 2,3,7,8-tetrachlorodibenzo-*p*-dioxin. *Chem. Biol. Interact.*, **10,** 199–214
103. Koster, A. Sj. and Noordhoek, J. (1982). Similarity of rat intestinal and hepatic microsomal 7-hydroxycoumarin-UDP-glucuronyltransferase: *In vitro* activation by Triton X-100, UDP-*N*-acetylglucosamine and $MgCl_2$. *Biochem. Pharmacol.*, **31,** 2701–4
104. Shirkey, R. J., Chakraborty, J. and Bridges, J. W. (1979). An improved method for preparing rat small intestine microsomal fractions for studying drug metabolism. *Anal. Biochem.*, **93,** 73–81
105. Borm, P., Mingels, M-J., Hulshoff, A., Frankhuijzen-Sierevogel, A. and Noordhoek, J. (1983). Rapid formation of *N*-hydroxymethylpentamethylmelamine by mitochondria from rat small intestinal epithelium. *Life Sci.*, **33,** 2113–9
106. Hülsmann, W. C., van den Berg, J. W. O. and de Jonge, H. R. (1973). Isolation of intestinal mucosa cells. *Meth. Enzymol.*, **32,** 665–73
107. Zakim, D., Goldenberg, J. and Vessey, D. A. (1973). Influence of membrane lipids on the regulatory properties of UDP-glucuronyltransferase. *Eur. J. Biochem.*, **38,** 59–63
108. Koster, A. Sj., Meewisse, C. P. J. and Noordhoek, J. (1984). Glucuronidation in rat intestinal epithelial cells. Dependence on glucose supply and resistance to inhibition by ethanol and fasting. *Arch. Toxicol.*, **55,** 123–6
109. Eade, O. E., Andre-Ukena, S. St. and Beeken, W. L. (1981). Comparative viabilities of rat intestinal epithelial cells prepared by mechanical, enzymatic and chelating methods. *Digestion*, **21,** 25–32
110. Harrison, D. D. and Webster, H. L. (1969). The preparation of isolated intestinal crypt cells. *Exp. Cell Res.*, **55,** 257–60
111. Weiser, M. M. (1973). Intestinal epithelial surface membrane glycoprotein synthesis I. An indicator of cellular differentiation. *J. Biol. Chem.*, **248,** 2536–41
112. Watford, M., Lund, P. and Krebs, H. A. (1979). Isolation and metabolic characteristics of rat and chicken enterocytes. *Biochem. J.*, **178,** 589–96
113. Routledge, P. A. and Shand, D. G. (1979). Presystemic drug elimination. *Ann. Rev. Pharmacol. Toxicol.*, **19,** 447–68
114. Ochsenfahrt, H. and Winne, D. (1969). Der Einfluss der Durchblutung auf die Resorption von Arzneimitteln aus dem Jejunem der Ratte. *Naun. Schmied. Arch. Pharmacol.*, **264,** 55–75
115. Windmueller, H. G. and Spaeth, A. E. (1981). Vascular autoperfusion of rat small intestine *in situ. Meth. Enzymol*, **77,** 120–9
116. Iwamoto, K. and Watanabe, J. (1983). Limited capacity of jejunal segments to effect glucuronidation and sulphation of aspirin and salicylamide in rats. *J. Pharm. Pharmacol.*, **35,** 821–2
117. Brown, B. R. (1972). Effects of inhalation anesthetics on hepatic glucuronide conjugation. *Anesthesiology*, **37,** 483–8
118. Aune, H., Bessesen, A., Olsen, H. and Mørland, J. (1983). Acute effects of halothane and enflurane on drug metabolism and protein synthesis in isolated rat hepatocytes. *Acta Pharmacol. Toxicol.*, **53,** 363–8
119. Aune, H., Hals, P.-A., Hansen, B. I. and Aarbakke, J. (1984). Effect of diethyl ether on the formation of paracetamol sulphate and glucuronide in isolated rat hepatocytes. *Pharmacology*, **28,** 67–73
120. Watkins, J. B. and Klaassen, C. D. (1983). Chemically-induced alteration of UDP-glucuronic acid concentration in rat liver. *Drug Metab. Disp.*, **11,** 37–40

121. Klippert, P. J. M., Hulshoff, A., Hofman, G. and Noordhoek, J. (1984). Disposition of pentamethylmelamine in the rat. Liver first-pass metabolism. *Cancer Res.* (In press.)
122. Borm, P. J. A., Frankhuijzen-Sierevogel, A. C., Weller, E. B. C. M. and Noordhoek, J. (1984). Absorption and metabolism of hexamethylmelamine and pentamethylmelamine in everted perfused gut segments of the rat. Correlation with *in vivo* data. *J. Pharm. Pharmacol.* (submitted)
123. Hartmann, F. and Bissell, D. M. (1982). Metabolism of heme and bilirubin in rat and human small intestinal mucosa. *J. Clin. Invest.*, **70**, 23–9

Section 6 Conjugation of Endogenous Compounds: A. Bilirubin

Chairman: K. P. M. Heirwegh

21
Bilirubin solubility in bile

M. C. CAREY AND M. D. BERMAN

There is now general agreement that unconjugated bilirubin (UCB) is the major pigment molecule in pigment gallstones, pigmented cholesterol gallstones and in biliary sludge. Precipitated UCB exists as covalently linked 'black' polymers or as one or more salts of calcium. By X-ray diffraction and polarizing microscopy, these salts and polymers are generally amorphous (non-crystalline). For bilirubin to precipitate from bile the physical–chemistry of the system should follow a logical sequence:

(1) Bile must first become supersaturated with UCB and/or its calcium salts; this could occur either from increased hepatic secretion of UCB or deconjugation of conjugated bilirubin within the biliary tree.
(2) A nucleating agent or matrix must be present to induce precipitation of UCB from the bile system when supersaturation is modest (metastable).
(3) A retention site must be available for precipitation to occur, and for aggregation of the precipitates to form macroscopic stones.

We have addressed the first of these issues by examining the physical–chemical conditions necessary for maintaining UCB in solution in bile. To achieve this aim, we have determined the phase equilibria of UCB in model bile systems composed of taurine conjugated bile salts (NaTC, NaTDC) – egg yolk lecithin and cholesterol monohydrate. Our experiments were conducted as a function of a number of additional physical–chemical variables of physiological importance, particularly $[Ca^{2+}]$ and $[H^+]$. Owing to several wellknown physical–chemical peculiarities of bilirubin such as: (1) its chemical lability, especially in the presence of light and O_2; (2) its high crystal lattice energy; (3) its tendency to form both addition and molecular compounds with a number of organic solvents; and (4) its low solubility in water and in bile at physiologic pH, classical phase equilibria techniques cannot be rigorously employed. Hence, to study the equilibrium physical state of UCB in this complex detergent system, both a titrimetric and dissolution approach were employed.

In the first method, we acidometrically titrated pure UCB with HCl in the presence of micellar systems containing NaTC or NaTDC, together with lecithin and cholesterol and approached equilibrium from the supersaturated state. By this means UCB was progressively protonated from the di-anionic form at high pH to the mono-anionic form at intermediate pH values and to the diacid form at low pH.

In the second method, we determined UCB solubilities in NaTC micelles ±10.0 mmol/l $CaCl_2$ by dissolution of crystalline UCB at integer pH values between pH 2 and 10 in the presence of 0.2 mol/l buffers. The results demonstrate satisfactory agreement between UCB solubilities by the titrimetric and dissolution methods in 2.5 g/dl NaTC at the precipitation pH (~60 μmol/l) and provide a wealth of important information on the solution chemistry of bilirubin in model bile systems. The data include metastable and equilibrium solubilities of UCB, metastable and equilibrium precipitation pH values, the mean apparent p*K* of bilirubin's 2 carboxyl groups and the influences of added lecithin, cholesterol, temperature variation, total bile salt concentration, urea concentration, NaCl and particularly $CaCl_2$ concentration. We have also demonstrated that protonated bilirubin and cholesterol monohydrate do not compete for bile salt micellar binding sites. Added lecithin decreases UCB solubility in NaTC and NaTDC systems by ~50% and UCB solubility increases linearly with total bile salt concentration. Calcium decreases micellar UCB solubilities, particularly at pH values when the bile pigment is fully or partially ionized.

Of great importance for our understanding of pigment gallstone formation is that the final phase diagrams predict zones of metastable and labile supersaturation with unconjugated bilirubin as functions of $[H^+]$, $[Ca^{2+}]$, total lipid concentration and the bile salt–lecithin–cholesterol ratio. When reliable analytical data from the literature are plotted on this phase diagram, the results show that 'pigment' biles are markedly supersaturated with UCB, whereas control biles from non-stone animals and 'cholesterol' stone patients are unsaturated with UCB. Thus the phase diagram provides a rational physical–chemical basis for pigment gallstone formation in man and in two mouse models. In all cases, [bilirubin], $[Ca^{2+}]$, $[H^+]$, total bile salt concentration and the bile salt–lecithin ratio, but not the cholesterol content of bile, are the critical variables. Recent refinements in the quantification of bilirubin and its conjugates in bile by HPLC and H^+ and Ca^{2+} by ion specific electrodes will enable the 'pigment' lithogenic potential of native bile and bile-rich duodenal fluid to be readily measured in man.

22
Enzymic conjugation of bilirubin* with glucuronic acid. Effect of reversible binding of bilirubin to albumin

K. P. M. HEIRWEGH, J. A. T. P. MEUWISSEN, J. CUYPERS, M. GOOSSENS, R. HENDERIX AND P. ADRIAENSEN

SUMMARY

Substrate saturation curves of the membrane-bound enzyme bilirubin UDP-glucuronyltransferase were established at variable concentrations of bilirubin, at a constant concentration of either rat serum albumin or horse serum albumin.

(1) The saturation curves resembled a rectangular hyperbola with rat serum albumin and a sigmoidal curve with horse albumin.

(2) Rate expressions were derived on the basis of mathematical models involving, in addition to the usual assumptions applied in enzyme kinetics, the following specific assumptions. A suspension of membrane-bound UDP-glucuronyltransferase can be represented as a biphasic system consisting of a phospholipid phase and an aqueous phase (the aqueous interior and exterior of the vesicles). The substrate, bilirubin, distributes between both phases according to a zero-order partition coefficient, all steps of mass transport being rapid compared to the enzymic conversion of substrate. The enzyme molecules contain a single type of independent catalytic site acting exclusively on unbound bilirubin. The substrate carrier present in the enzymic system may bear either a single class or two classes of independent binding site.

(3) Simulation experiments and mathematical analysis of the reaction-rate expressions demonstrated that, even when the enzyme and carrier molecules each have a single class of substrate-binding site, the saturation curves can be

* In agreement with the proposal of the joint commission of IUPAC and IUB, bilirubin-IXα will be denoted as bilirubin, unless it is desirable to stress the isomeric structure.

either hyperbolic or sigmoidal. The type of curve obtained depends primarily on the relative binding affinity K of enzyme and carrier.

(4) The rate expression for a carrier with a single class of independent substrate-binding site is expressed by a four-parameter equation. The parameters were the maximal reaction rate (V_{max}) and the apparent $K_M(K_M^{app})$ of the enzyme, and the molar binding capacity (Bc) and the apparent binding affinity ($\bar{K}^{app}$) of the carrier.

(5) The kinetic data obtained in the presence of rat albumin could be fitted satisfactorily to the latter type of fitting function. The data allowed determination only of three parameter values or functions of parameters, e.g. V_{max}, Bc and K.

(6) Fitting of the kinetic data obtained in the presence of horse serum albumin required the assumption that the albumin preparation used contains two classes of independent bilirubin-binding site.

(7) The advantages and disadvantages of performing enzymic assays in the presence or absence of a substrate carrier, and the significance of observing hyperbolic or sigmoidal substrate saturation curves in the presence of carrier protein are discussed.

INTRODUCTION

In the present communication, it is our intention to outline how the physical chemistry of the poorly water-soluble pigment, bilirubin, can be brought to bear on the design of enzymic assays of bilirubin UDP-glucuronyltransferase and on the interpretation of the kinetic results. Since several points to be made apply to most types of poorly water-soluble substrate we will begin this presentation by some considerations which appear to be of general validity.

Enzymic assays with poorly water-soluble substrates may meet with considerable theoretical and technical difficulties[1,2], due to the presence of one or several physically ill-defined forms of the substrate, linked to other chemical species by often ill-definable or unrecognized reactions. For correct analysis and interpretation of kinetic data, all chemical reactions operating on reagents and products must be known. If so, a complete set of reaction equations can be formulated and formulae linking the reaction-rate to the concentrations of reactants and products can be derived.

Poorly water-soluble substrates are usually acted upon by membrane-bound enzymes. To a first approximation such systems can be treated as biphasic systems in that they are composed of two physically distinct regions: the aqueous environment (the interior and exterior of the vesicles) and the phospholipid phase[3–5]. The concentrations of substrate in these phases are generally different. In the simplest biphasic enzyme system conceivable, the substrate is present in at least three forms: substrate dissolved in the aqueous and lipid phases, and enzyme-bound substrate. The latter form can usually be neglected. Furthermore, each form may exist as a number of different species (neutral and ionized). Depending on the location of the enzymic sites, only the fraction of unbound substrate present in the compartment containing the enzymic sites will be kinetically active. Provided all steps of mass transport (e.g. entrance and release from the membranes and diffusion in the plane of the membranes) are rapid compared to the enzymic conversion step, the formulation, for biphasic systems, of the reaction-rate as a function of the concentrations of reactants and products is relatively easy[3–5]. For single-enzyme reactions, the rate expressions then are formally the same as for the corresponding single-phase systems when the total concentrations are used as the concentration variables (K. P. M. Heirwegh, unpublished work). However, kinetic coefficients derived from kinetic data are functions of the corresponding true kinetic coefficients and of variables such as the concentration of membrane phospholipid.

Depending on the composition of the system and on the way it is assembled, additional pools of substrate may exist. Poorly water-soluble substances may dimerize, form colloids, precipitate, adsorb to glass walls, etc. and will bind to added or endogenous binding protein. If the concentration of the kinetically active substrate species is linked to any other forms by rapid and reversible reactions, such as may be the case for dimerization and binding to protein, kinetic treatment of such systems is still feasible[3,4]. It may be noted that the occurrence of a slow step does not necessarily render the kinetics unduly complicated. In a reaction system containing membrane-bound sialidase and ganglioside G_{DIa}, the value of K_M^{app} for the ganglioside decreased linearly with increasing membrane fluidity, suggesting relatively slow diffusion of the substrate in the plane of the membrane[6]. This kinetic system could still be represented by a relatively simple kinetic equation[6]. On the other hand, dissolution of precipitated substrate or desorption from glass walls, or an ill-defined equilibrium such as colloid formation may render kinetic interpretation impossible.

Various approaches can be applied to introduce poorly water-soluble substances into the reaction system. Frequently, substrate is dissolved first in a water-miscible organic solvent. Apart from possible perturbation of membranes[7], one should consider the possibilities that, on addition of the concentrated substrate solution to the more dilute reaction mixture, the substrate will come out of solution, form dimers, adsorb to the walls of the reaction vessel, etc. In contrast, it may be possible to take account of allosteric interaction of the organic solvent with the enzymic sites and of competitive binding of the solvent as an inhibitor or alternative substrate. In studies of the spectral changes of cytochrome P-450 induced by added substances, the effects of added solvent interacting at an allosteric, ligand-binding or substrate-binding site have been treated mathematically[8]. This treatment could be useful as a guide for assessing similar effects on enzyme-catalysed reactions. The use of detergent to dissolve the substrate may produce a number of ill-defined reactions including perturbation of membranes[7].

To avoid the addition of a co-solvent or detergent, the substrate can be evaporated as a thin film and then be treated with the membrane preparation[9], or, if applicable, the substrate can be added as a salt solution to the reaction mixtures. Here also, part of the substrate may be present in the system as dimers, as colloidal material or as a precipitate. For example, since at near-neutral pH the solubility of bilirubin is very low with a concomitant tendency to colloid formation[10–12] and precipitation, one must check for the absence of colloids from the final reaction mixtures.

Provided side reactions can be neglected or can be taken into account, this direct introduction of the substrate into the reaction mixtures is attractive, since the procedure leads to relatively simple kinetic expressions. However, the rather limited total concentration of poorly water-soluble substrate that can be achieved is a serious drawback. Indeed, in particular with purified enzymes, the storage capacity for rapidly accessible substrate may be quite small, so that it may be difficult or impossible to maintain the pseudo steady-state regime long enough for accurate measurement of the initial velocity. It is of crucial importance, therefore, to demonstrate constancy of the reaction rate over the period of observation. In assays of the activity of mixed-function oxidase acting on benz(a)pyrene, slow conversion rates with a considerable time lag were due to rate-limiting mobilization of precipitated substrate[13]. The time lag was removed and the reaction rate increased by performing the assays at higher enzyme concentration (i.e. increased phospholipid concentration) or by adding albumin. In both cases the store of rapidly available substrate is increased. The presence of endogenous binding protein (e.g. adsorbed to insufficiently washed microsomal material) or the addition of such protein to inhibit an undesirable reaction (e.g. precipitation of substrate or adsorption to the walls of the reaction vessel) will of course affect the kinetics of the reaction system. Rarely, if at all, are such binding effects taken into account in formulating rate expressions. Since the substrate saturation curves may still superficially resemble rectangular hyperbolae[4], interference in the kinetic system by the substrate binder, although affecting the expressions for the kinetic coefficients, may not be easily diagnosed. Alternatively, the substrate or an effector may be bound so strongly that sigmoidal reaction rate–concentration curves are observed, erroneously suggesting an allosteric mechanism[4].

Therefore, deliberate combination of the substrate with protein, binding the substrate reversibly and releasing it rapidly to the aqueous environment, may offer several advantages. At a total substrate/binding site ratio below one, the unbound concentration of substrate will be buffered at a low value, thus avoiding peak concentrations at which slowly reversible reactions such as colloid formation or precipitation could occur. Also, the storage capacity of the system can be varied between rather wide limits by varying the concentration of binder, thus facilitating determination of initial reaction rates. Therefore, reaction systems containing binding protein may be of value for assaying enzymes acting upon poorly water-soluble substrates. To obtain the kinetic coefficients from the rate data one could change (1) the substrate concentration at constant concentration of binder, (2) the concentration of binder at constant substrate concentration, or (3) the concentrations of both substrate and binder, keeping their proportion constant. The latter two approaches suffer from the risk that at varying concentrations of binding protein, variable removal of some membrane components and/or binding of endogenous regulating components may occur. The first approach has been explored experimentally in the present study.

MATERIALS AND METHODS

Materials

Thin-layer plates (Silica gel 60) were obtained from Merck A.-G., Darmstadt, Germany. Bilirubin (from bovine gallstones) was obtained from Sigma Chemical Co., St. Louis, MO, USA. TLC analyses on silica gel plates with $CHCl_3$-methanol (85 : 15, v/v) or toluene/ethyl acetate (85 : 15, v/v) as the developing solvent, indicated a single yellow band (IIIα, IXα and XIIIα isomers of bilirubin) and the absence of colourless fluorescent bands[14]. By TLC analysis with $CHCl_3$/acetic acid (99 : 1, v/v)[15] the preparation was shown to contain less than 7.2% of the IIIα and XIIIα isomers (bilirubin-IXα, about 93%). The preparations of rat (lot no. 27), bovine and horse serum albumin (lot no. 5) were Pentex^R fraction-V products from Miles Laboratories, Inc., Kankakee, ILL, USA. In the rat and horse serum albumin preparations only a single band was detected by electrophoresis in polyacrylamide gels containing sodium dodecyl sulphate[16]. Other products were as specified previously[17-19].

Methods

Washed microsomes in 0.25 mol/l sucrose, 1 mol/l Na_2EDTA, pH 7.4 (20–25 mg of protein/ml) were prepared according to the method of de Duve, Pressman, Gianetto, Wattiaux and Appelmans[20] as described previously[17]. Small portions (4 ml) were frozen rapidly at the temperature of acetone saturated with solid CO_2 and stored at −25°C until used. Enzymic assay of UDP-glucuronyltransferase activity with microsomal material, bilirubin (in the presence of serum albumin) as the acceptor substrate, UDP-glucuronate as the glycosyl donor, and UDP-*N*-acetylglucosamine as an enzyme activator, were modelled on previous work[17,18]. Enzymic incubation was at 37°C in incubation mixtures containing the following components: NAD^+ (1.03 mmol/l), saccharo-1,4-lactone (5 mmol/l), UDP-*N*-acetylglucosamine (4.5 mmol/l), *Hepes* [4-(2-hydroxyethyl)-1-piperazine-ethanesulphonic acid]/NaOH (80 mmol/l NaOH), $MgCl_2$ (6.75 mmol/l), UDP-glucuronic acid (5 mmol/l) and microsomal material (5 mg of protein/ml), in a final volume of 1 ml. Concentrations indicated in parentheses are final concentrations in the incubation mixtures (final pH 7.53 ± 0.01). As a routine, samples of the albumin/bilirubin mixtures, added to the incubation mixtures, and of the final mixtures were checked spectrophotometrically for the absence of colloidal bilirubin[21]. The final concentrations of bilirubin and albumin are given in the legend for Figure 22.1. Further details about the procedures used for preparing the incubation mixtures and for performing the enzymic assays can be found elsewhere[19]. The total concentration of conjugated bilirubin synthesized (BX, monoconjugates; BX_2, diconjugate) was determined by the method of Van Roy and Heirwegh[18] as outlined elsewhere[19].

Values of the initial reaction rates: $(dB_t/dt)_{t=0}$, where B_t is the initial total concentration of bilirubin, were obtained by a linear least-squares fit of the rate of product formation, $d(BX+BX_2)/dt$ against reaction time t. The concentrations of bilirubin in the bilirubin/albumin mixtures were determined by the *p*-iodoaniline diazo method[22]. Albumin concentration was determined by the method of Lowry, Rosebrough, Farr and Randall[23] using bovine serum albumin as a standard.

DESCRIPTION OF A SIMPLE BIPHASIC MODEL

In contrast to the use of volume fractions and molar concentrations in previous biphasic models[3,4], mole fractions (X) are more appropriate for kinetic and thermodynamic treatment of condensed systems[24].

A single-substrate (B), single-product (P) enzymic reaction, in the absence of product inhibition, is represented by

$$B^i + E^i \rightleftharpoons EB^i \rightleftharpoons EP^i \rightleftharpoons E^i + P^i \qquad [1]$$

where E, EB and EP denote the catalytic site, enzyme-substrate and enzyme-product complex, respectively. The reactions occur in a homogeneous compartment i which, depending on the location of the enzymic sites, can be the aqueous phase (i = aq) or the phospholipid phase (i = m). Provided rapid and reversible reactions or steps of mass transport link the exchangeable chemical species B^i and P^i, intervening in reactions [1], to the same species in the other compartment or to different species in compartment i, the kinetic expressions are formally the same as for single-phase systems of corresponding complexity (K. P. M. Heirwegh, unpublished work). Thus, for the system described, the initial reaction rate v_o, in the absence of product ($X_p^i = 0$), is given by

$$v_0 = V_{max} \cdot X_b^i \cdot \bar{K}_M / (1 + X_b^i \cdot \bar{K}_M). \qquad [2]$$

X_b^i and X_p^i is the local concentration of unbound substrate and product, respectively. V_{max} is the maximal reaction rate. $\bar{K}_M = 1/K_M$, where K_M is the Michaelis–Menten coefficient for substrate B.

Since the local concentration X_b^i is unknown, it is necessary to express it as a function of the total substrate concentration, B_t. The total concentration J_t of any substance J is defined as the total number of moles of J present in the system divided by the chemical content of the aqueous phase. In deriving the required relationship, one has to take into account the various reactions which occur in the system. We assume that distribution of the substrate between the membrane phospholipid and the aqueous phase can be described by a linear partition equilibrium[3–5].

$$B^{aq} \rightleftharpoons B^m, \qquad [3]$$

characterized by the partition coefficient P_b

$$P_b = X_b^m / X_b^{aq}. \qquad [4]$$

Reversible binding to a single class of binding site of a binder C, present in the aqueous phase,

$$B^{aq} + C^{aq} \rightleftharpoons BC^{aq} \qquad [5]$$

is described by the equilibrium equation

$$\bar{K} = X_{bc}^{aq} / (X_b^{aq} \cdot X_c^{aq}) \qquad [6]$$

where $\bar{K}$ is the affinity constant. In previous modelling of biphasic systems[4] use was made of a distribution function F_k that is characteristic for each species which partitions between the phases. If unbound substrate B is present in several molecular forms (e.g. neutral and ionized) in a compartment which contains binding sites, binding reactions may have to be formulated for each of these forms. For example, if the substrate is an acid AH, either AH or A^- or both species may serve as substrate for the enzyme or as a ligand for the carrier. For each exchangeable molecular species that intervenes in a reaction, the distribution function F_k is obtained from the following equation:

$$1/F_k = n_k^{aq}/[\sum_k n_{b,k}^{aq} + \sum_k n_{b,k}^{m}]. \qquad [7]$$

n_k^{aq} represents the number of moles of B present in the aqueous phase as the species intervening in the reaction considered. The summations extend over all unbound forms of B. In what follows we will suppose that a single and the same form of B is involved in binding to the enzyme E and to the carrier C. Taking into account differential partition of neutral and variously charged types of molecules, distribution functions for various types of species have been established (K. P. M. Heirwegh, unpublished work). They depend on the phospholipid concentration and pH of the system, and on the partition coefficients and pK_as of the various species of B.

Neglecting enzyme-bound substrate, one obtains from the mass balance on substrate the following equation

$$R = B_t/C_t = x + m\cdot N\cdot C_t\cdot \bar{K}^{app}\cdot x/(1 + C_t\cdot \bar{K}^{app}\cdot x) \qquad [8]$$

with

$$x = F_b\cdot X_b^{aq} = F_b\cdot X_b^{m}/P_b \qquad [9]$$

and

$$\bar{K}^{app} = \bar{K}/F_b \qquad [10]$$

B_t and C_t is the total concentration of substrate and of carrier, respectively. m indicates the number of binding sites per mole of binding protein and N the fraction of sites available for binding. The product $m\cdot N\cdot C_t$ represents the effective binding capacity of the carrier. Making use of equation [9], the expression for the reaction rate [2] is rewritten in the more general form

$$v_0 = V_{max}\cdot C_t\cdot \bar{K}_M^{app}\cdot x/(1 + C_t\cdot \bar{K}_M^{app}\cdot x) \qquad [11]$$

with

$$\bar{K}_M^{app} = \bar{K}_M/F_b \quad \text{aqueous-faced enzymic sites} \qquad [12]$$

$$\bar{K}_M^{app} = \bar{K}_M\cdot P_b/F_b \quad \text{lipid-faced enzymic sites} \qquad [13]$$

Equations [8] and [11] describe the biphasic system considered. Elimination of x from equation [8] and substitution into equation [11] yields

$$v_0 = V_{max}\cdot \bar{K}_M^{app}\cdot t/(2\cdot \bar{K}^{app} + \bar{K}_M^{app}\cdot t)$$

with

$$t = v + (v^2 + 4\cdot R\cdot C_t\cdot \bar{K}^{app})^{1/2}$$

and

$$v = R\cdot C_t\cdot \bar{K}^{app} - m\cdot N\cdot C_t\cdot \bar{K}^{app} - 1 \qquad [14]$$

At constant pH and phospholipid concentration, only values of $\bar{K}^{app}$ and $\bar{K}_M^{app}$ can be derived from substrate-saturation curves, not the factor F_b. Development of a rate equation, similar to equation [14], for a system containing a carrier with two classes of independent substrate-binding site is straightforward (K. P. M. Heirwegh, unpublished work).

In the present experimental set-up the bilirubin concentration B_t was varied at constant carrier concentration C_t. Data pairs (R, v_0) were fitted to the function $v_0 = f(R, V_{max}, \bar{K}_M^{app}, m\cdot N, \bar{K}_{app})$ for a system containing a carrier with a single class of binding site (eqn. [8]), and to a function $v_0 = f(R, V_{max}, \bar{K}_M^{app}, m_1 \cdot N_1, \bar{K}_1^{app}, m_2 \cdot N_2, \bar{K}_2^{app})$ for a carrier with two classes of independent binding site (full equation not shown). R, the dimensionless concentration ratio B_t/C_t was used as the supposedly error-free independent variable. The reaction rate values were divided by an arbitrary but known constant with the same dimensions as the measured rate values, permitting us to perform the calculations on dimensionless numbers. The constant factor was chosen in such a way that the dependent variable covered the range zero to one. A program based on a gradient-expansion algorithm (E04FDF from the NAG library, Numerical Algorithm Group, Ltd., Oxford) was employed for fitting the data pairs (R, v_0) to the fitting functions. Comparative results were also obtained by applying the Bootstrap method[25] and the PAR routine from the BMDP Statistical Software package (1981 edition; University of California, Berkely, USA).

RESULTS AND DISCUSSION

The enzyme activity–bilirubin concentration curves we obtained are shown in Figure 22.1, for rat and horse albumin as the substrate carrier. The curve

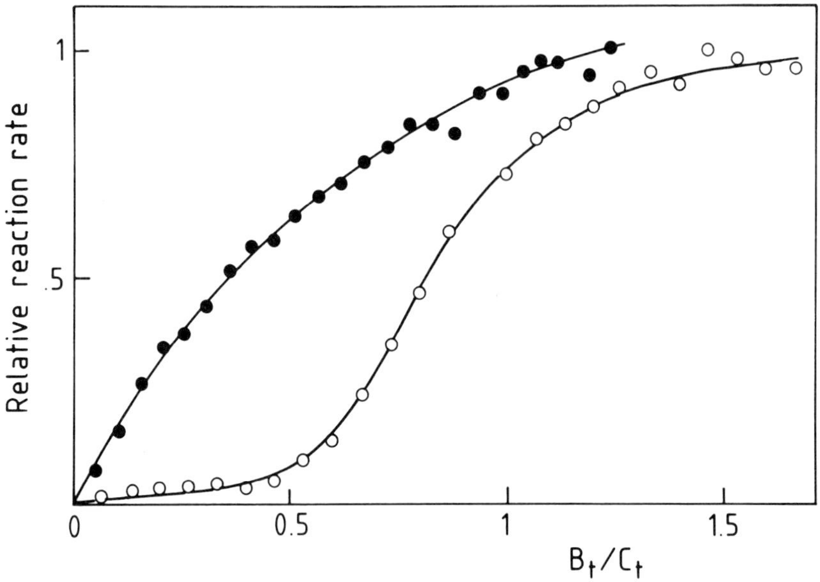

Figure 22.1 Initial reaction rate of microsomal UDP-glucuronyltransferase as a function of the bilirubin/albumin concentration ratio. The enzyme activity was assayed as outlined in the Methods section in the presence of serum albumin at constant final concentration. (●), 3.80–91.3 μmol/l bilirubin and 73.7 μmol/l rat serum albumin (MW63 650); (○), 5.41–135 μmol/l bilirubin and 81.3 μmol/l horse serum albumin (MW68 600). The rate data are expressed in arbitrary dimensionless units by assigning to the highest value the dimensionless number 1. Redrawn by permission from *Biochem. Soc. Trans.*, **12,** 11–3, copyright © 1984 The Biochemical Society, London

obtained with rat albumin resembles a rectangular hyperbola. The finding of a sigmoidal saturation curve in the presence of horse serum albumin does not necessarily imply an underlying allosteric mechanism. Indeed, as shown by simulation experiments[4], hyperbolic and sigmoidal curves can be observed for enzyme systems containing a single type of enzymic site and a carrier with a single class of binding site, the type of curve being found depending primarily on the relative binding affinity K

$$K = \bar{K}_M^{app}/\bar{K}^{app}. \quad [15]$$

The significance of the relative affinity K in determining the shape of the saturation curves can be demonstrated by standard algebraic analysis of rate equations such as equation [14]. For a system containing a carrier with a single class of binding site, the tangent to the v_0/R curves near the origin of R is given by

$$(\mathrm{d}r/\mathrm{d}R)_{R=0} = C_t \cdot \bar{K}_M^{app}/(1+m \cdot N \cdot C_t \cdot \bar{K}^{app}) \quad [16]$$

with $r = v_0/V_{max}$. The product $m \cdot N \cdot C_t \cdot \bar{K}$, which equals the binding activiy Ba of the carrier[26,27], is about 964 and 5600 for the experiment with rat and horse albumin, respectively. The apparent binding activity Ba^{app} (= $m \cdot N \cdot C_t \cdot \bar{K}^{app}$), which equals Ba/F_b (with $F_b > 1$), probably is still considerably higher than one. Calculation of Ba^{app} is impossible for the present experiments since the value of the distribution function F_b cannot be estimated at constant enzyme concentration. When the apparent binding activity is significantly larger than one, equation [16] becomes

$$(\mathrm{d}r/\mathrm{d}R)_{R=0} = K/(m \cdot N) \qquad \text{at } Ba^{app} \gg 1. \quad [17]$$

The parameter m·N is generally close to one. For $m \cdot N = 1$, the saturation curves start off with a slope value equal to one, when enzyme and carrier bind the substrate with equal affinity ($K = 1$). When the carrier binds the ligand more strongly ($K < 1$), the slope value is less than one, and vice versa. The shape of the saturation curves is determined by the second derivative $\mathrm{d}^2r/\mathrm{d}R^2$. Near the origin of R

$$(d^2r/\mathrm{d}R^2)_{R=0} = k' \cdot [Ba^{app} - (1+Ba^{app}) \cdot K] \quad [18]$$

where k' is a positive function. The second derivative can be positive (concave upward start-off; sigmoidal curve), zero (linear start-off) or negative (concave downward start-off; hyperbolic curve) (K. P. M. Heirwegh, unpublished work). When the apparent binding activity is relatively high ($Ba^{app} \gg 1$), the shape of the saturation curves is determined only by the relative binding affinity K: at $K > 1$, hyperbolic saturation curve; at $K < 1$, sigmoidal saturation curve.

Fitting of (R, v_0) data pairs obtained with rat serum albumin as the substrate carrier could be performed satisfactorily with equation [14], $v_0 = f(R, V_{max}, \bar{K}_M^{app}, m \cdot N, \bar{K}^{app})$, which implies a carrier with a single type of binding site. Apparently, the four parameters to be determined are not independent, since fitting with a variety of starting values showed that the parameters $m \cdot n$ and V_{max} each converged to a stable value (Table 22.1) whereas $\bar{K}_M^{app}$ and $\bar{K}^{app}$ yielded quite disparate values. Although calculation of the affinity ratio K from the latter parameter values showed that K in all cases assumed a reproduc-

Table 22.1 The activity of bilirubin UDP-glucuronyltransferase in the presence of rat serum albumin. Non-linear fit assuming a single class of binding sites

		Program		
		E04FDF	*Bootstrap*	*PAR*
Exact solution				
$v_0 = f(R, V_{max}, \bar{K}_M^{app}, m \cdot N, \bar{K}^{app})$				
	V_{max}:	0.98 ± 0.01*		
	$m \cdot n$:	1.20 ± 0.08*		
	K:	2.18		
Approximate solution				
$v_0 = f(R, P_1, P_2)$**				
	P_1:	0.583 ± 0.015	0.582 ± 0.020	0.583 ± 0.019
	P_2:	0.550 ± 0.012	0.550 ± 0.014	0.550 ± 0.017

* These estimates of the standard deviation have to be regarded with caution because of the interdependence of the four parameters

** The parameters P_1 and P_2 are defined by equation [18]

ible value, 2.18, it is not possible to express the exact equation [14] as a function of the three parameters, $m \cdot N$, V_{max} and K. However, in general, simulated curves calculated from the values of $m \cdot N$ and V_{max}, and from any pair of values of $\bar{K}_M^{app}$ and $\bar{K}^{app}$ fitted the data quite well.

Since the binding affinity of rat serum albumin for bilirubin is rather high $(1.1 \times 10^7\ \text{mol/l})^{-1}$ at 4°C)[26,27], it seemed of interest to consider the possibility that, for the value of C_t and range of values of B_t/C_t used, the unbound fraction of bilirubin is small compared to the bound fraction. Neglecting the first term on the right-hand side of equation [8], solving for x, and substituting this value into equation [11] yields

$$\begin{aligned} v_0 &= R/[m \cdot N/(K \cdot V_{max}) + (K-1)/(K \cdot V_{max}) \cdot R] \\ &= R/(P_1 + P_2 \cdot R) \qquad \text{for } x \ll R. \end{aligned} \qquad [19]$$

Only two parameter relationships can be derived from this equation. Quite accurate and concordant values of P_1 and P_2 were obtained by the gradient-expansion method, the PAR routine and the Bootstrap method (Table 22.1). There was little to choose beween simulated curves obtained with the exact equation or with equation [19]. Since the experimental curve for rat albumin resembled a rectangular hyperbola it follows from the satisfactory fit obtained with equation [19] that K must be larger than one. The assumption $x \ll R$, underlying equation [19], is always verified at constant carrier concentration for R values that are close enough to zero. For systems with K larger than 1 it thus will always be possible to delineate a range of R values between zero and some finite value of R for which equation [19] can be applied. At higher values of R, the assumption $x \ll R$ must gradually break down, becoming quite untenable when the carrier is nearly saturated. At this stage, the first term of equation [8] will increase linearly with R, the second term, which is related to the bound fraction, remaining nearly unchanged.

Establishment of a fitting function for the experiment with horse serum albumin involved the postulate that the albumin preparation used contains two classes of independent binding site. After having set up a balance equation, classes of independent binding site. After having set up a balance equation, similar to equation [8], and introduction of the x variable into equation [11], a fitting function $v_0 = f(R, V_{max}, \bar{K}_M^{app}, m_1N_1, \bar{K}_1^{app}, m_2N_2, \bar{K}_2^{app})$, containing a cubic root was derived. Due to interdependence of the six parameters, no satisfactory fit to the exact equation was obtained. It could be shown, however, that the relative affinities $\bar{K}_M^{app}/\bar{K}_1^{app}$ and $\bar{K}_M^{app}/\bar{K}_2^{app}$ are of key importance in describing the saturation curves and in fitting data pairs to the fitting functions, as was observed for the parameter $K = \bar{K}_M^{app}/\bar{K}^{app}$ in the analysis of kinetic systems containing a carrier with a single type of binding site. Further work is in progress.

From a practical point of view, it may be of interest to inquire what could be the significance of a saturation curve, having, apparently, the shape of a rectangular hyperbola, for an enzymic system containing a substrate-binding protein at constant concentration? Suppose, for example, that a $1/v_0$ versus $1/B_t$ plot has yielded a curve which cannot be distiguished significantly from a straight line. Two interpretations seem to be possible. First, the binding activity of the carrier may be so weak that the bound fraction of substrate is negligible compared to the total unbound fraction (aqueous and lipid phase). In this case, the saturation curve can be described exactly by a rectangular hyperbola and the fit would yield V_{max} and $\bar{K}_M^{app}$. Alternatively, as shown by equation [19], an apparently rectangular hyperbola could also be observed if the relative binding affinity K is larger than one, provided the apparent binding activity Ba^{app} is sufficiently high to render the unbound fraction of substrate small compared to the bound fraction ($x \ll R$) over an experimentally accessible range of R values.

To show the effect of using the function of a rectangular hyperbola to fit experimental data for the latter case, equation [19] can be written in the alternative form

$$v_0 = V_{max} \cdot [K/(K-1)] \cdot B_t/[m \cdot N \cdot C_t/(K-1) + B_t]. \qquad [20]$$

If reaction rate data, such as obtained in our experiment with rat albumin, were fitted in the usual way to a rectangular hyperbola, i.e. a fit of v_0 against B_t, one would obtain the following expressions for the observed V_{max} and K_M.

$$V_{max}^{obs} = V_{max} \cdot [K/(K-1)] \qquad [21]$$
$$K_M^{obs} = m \cdot N \cdot C_t/(K-1). \qquad [22]$$

When the relative affinity K is sufficiently large ($K \gg 100$) the true value of V_{max} would be obtained but the observed K_M would be equal to $K_M \cdot (m \cdot N \cdot C_t \cdot \bar{K}^{app})$ or $K_M \cdot Ba^{app}$.

In a kinetic system containing endogenous carrier material or when binding protein is added, e.g. to inhibit precipitation of substrate or adsorption to the walls of the reaction vessel, determination of the kinetic coefficients from a saturation curve conforming apparently to a rectangular hyperbola, will suffer from the same uncertainties as discussed above. On the other hand, before a sigmoidal saturation curve is interpreted to indicate an allosteric mechanism, one has to rule out carefully the possibility that the kinetic response at small values of R is being kept low by the presence in the system of even small concentrations of strongly binding material.

ACKNOWLEDGEMENTS

The authors are grateful to Prof G. J. Dutton (Dundee, Scotland) for stimulating discussions and to the Nationaal Fonds voor Geneeskundig Wetenschappelijk Onderzoek of Belgium for financial support towards the expenses of the experiments.

References

1. Hansen, A. R. and Fouts, J. R. (1972). Some problems in Michaelis–Menten kinetic analysis of benzpyrene hydroxylase in hepatic microsomes from polycyclic hydrocarbon-pretreated animals. *Chem. Biol. Interact.*, **5**, 167–82
2. Hook, G. E. R., Bend, J. R. and Fouts, J. R. (1973). The effect of some biphenyl solubilizing and suspending agents on biphenyl 4-hydroxylase of rabbit liver microsomes. *Chem. Biol. Interact.*, **7**, 205–22
3. Parry, G., Palmer, D. N. and Williams, D. J. (1976). Ligand partitioning into membranes: its significance in determining K_M and K_S values for cytochrome P-450 and other membrane bound receptors and enzymes. *FEBS Lett.*, **67**, 123–9
4. Heirwegh, K. P. M., Campbell, M. and Meuwissen, J. A. T. P. (1978). Compartmentation of membrane-bound enzymes. Some basic concepts and consequences for kinetic studies. In Aitio, A. (ed.). *Conjugation Reactions in Drug Biotransformation*, pp. 191–202. (Amsterdam: Elsevier/North-Holland Biomedical Press)
5. Ragan, C. I. (1978). The role of phospholipids in the reduction of ubiquinone analogues by the mitochondrial reduced nicotinamide-adenine dinucleotide-ubiquinone oxidoreductase complex. *Biochem. J.*, **172**, 539–47
6. Scheel, G., Acevedo, E., Conzelmann, E., Nehrkorn, H. and Sandhoff, K. (1982). Model for the interaction of membrane-bound substrates and enzymes. *Eur. J. Biochem.*, **127**, 245–53
7. Dutton, G. J., Wishart, G. J., Leakey, J. E. A. and Goheer, M. A. (1976). Conjugation with glucuronic acid and other sugars. In *Drug Metabolism – From Microbe to Man*, pp. 71–90. (London: Taylor & Francis, Ltd.)
8. Backes, W. L. and Canady, W. J. (1981). Methods for the evaluation of hydrophobic substrate binding to cytochrome P-450. *Pharm. Ther.*, **12**, 133–58
9. Zakim, D. and Vessey, D. A. (1977). Membrane-bound estrone as substrate for microsomal UDP-glucuronyltransferase. *J. Biol. Chem.*, **252**, 7534–7
10. Jirsa, M. and Sponar, J. (1956). Das Absorptionsspektrum, der physikalische Zustand und die Geschwindigkeit der Diazoreaktion des Bilirubins. *Z. Ges. Inn. Med.*, **11**, 519–22
11. Brodersen, R. (1980). Binding of bilirubin to albumin. *CRC Crit. Rev. Clin. Lab. Sci.*, **11**, 305–99
12. Brodersen, R. (1982). Physical chemistry of bilirubin: binding to macromolecules and membranes. In Heirwegh, K. P. M. and Brown, S. B. (eds.). *Bilirubin.* Vol. I, *Chemistry*, pp. 75–123. (Florida: CRC Press)
13. Alvares, A. P., Shilling, G., Garbut, A. and Kuntzman, R. (1970). Studies on the hydroxylation of 3,4-benzpyrene by hepatic microsomes – Effect of albumin on the rate of hydroxylation of 3,4-benzpyrene. *Biochem. Pharmacol.*, **19**, 1449–55
14. McDonagh, A. F. (1979). Bile pigments: Bilatrienes and 5,15-biladienes. In Dolphin, D. (ed.). *The Porphyrins*, Vol. 6, *Biochemistry*, part A, pp. 293–490. (New York, San Francisco, London: Academic Press)
15. McDonagh, A. F. and Assisi, F. (1972). The ready isomerization of bilirubin IX-α in aqueous solution. *Biochem. J.*, **129**, 797–800
16. Laemmli, U. K. (1970). Cleavage of structural proteins during the assembly of the head of bacteriophage T4. *Nature*, **227**, 680–5
17. Heirwegh, K. P. M., Van De Vijver, M. and Fevery, J. (1972). Assay and properties of digitonin-activated bilirubin uridine disphosphate glucuronyltransferase from rat liver. *Biochem. J.*, **129**, 605–18

18. Van Roy, F. D. and Heirwegh, K. P. M. (1968). Determination of bilirubin glucuronide and assay of glucuronyltransferase with bilirubin as acceptor. *Biochem. J.*, **107,** 507–18
19. Heirwegh, K. P. M. (1984). Effects of binding of amphipathic compounds to carrier proteins on their enzymic biotransformation by membrane-bound enzymes. *Biochem. Soc. Trans.*, **12,** 11–3
20. de Duve, C., Pressman, B. C., Gianetto, R., Wattiaux, R. and Appelmans, F. (1955). Tissue fractionation studies. 6. Intracellular distribution patterns of enzymes in rat-liver tissue. *Biochem. J.*, **60,** 604–17
21. Brodersen, R. (1979). Bilirubin. Solubility and interaction with albumin and phospholipid. *J. Biol. Chem.*, **254,** 2364–9
22. Van Roy, F. P., Meuwissen, J. A. T. P., De Meuter, F. and Heirwegh, K. P. M. (1971). Determination of bilirubin in liver homogenates and serum with diazotized *p*-iodoaniline. *Clin. Chim. Acta*, **31,** 109–18
23. Lowry, O. H., Rosebrough, N. J., Farr, A. L. and Randall, R. J. (1951). Protein measurements with the Folin phenol reagent. *J. Biol. Chem.*, **193,** 265
24. Tanford, Ch. (1980). *The Hydrophobic Effect. Formation of Micelles and Biological Membranes.* 2nd Edn. (New York: Wiley & Sons)
25. Diaconis, P. and Efron, B. (1983). Computer-intensive methods in statistics. *Sci. Am.*, **248,** 96–108
26. Meuwissen, J. A. T. P. (1984). Transport of Bilirubin-IXα in Liver and Blood. A biophysical and biochemical Approach. *PhD Thesis*, University of Leuven, Belgium
27. Meuwissen, J. A. T. P. and Heirwegh, K. P. M. (1982). Aspects of bilirubin transport. In Heirwegh, K. P. M. and Brown, S. B. (eds.). *Bilirubin*, Vol. 2, *Metabolism*, pp. 39–83. (Boca Raton: CRC Press)

23
Studies on substrate specificity of microsomal bilirubin-IXα UDP-glucuronyltransferase in rat liver

N. BLANCKAERT AND F. VANSTAPEL

Hepatic esterification is an essential step in the elimination of bilirubin-IXα from the body. In most mammals, this conjugation occurs predominantly with glucuronic acid and to a minor extent with glucose and xylose (for a comprehensive review, *see* Ref. 1). Some species, including man, rat, dog, and cat, excrete the esterified bilirubins in bile in both mono-esterified and di-esterified forms. The monoconjugated pigment found in bile comprises two isomeric forms, i.e. the C-8 and C-12 isomers, esterified at the propionic acid side-chain attached at C-8 or C-12, respectively, of the unsymmetrically substituted bilirubin-IXα molecule (Figure 23.1)[2,3]. Formation of the two isomeric bilirubin-IXα monoglucuronides as well as of bilirubin-IXα diglucuronide is catalysed by a hepatic microsomal UDP-glucuronyltransferase system[4–8].

Since several distinct forms of the UDP-glucuronyltransferase have been shown to exist in rat liver microsomes[9], the question arises whether or not formation of the two isomeric monoglucuronides and conversion of the monoglucuronides to diglucuronide depends on separate enzyme forms and/or different substrate-binding sites. Furthermore, how do synthetic structural variants of bilirubin-IXα and major xenobiotic substrates of the hepatic UDP-glucuronyltransferase system interact with glucuronidation of bilirubin-IXα? Evidence suggesting that a UDP-glucuronyltransferase form exhibiting a high degree of specificity toward bilirubin exists in rat liver comes from the observation that a homozygous mutant rat strain, the so-called homozygous Gunn rat (Gunn rat), is unable to form bilirubin glucuronides *in vivo*, and has no detectable hepatic UDP-glucuronyltransferase activity towards bilirubin-IXα and bilirubin-IXα monoglucuronides[4,5,7]. In contrast, glucuronidation of the other major substrates for UDP-glucuronyltransferase, such as *p*-nitrophenol, morphine, and 4-methylumbelliferone appears to be either normal or only partially defective in the Gunn rat strain[10].

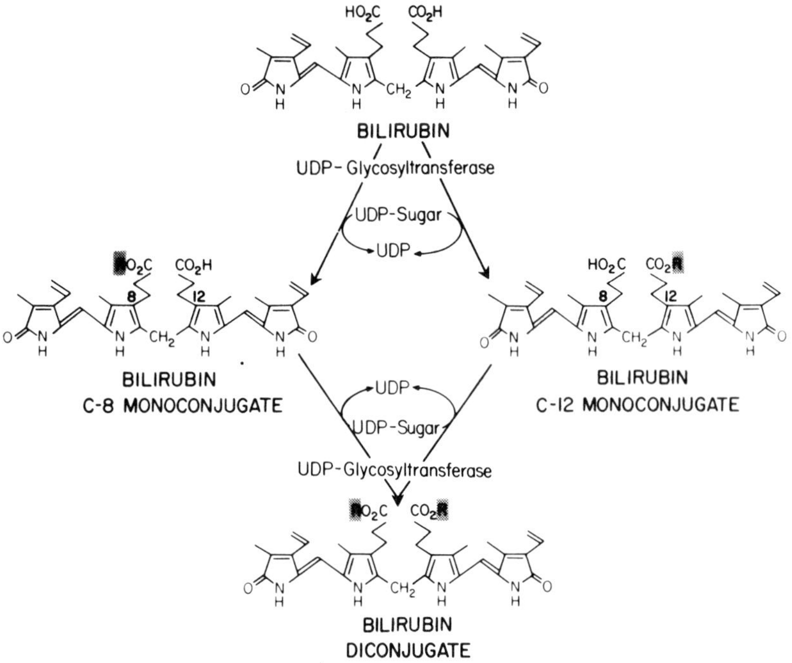

Figure 23.1 Hepatic esterification of bilirubin-IXα. R represents a glycosyl moiety transferred from a UDP-sugar to the propionic acid side-chain attached at either carbon 8 (C-8) or carbon 12 (C-12) of bilirubin. This transfer reaction is catalysed by a hepatic UDP-glucuronyltransferase system

In the present studies, we have investigated the interaction of various compounds with bilirubin-IXα UDP-glucuronyltransferase using the following two complementary criteria. (1) Is the compound glucuronidated in normal rat liver, and, if so, is this glucuronidation totally defective in the Gunn rat? Confirmative answers to both questions suggests that glucuronidation of the compound solely depends on the bilirubin-conjugating form of UDP-glucuronyltransferase. (2) Does the investigated substance competitively inhibit the glucuronidation of bilirubin-IXα by microsomal preparations from normal rat liver?

MATERIALS AND METHODS

Materials

The following chemicals were obtained from the sources indicated: UDP-glucuronic acid (UDPGlcUA), UDP-*N*-acetylglucosamine (UDPGlcNAc), HEPES, bilirubin-IXα, NAD^+, glucaro-1,4-lactone, testosterone, 4-nitrophenol, chloramphenicol (Sigma, St. Louis, MO); 3-[(3-cholamidopropyl) dimethylammonio]-2-hydroxy-1-propane-sulphonate (CHAPSO, Biorad, Richmond, CA); δ-amino[4-^{14}C]laevulinic acid, 58 mCi/mmol (New England Nuclear, Boston, MA); morphine sulphate (Mallinckrodt, St. Louis, MO); mesobilirubin-IXα, 'bilirubin conjugate', corresponding with a mixture of mono- and ditaurylconjugates of bilirubin-IXα (Porphyrin Products, Logan, UT).

Thin-layer chromatography (TLC) was performed on glass plates pre-coated with silica-gel 60 (5763/0025 and 5762/0025, from EM Laboratories, Elmsford, NY).

Liver microsomes were prepared from fasted (12 h) male Sprague-Dawley rats, 300–350 g body weight (normal rats), and from male homozygous Gunn rats (j/j; 300–350 g body weight) raised at the University of California, School of Medicine, San Francisco.

Methods

The following bile pigments were prepared as previously described: [^{14}C]-bilirubin-IXα with a specific radioactivity of 46 800 dpm/nmole[11]; bilirubin-IIIα and bilirubin-XIIIα[12]; bilirubin-IXβ, -IXγ, -IXδ[13]; bilirubin-IXα C-8 and C-12 monoamides[2]; biliverdin-IXα dimethyl ester[14]; biliverdin-IXα[15]. Dimethoxybilirubin-IXα and dimethoxybilirubin-IXα monomethyl esters were obtained respectively by complete and partial saponification[3] of dimethoxybilirubin-IXα dimethyl ester. The latter product was prepared by methylation of bilirubin-IXα with ethereal diazomethane[16] and isolated as described elsewhere[3]. Dimethoxybilirubin-IXα and dimethoxybilirubin-IXα monomethyl ester were purified by TLC using chloroform/methanol (9 : 1 v/v). Analytical separation of dimethoxybilirubin-IXα and its mono- and dimethyl esters was performed with toluene/ethanol (25 : 2, v/v). Biliverdin-IXα monomethyl ester was prepared by partial saponification[3] of the corresponding dimethyl ester. Analytical separation of biliverdin-IXα and its mono- and dimethyl esters was carried out with chloroform/methanol/water (40 : 9 : 1 v/v/v). Commercially obtained mesobilirubin-IXα and the biosynthetic [^{14}C]-bilirubin-IXα were purified by TLC using chloroform/methanol/g-acetic acid (97 : 2 : 1 v/v/v). The commercial bilirubin tauryl conjugate preparation was subjected to TLC using chloroform/methanol/water (10 : 5 : 1 v/v/v). Two major bands were obtained and identified: one was a mixture of the C-8 and C-12 monotauryl conjugates, the other was bilirubin-IXα ditauryl conjugate.

Microsomal fractions of rat liver were prepared as previously described from animals pretreated with sodium phenobarbital (1 g/l) in the drinking water for 7 days[4]. Protein and total bilirubin concentrations were measured respectively by the methods of Lowry *et al.*[17] and Novros *et al.*[18].

Incubation mixtures employed for qualitative analysis of the reaction products contained the following components: rat liver microsomes resuspended in 0.25 mol/l sucrose containing 1 mmol/l EDTA; HEPES buffer, pH 7.8 (0.140 mol/l); CHAPSO (5 mmol/l); $MgCl_2$ (6.25 mmol/l); NAD^+ (10 mmol/l); glucaro-1,4-lactone (1 mmol/l); UDPGlcUA (0 or 5 mmol/l); ~100 μmol/l of one of the bile pigments listed in Table 23.1. The concentration of rat liver microsomal protein was 3 mg/ml. The reaction mixtures were incubated at 37°C for 90 min, and the reaction products were analysed by either the ethyl anthranilate diazo-method[19] or the alkaline methanolysis procedure combined with TLC[3].

Structure elucidation of the ethyl anthranilate azo derivatives was performed according to published procedures[20] and comprised a series of chemical tests including acetylation, methylation, and alkaline methanolysis or ethanolysis with chromatographic analysis of the reaction products at each derivatization stage. Ethyl anthranilate azo pigments are designated as proposed by Bergstrom and Blumenthal (Figure 23.2)[21]. Incubation mixtures used for the study of the enzyme kinetics in the presence and absence of a potential inhibitor had the same composition except that [^{14}C-]bilirubin-IXα at five different concentrations (1–10 μmol/l) was used as an enzyme substrate, and the microsomal protein concentration was lowered to 0.25 mg/ml. Assay of initial rates of formation of individual reaction products was carried out as described elsewhere[22]. Lineweaver–Burk double-reciprocal plots were constructed for estimation of K_m, V_{max}, and K_I values.

RESULTS

Glucuronidation of bilirubins by microsomal fractions of rat liver

Under conditions leading to the conversion of over 80% of the bilirubin-IXα substrate into glucuronidated pigment by normal rat liver microsomes, glucuronide formation was undetectable with Gunn rat liver microsomes incubated with any one compound of a series of bile pigments (Table 23.1). In

Table 23.1 Glucuronidation *in vitro* of various bile pigments by microsomal fractions from liver of normal rats and homozygous Gunn rats

Tested compound	*Concentration* (μmol/l)	*Glucuronidation* *Normal rat*	*Gunn rat*
Bilirubin-IXα (BR)	100	+*	–
Bilirubin-IIIα	100	+*	–
Bilirubin-XIIIα	100	+*	–
Bilirubin-IXβ	100	+*	–
Bilirubin-IXδ	100	+*	–
Bilirubin-IXγ	100	+	–
BR C-8 monoamide	112	+	–
BR C-12 monoamide	110	+	–
BR monotauryl conjugate	100	+	–
Biliverdin-IXα	200	+	–
Dimethoxybilirubin-IXα	100	+	–

* Indicates that mono- and diglucuronidated reaction products were demonstrated

contrast, all tested bilirubins and biliverdin-IXα were glucuronidated by the microsomal fractions of normal rat liver. Azopyrromethene (Azpm) monoglucuronide was identified in the incubation mixtures containing UDP-glucuronic acid, but was absent in controls without added UDP-glucuronic acid when bilirubin-IXα C-8 or C-12 monoamide, bilirubin-IXα monotauryl conjugate, bilirubin-IIIα or -XIIIα, mesobilirubin-IXα, or bilirubin-IXγ was used as substrate. Incubation mixtures containing UDP-glucuronic acid and bilirubin-IXβ or -IXδ yielded two glucuronidated Azpm fractions. The predominant one was identified as the monoglucuronide, Azpm-3,7[Glc]; the second one corresponded with the diglucuronide, Azpm-3[GlcU],7[GlcU] (Figure 23.2). Interestingly, the alternative isomeric monoglucuronide, Azpm-3[GlcU],7, was not formed during enzymic incubation.

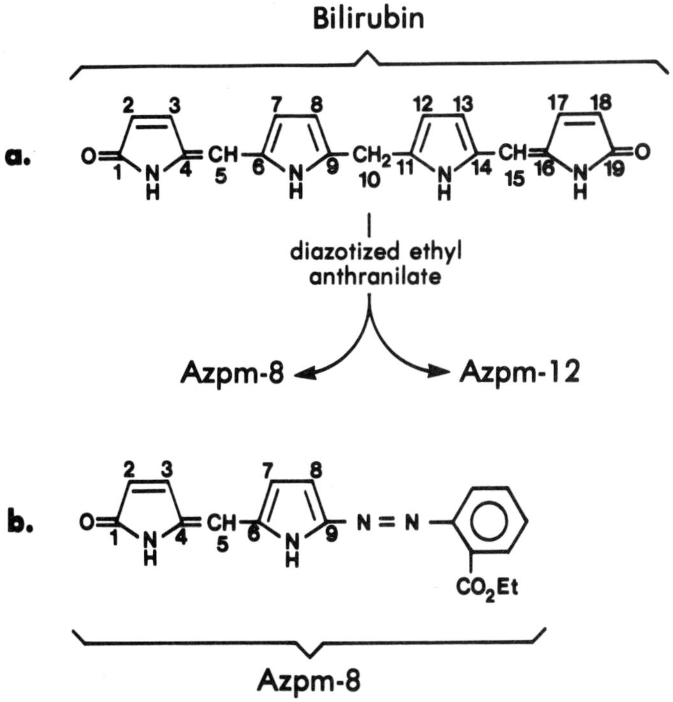

Figure 23.2 Structural features of bilirubins and their ethyl anthranilate azo derivatives. Panel **(a)** shows the tetrapyrrolic structure and numbering of the skeletal carbon atoms of bilirubin molecule. Diazotized ethyl anthranilate cleaves the tetrapyrrole into two dipyrrolic axopyrromethene derivatives (Azpm), one of which is shown in panel (**b**)

Qualitative analysis of the reaction products in the incubation mixtures could not be performed by the diazo-method when biliverdin-IXα or dimethoxybilirubin-IXα was used as substrate. The former compound is diazo-negative; the latter one yielded remarkably unstable azo derivatives. Therefore, enzymic reactions mixtures were analysed by the alkaline methanolysis method and TLC of the reaction products using the corresponding monomethyl esters and dimethyl ester as chromatographic reference compounds. Enzymic formation of a monoglucuronidated derivative was demonstrated for both biliverdin-IXα and dimethoxybilirubin-IXα while diglucuronide production remained undetectable by TLC in both cases.

Kinetic analysis of glucuronidation *in vitro* of bilirubin-IXα in the presence and absence of possible inhibitors

Using CHAPSO-disrupted microsomes and five different concentrations of bilirubin-IXα between 1 and 10 μmol/l, Michaelis–Menten kinetics were observed for formation of the C-8 isomer and C-12 isomers of monoglucuronide (Figure 23.3). Formation of diglucuronide at rates between 10% and 15% of the rate of monoglucuronide production was observed in all incubation mixtures. However, the assay conditions were optimized for estimating initial rates of monoglucuronide formation, and diglucuronide production rates were so small that accurate measurement of initial velocities was impossible.

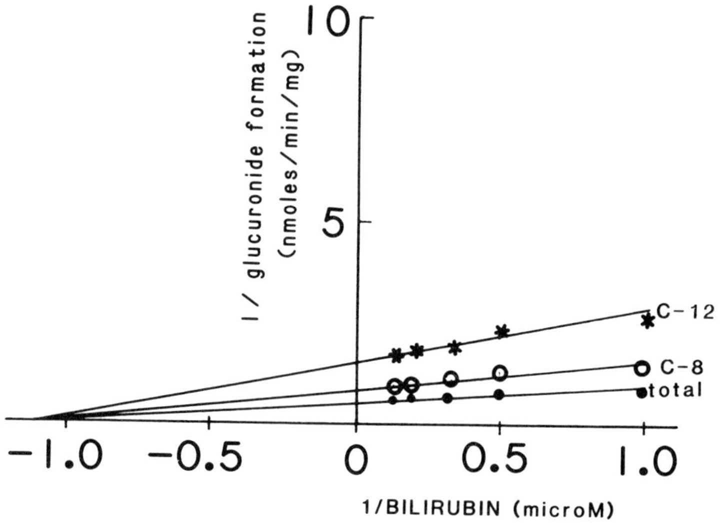

Figure 23.3 Lineweaver–Burk plots of UDP-glucuronyltransferase activities at various concentrations of bilirubin-IXα. C-12 (*) and C-8 (○) refer to initial rates of formation of the individual C-12 and C-8 isomers of bilirubin-IXα monoglucuronide. Total (●) refers to total monoglucuronide production

In the absence of inhibitor, K_m values for total monoglucuronide formation varied between 0.5 and 1.1 μmol/l with V_{max} values between 1.6 and 1.9 nmol of bilirubin-IXα monoglucuronides/min per mg microsomal protein (Table 23.2). A pattern typical for competitive inhibition (Figure 23.4) was obtained with all tested bile pigments (Table 23.2). Chloramphenicol, 4-nitrophenol, morphine, and testosterone gave inhibition which was discernible only at relatively high inhibitor concentrations (at least 500 μmol/l, compared to 1 μmol/l bilirubin-IXα) and, respectively, amounted to 14%, 18%, 38%, and 61% at the highest tested concentration (1000 μmol/l, 500 μmol/l, 2000 μmol/l, and 500 μmol/l, respectively), but was not of a competitive nature.

The K_m values of the formation of C-8 and C-12 isomers of bilirubin-IXα monoglucuronide were identical, and competitive inhibition exerted by the various bile pigments did not affect the ratio of C-8 monoglucuronide to C-12 monoglucuronide in the incubation mixture.

DISCUSSION

At present it is generally accepted that glucuronidation of a large number and variety of endogenous and xenobiotic compounds is catalysed by a family

Table 23.2 Kinetic constants of bilirubin-IXα UDP-glucuronyltransferase of normal rat liver microsomes in the presence and absence of potential inhibitors

Tested inhibitor	*Concentration* (μmol/l)	*Without inhibitor* K_m	*Without inhibitor* V_{max}	*With inhibitor* V_{max}	*With inhibitor* K_I
Bilirubin-IIIα	10	0.8	1.6	1.6	1.0
Bilirubin-XIIIα	10	0.9	1.8	1.5	1.2
Mesobilirubin-XIα	20	0.9	1.6	1.9	1.3
Dimethoxybilirubin-IXα	20	0.9	1.8	1.8	1.0
Biliverdin-IXα	50	1.1	1.9	1.4	13.7

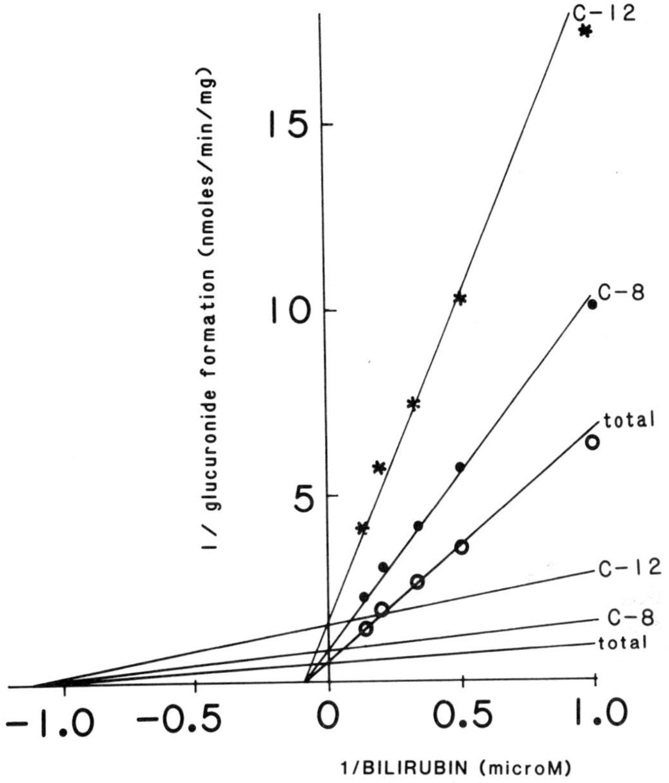

Figure 23.4 Lineweaver–Burk plots showing inhibition of bilirubin-IXα UDP-glucuronyltransferase activity by bilirubin-XIIIα. C-12(*) and C-8(●) refer to initial rates of formation of the individual C-12 and C-8 isomers of bilirubin-IXα monoglucuronide. Total (○) refers to total monoglucuronide production. The concentration of bilirubin-XIIIα was 10 μmol/l

of closely related UDP-glucuronyltransferase forms. Several distinct UDP-glucuronyltransferases appear to exist in rat liver, and criteria used to distinguish these forms include, *inter alia*, physical separation and developmental, induction and kinetic differences. An important endogenous substrate of the UDP-glucuronyltransferase system is the natural breakdown product of haem, bilirubin-IXα. Detoxication and efficient disposal of this catabolite hinges upon esterification of at least one of the pigment's two propionic acid side-chains with glucuronic acid. Nature appears to have allotted a specific transferase form to this crucial glucuronidation reaction. Evidence supporting this view comes from the finding that the mutant Gunn rat strain is completely unable to glucuronidate bilirubin-IXα, while UDP-glucuronyltransferase activity towards other substrates is unimpaired or only slightly reduced[10,23,24]. Furthermore, conversion *in vitro* and *in vivo* of monoglucuronide into diglucuronide is completely defective in the Gunn rat[4,5,7]. Collectively, these findings suggest that a single enzyme form and/or substrate-binding site is responsible for the four glucuronidation reactions involved in the formation of bilirubin-IXα glucuronides. Our recent observation that highly purified bilirubin-IXα UDP-glucuronyltransferase from normal rat liver is able to catalyse diglucuronide formation from bilirubin-IXα as well as from bilirubin-IXα monoglucuronides supports this view[25].

The present study was an attempt to further delineate the substrate specificity of the substrate binding site of bilirubin-IXα UDP-glucuronyltransferase. Two complementary operational criteria were used to decide whether a compound was glucuronidated by bilirubin-IXα UDP-glucuronyltransferase or by another enzyme form. Our findings indicate that a wide variety of bile pigments including congeners of bilirubin-IXα with modified side-chain composition or sequence, or with a modified skeletal structure compared to the natural IXα pigment are effectively glucuronidated by microsomal fractions of normal rat liver and depend for this on the bilirubin-IXα-conjugating enzyme form. Furthermore, the observation that these compounds compete with bilirubin-IXα for binding at the enzyme's active site indicates that a single substrate-binding site is responsible for their glucuronidation. Glucuronidation at this active site seems to be defective in the homozygous Gunn rat. Also, the fact that an identical K_m value was found for the formation of the C-8 and the C-12 isomers of bilirubin-IXα monoglucuronides in the presence, as well as in the absence, of an inhibiting bile pigment indicates that a single bilirubin-binding site is responsible for both reactions. Whether or not the same enzymatic site is involved in the conversion of monoglucuronides to diglucuronide remains to be elucidated.

ACKNOWLEDGEMENTS

We thank Ms L. Hammaker and Mr K. Pua for their excellent technical assistance, and Ms D. Fedorchak and Mr M. Karasik for excellent editorial assistance. F. V. is indebted to the Fund for Scientific Research, Belgium, for a travel grant. This work was supported by NIH grant AM-11275 and the Liver Core Center Grant NIH AM-26743.

References

1. Blanckaert, N. and Schmid, R. (1982). Physiology and pathophysiology of bilirubin metabolism. In Zakim, D. and Boyer, T. D. (eds.). *A Textbook of Hepatology*, pp. 246–96. (Philadelphia: W. B. Saunders)

2. Jansen, F. H. and Billing, B. H. (1971). The identification of monoconjugates of bilirubin in bile as amide derivatives. *Biochem. J.*, **125,** 917–9
3. Blanckaert, N. (1980). Analysis of bilirubin and bilirubin mono- and diconjugates. Determination of their relative amounts in biological samples. *Biochem. J.*, **185,** 115–28
4. Blanckaert, N., Gollan, J. L. and Schmid, R. (1979). Bilirubin diglucuronide synthesis by a UDP-glucuronic acid-dependent enzyme system in rat liver microsomes. *Proc. Natl. Acad. Sci. USA*, **76,** 2037–41
5. Blanckaert, N., Gollan, J. L. and Schmid, R. (1980). Mechanism of bilirubin diglucuronide formation in intact rats. *J. Clin. Invest.*, **65,** 1332–42
6. Gordon, E. R. and Goresky, C. A. (1980). The formation of bilirubin diglucuronide by rat liver microsomal preparations. *Can. J. Biochem.*, **58,** 1302–10
7. Sieg, A., Van Hees, G. P. and Heirwegh, K. P. M. (1982). Uridine diphosphate-glucuronic acid-dependent conversion of bilirubin monoglucuronides to diglucuronide in presence of plasma membranes from rat liver is nonenzymic. *J. Clin. Invest.*, **69,** 347–57
8. Gordon, E. R., Sommerer, U. and Goresky, C. A. (1983). The hepatic microsomal formation of bilirubin diglucuronide. *J. Biol. Chem.*, **258,** 15028–30
9. Burchell, B. (1981). Identification and purification of multiple forms of UDP-glucuronyltransferase. *Rev. Biochem. Toxicol.*, **3,** 1–32
10. MacKenzie, P. I. and Owens, I. S. (1983). Differences in UDP-glucuronosyltransferase activities in congenic inbred rats homozygous and heterozygous for the jaundice locus. *Biochem. Pharmacol.*, **32,** 3777–81
11. Ostrow, J. D., Hammaker, L. and Schmid, R. (1961). The preparation of crystalline bilirubin-C^{14}. *J. Clin. Invest.*, **40,** 1442–52
12. McDonagh, A. F. and Assisi, F. (1971). Commercial bilirubin: a trinity of isomers. *FEBS Lett.*, **18,** 315–7
13. Blanckaert, N., Heirwegh, K. P. M. and Compernolle, F. (1976). Synthesis and separation by thin-layer chromatography of bilirubin-IX isomers. Their identification as tetrapyrroles and dipyrrolic ethyl anthranilate azopigments. *Biochem. J.*, **155,** 405–17
14. Bonnett, R. and McDonagh, A. F. (1973). The meso-reactivity of porphyrins and related compounds. Part VI. Oxidative cleavage of the haem system. The four isomeric biliverdins of the IX series. *J. Chem. Soc. Perkin Trans.*, **1,** 881–8
15. McDonagh, A. F. and Palma, L. A. (1980). Preparation and properties of crystalline biliverdin-IXα. *Biochem. J.*, **189,** 193–208
16. Kuenzle, C. C., Weibel, M. H. and Pelloni, R. R. (1973). The reaction of bilirubin with diazomethane. *Biochem. J.*, **133,** 357–68
17. Lowry, O. H., Rosebrough, N. J., Farr, A. L. and Randall, R. J. (1951). Protein measurement with the Folin phenol reagent. *J. Biol. Chem.*, **193,** 265–75
18. Novros, J. S., Thomas, T. R. and Knoblock, E. C. (1979). Improved method for accurate quantitation of total and conjugated bilirubin in serum. *Clin. Chem.*, **25,** 1891–9
19. Heirwegh, K. P. M., Van de Vijver, M. and Fevery, J. (1972). Assay and properties of digitonin-activated bilirubin uridine diphosphate glucuronyltransferase from rat liver. *Biochem. J.*, **129,** 605–18
20. Heirwegh, K. P. M. and Blanckaert, A. (1982). Analytical chemistry of rubins. In Heirwegh, K. P. M. and Brown, S. B. (eds.). *Bilirubin*, Vol. I, *Chemistry*, pp. 125–51. (Boca Raton, FL: CRC Press)
21. Bergstrom, D. E. and Blumenthal, S. G. (1982). Abbreviations and symbols for bile pigments and their azopyrromethene derivatives. In Lightner, D. A. (ed.). *Structure, Photochemistry, and Organic Chemistry of Bilirubin*, pp. 1–58. Submitted to the *IUPAC-IUB Joint Commission on Biochemical Nomenclature*
22. Vermeir, M., Vanstapel, F. and Blanckaert, N. (1984). Radioassay of UDP-glucuronyltransferase-catalyzed formation of bilirubin monoglucuronides and bilirubin diglucuronide in liver microsomes. *Biochem. J.*, **222** (In press)
23. Schmid, R., Axelrod, J., Hammaker, L. and Swarm, R. L. (1958). Congenital jaundice in rats, due to a defect in glucuronide formation. *J. Clin. Invest.*, **37,** 1123–30
24. Blanckaert, M., Fevery, J., Heirwegh, K. P. M. and Compernolle, F. (1977). Characterization of the major diazo-positive pigments in bile of homozygous Gunn rats. *Biochem J.*, **164,** 237–49
25. Burchell, B. and Blanckaert, N. (1984). Bilirubin mono- and diglucuronide formation by purified rat liver microsomal bilirubin UDP-glucuronyltransferase. *Biochem. J.*, **222** (In press)

24
Differential regulation of bilirubin UDP-glucuronyltransferase activity in hepatic subcellular membranes

J. L. GOLLAN AND S. C. HAUSER

ABSTRACT

This study defines the subcellular location of hepatic bilirubin UDP-glucuronyltransferase and examines the regulation of enzyme activity in different intracellular membranes. Purity of membrane fractions isolated from rat liver was assessed by electron microscopy and marker enzymes. The formation rates of bilirubin diglucuronide and monoglucuronides (C-8 and C-12 isomers) were determined by radiochemical assay of bilirubin UDP-glucuronyltransferase, using a physiologic substrate concentration of [^{14}C] bilirubin. The majority of enzyme activity was found in smooth and rough endoplasmic reticulum, with small amounts in the nuclear envelope and Golgi membranes. No measurable activity was found in plasma membranes or in cytosol. The regulation of bilirubin UDP-glucuronyltransferase activity differed amongst intracellular membranes; enzyme activity measured in the presence of the physiologic activator, UDP-*N*-acetylglucosamine, exhibited latency in smooth endoplasmic reticulum and Golgi membranes, but not in rough endoplasmic reticulum and the nuclear envelope. Since the rough membranes comprise 60% of hepatocyte endoplasmic reticulum, and bilirubin UDP-glucuronyltransferase activity *in vitro* is maximal in this membrane fraction under presumed physiologic conditions, the rough endoplasmic reticulum would appear to be the major site of bilirubin glucuronidation in hepatocytes.

INTRODUCTION

Bilirubin conjugation results in the formation of bilirubin monoglucuronides (C-8 and C-12 BMG isomers) and bilirubin diglucuronide (BDG), the principal pigments excreted in human and rat bile. Formation of both BMG and BDG from bilirubin is catalysed by bilirubin UDP-glucuronyltransferase, which is found in rat liver microsomal preparations[1,2]. However, the intracellular location of bilirubin UDP-glucuronyltransferase in hepatocytes has not been clearly defined. It has been suggested that the enzyme resides in smooth endoplasmic reticulum[3,4], although several investigators have demonstrated enzyme activity in both smooth and rough endoplasmic reticulum fractions of rat liver. Some studies have documented greater bilirubin UDP-glucuronyltransferase activity in smooth than in rough endoplasmic reticulum[5], while others have reported the opposite[6]. We postulated that hepatic bilirubin UDP-glucuronyltransferase, like other multifunctional enzymes (e.g. glutathione S-transferases, galactosyltransferases and glucose-6-phosphatase), may be located in a variety of subcellular membranes[7–10]. Since the UDP-glucuronyltransferases are membrane-bound enzymes and their activity is modulated by the phospholipid composition and the physical properties of the membrane[11,12], we also considered that the regulation of bilirubin UDP-glucuronyltransferase activity may vary in different subcellular membranes.

In previous studies, conventional assays have been used to measure bilirubin UDP-glucuronyltransferase activity. However, these assays employ unphysiologic conditions, such as bilirubin substrate concentrations greatly in excess of those present in normal liver[1], perturbation of the liver membrane preparations with detergents, or omission of the allosteric effector, UDP-*N*-acetylglucosamine (UDP-GlcNAc), from the assay mixture. Recently, we have developed a new radiochemical assay for bilirubin UDP-glucuronyltransferase activity which overcomes the problems associated with conventional assays[13], and accurately measures the rates of formation of BDG as well as both the C-8 and C-12 BMG isomers[14]. In the present study, this assay has been applied systematically to define the intracellular sites and regulation of bilirubin UDP-glucuronyltransferase activity, using preparations of smooth and rough endoplasmic reticulum, Golgi and plasma membranes, nuclear envelope and cytosol isolated from rat liver.

MATERIALS AND METHODS

Materials

Male Sprague-Dawley rats weighing 200–300 g were used. The animals were allowed free access to standard rat chow and water, except where indicated for specific methods.

[^{14}C]bilirubin (2.6–15.8 Ci/mol) was prepared biosynthetically[15] from the bile of rats infused intravenously with δ[4-^{14}C]-aminolaevulinic acid (40–60 Ci/μmol). UDP-glucuronic acid (ammonium salt), UDP-*N*-acetylglucosamine (sodium salt), β-nicotinamide adenine dinucleotide (grade III), digitonin, deoxyribonuclease I (type I), D-saccharic acid 1,4-lactone, and bovine serum albumin (fatty acid-free, fraction V) were all obtained from Sigma Chemical Co. All other reagents were the highest analytical grade available. For thin-layer chromatography, glass plates precoated with silica gel were used (silica gel 60).

Cell fractionation procedures

Smooth and rough endoplasmic reticulum

Smooth and rough endoplasmic reticulum were obtained using a modification of the procedure described by Eriksson, DePierre and Dallner[16]. Because of the possible effects of anaesthesia on bilirubin UDP-glucuronyltransferase and the isolated membranes, animals were sacrificed by decapitation and the liver was rapidly resected. For each experiment, three to five livers obtained from fasted rats were rinsed in cold 1.15 g/100 ml KCl, sliced into small pieces, and homogenized in 0.25 mol/l sucrose (1 g liver/3.0 ml). The pooled liver homogenate was centrifuged at 41 000 *g* for 7 min, and the supernate was collected and layered onto a discontinuous sucrose–caesium chloride gradient as described. The smooth and rough fractions were collected, washed with 0.25 mol/l sucrose containing 1 mmol/l disodium EDTA, pH 7.3, pelleted at 40 000 *g* for 30 min, resuspended and repelleted in the same manner. These preparations (as well as the other fractions described below) were assayed for bilirubin UDP-glucuronyltransferase activity immediately following preparation (fresh) or were frozen (−70°C) immediately after preparation and assayed for bilirubin UDP-glucuronyltransferase activity within 48 hours.

Golgi membranes

Golgi membranes were prepared for each experiment by the method of Hino *et al.*[17] from three or four pooled livers obtained from non-fasted rats. The procedure was modified as follows: each rat was lightly anaesthetized with ether, the abdomen rapidly opened and the liver perfused *in situ* with ice-cold 1.15 g/100 ml KCl. The final Golgi fraction (designated 'BY' by Hino *et al.*[17]) was centrifuged as described and the supernate was centrifuged at 49 000 *g* for 10 min. The pellet obtained from this spin was resuspended in a small volume of buffer (0.5 mol/l sucrose, 50 mmol/l Tris-maleate, 1 g/100 ml dextran, pH 6.75).

Isolated nuclei and nuclear envelope

Livers obtained after decapitation from three or four fasted rats were pooled and hepatocyte nuclei were isolated as described by Blobel and Potter[18]. In all experiments, the nuclei were examined by phase-contrast microscopy, and if extranuclear membrane contamination was not observed, the pellet was resuspended in $CaCl_2$ buffer and centrifuged at 3000 *g* for 10 min. Nuclear envelope was then prepared from the nuclear pellet by DNAse digestion according to the method of Kay *et al.*[19].

Plasma membranes

Plasma membranes were isolated by two different approaches in order to prepare fractions relatively free of or enriched in bile canaliculi. Two livers from fasted rats were pooled for each experiment, and the membranes were isolated according to Song *et al.*[20] ('canalicular-enriched') or with the modifications of Yousef *et al.*[21] to isolate a relatively 'canalicular-free' preparation.

Cytosol

Two fasted rats were decapitated and their livers homogenized in 0.25 mol/l sucrose containing 1 mmol/l disodium EDTA, pH 7.3 (1 g liver/3.0 ml buffer). The homogenate was centrifuged at 41 000 *g* for 7 min and the supernate was decanted and centrifuged at 100 000 *g* for 2 h. The supernate from this last centrifugation was the cytosol fraction.

Bilirubin UDP-glucuronyltransferase activity

Bilirubin UDP-glucuronyltransferase activity was determined in rat liver membrane preparations and cytosol by radiochemical assay[13]. Assay mixtures (total volume 1.2 ml) were prepared on ice in glass-stoppered tubes containing the following constituents: 0.4 ml triethanolamine-HCL buffer, pH 7.6 (0.167 mol/l HCL), 2 mmol/l $MgCl_2$, 8.3 mmol/l D-saccharic acid 1,4-lactone, 1.7 mmol/l β-nicotinamide adenine dinucleotide, 20 mmol/l UDP-glucuronic acid, 1 mmol/l UDP-*N*-acetylglucosamine, 0.2 ml water, and 0.5 ml of the membrane preparation or cytosol (containing 1.0–3.6 mg protein) in 0.25 mol/l sucrose–1 mmol/l disodium EDTA (pH 7.3). After a 2-minute preincubation at 38.2°C in a shaking water-bath, the reaction was started by the addition of 0.1 ml of a solution containing [^{14}C]bilirubin (15 μmol/l dissolved in 15–30 μl of 0.05 mol/l NaOH, to which bovine serum albumin (7.5 μmol/l) had been added). Incubations were performed under argon in dim light for up to 5 min, and aliquots (0.1–0.2 ml) were removed at 0.5–1.0 min intervals and promptly mixed with 6 ml cold methanol. To enable the location of the radiolabelled pigment bands to be visualized on thin-layer plates, 15 μl of a mixture consisting of bilirubin dissolved in dimethylsulphoxide (1 mg/ml) and an equal volume of rat bile enriched in bilirubin glucuronides (i.e. bile collected from a rat infused intravenously with 5 μmol h^{-1} 100 g body weight^{-1} bilirubin) were added to the cold methanol mixture. The radiolabelled reaction products, bilirubin diglucuronide and the C-8 and C-12 isomers of bilirubin monoglucuronides, were converted to their corresponding di- and monomethyl esters by alkaline methanolysis[14]. The pigment-containing extracts obtained by alkaline methanolysis were stored at −70°C under argon for a maximum of 48 h. Pigment fractions were separated by thin-layer chromatography on silica gel plates, using a mixture of chloroform, methanol and glacial acetic acid (96 : 2 : 2) containing 0.5 g/100 ml butylated hydroxytoluene. Bilirubin and the transesterified reaction products separated into discrete bands, which were scraped from the plates into scintillation vials. Soluene-350 (0.5 ml), isopropyl alcohol (0.1 ml) and 30 g/100 ml hydrogen peroxide (0.1–0.2 ml) were added to each vial, and after a minimum of 2 hours, 5 ml of Dimilume or Dimiscent was added prior to counting.

Control incubations without UDP-glucuronic acid in the assay mixture consistently yielded greater than 95% of total radioactivity in the unconjugated bilirubin band. The rates of formation of the individual BMG isomers, total BMG, BDG and total glucuronides were calculated from the initial period during which the reaction was linear, on a Hewlett Packard 9845B system with graphics, and were expressed as pmol min^{-1} mg^{-1} of membrane protein. Protein was determined according to the method of Lowry *et al.*[22] using bovine serum albumin as standard. For analysis of the data, the Student's *t*-test was performed on paired (SER and RER) or unpaired (all other experiments) data.

RESULTS

Subcellular distribution of bilirubin UDP-glucuronyltransferase activity

Maximal bilirubin UDP-glucuronyltransferase activity was determined in membrane preparations which had been activated by preincubation for 30 min on ice with digitonin, 1 mg/mg protein[23], immediately prior to assay. Bilirubin UDP-glucuronyltransferase activity in nuclear envelope and Golgi membranes was shown to be maximal at this concentration of digitonin. It was also demonstrated that there were no differences in bilirubin UDP-glucuronyltransferase activity determined in freshly prepared subcellular fractions or in the same preparations after storage for 48 h at −70°C.

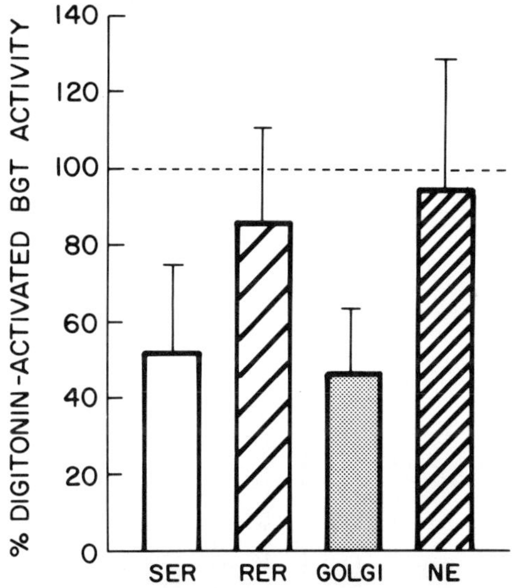

Figure 24.1 Maximal bilirubin UDP-glucuronyltransferase (BGT) activity in digitonin pretreated subcellular membranes. Enzyme activity (±SD) in digitonin-activated preparations of smooth and rough endoplasmic reticulum (SER and RER, $n=8$), Golgi membranes (GOLGI, $n=4$), and nuclear envelope (NE, $n=5$) prepared from rat liver. Significant differences were observed for SER vs GOLGI, $p<0.02$, RER vs GOLGI, $p<0.05$; SER vs NE and RER vs NE, $p<0.001$; GOLGI vs NE, $p<0.005$. There was no significant difference between the activity in SER and RER. (With permission from Hauser, S. C. *et al.*[31])

Bilirubin UDP-glucuronyltransferase activity was not detected in the cytosolic fraction ($n=2$), or in the bile-canalicular enriched ($n=2$) or the relatively bile-canalicular free ($n=2$) plasma membranes. In contrast, significant hepatic bilirubin UDP-glucuronyltransferase activity was found in all SER, RER, Golgi and nuclear envelope preparations (Figure 24.1). Maximal activity (pmol min^{-1} mg $protein^{-1}$) in digitonin-activated SER and RER (mean values 1708 and 1354, respectively) were comparable and exceeded those in Golgi membranes (956; $p<0.02$ and $p<0.05$, respectively), and nuclear envelope (352; $p<0.001$). The rates of bilirubin diglucuronide synthesis as a percentage of total conjugates formed were similar for all membrane preparations with and without UDP-GlcNAc or digitonin pretreatment (mean, 12–21%). Similarly, the C-8/C-12 BMG isomer ratios (mean, 1.8–2.8) were comparable in all membrane fractions, regardless of the assay conditions.

Regulation of bilirubin UDP-glucuronyltransferase activity in different subcellular membranes

The activity of bilirubin UDP-glucuronyltransferase in RER ($n=8$) and nuclear envelope ($n=11$) determined under assay conditions containing UDP-GlcNAc was unchanged by digitonin pretreatment of the membranes (Figure 24.2). Thus, maximal bilirubin UDP-glucuronyltransferase activity was evident in these membrane preparations when assayed in the presence of UDP-GlcNAc and without detergent activation. However, mean bilirubin UDP-glucuronyltransferase activities in SER ($n=8$) and Golgi membranes ($n=11$) treated with UDP-GlcNAc were only 52% and 47%, respectively ($p<0.005$), of that observed in the same preparations after preincubation with digitonin (Figure 24.2).

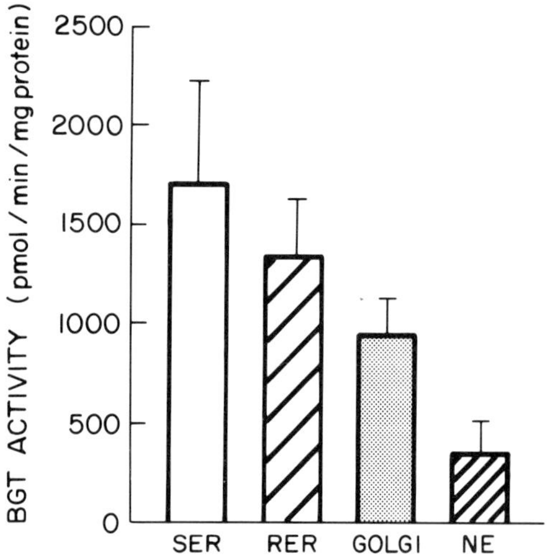

Figure 24.2 Bilirubin UDP-glucuronyltransferase activity in hepatic subcellular preparations assayed in the presence of UDP-*N*-acetylglucosamine (UDP-GLcNAc) and expressed as a percentage of maximal digitonin-activated enzyme activity (*see* Figure 24.1). Digitonin pretreatment did not alter bilirubin UDP-glucuronyltransferase (BGT) activity in RER ($n=8$) or nuclear envelope (NE; $n=11$). However, enzyme activity was increased significantly in digitonin pretreated SER ($p<0.005$; $n=8$) and Golgi membranes (GOLGI; $p<0.005$; $n=11$). (With permission from Hauser, S. C. *et al.*[31])

Moreover, bilirubin UDP-glucuronyltransferase activity measured in the absence of digitonin pretreatment was unaltered by exposing microsomes to either hypotonic sucrose or caesium chloride (i.e. conditions encountered during the preparation of SER and RER). In addition, when the UDP-GlcNAc concentration in the assay mixture was increased from 1 mmol/l to 5 mmol/l, bilirubin UDP-glucuronyltransferase activity in Golgi membranes or microsomes was unchanged.

For both SER and RER, bilirubin UDP-glucuronyltransferase activity in UDP-GlcNAc-treated preparations (880 and 1086, respectively; $n=5$) exceeded that in native untreated preparations, which were assayed under identical conditions, but without UDP-GlcNAc (416 and 752; $n=5$; $p<0.05$ and $p<0.01$, respectively; Figure 24.3). In the native preparations, enzyme activity was greater in RER and SER ($p<0.05$). In all experiments in which RER and SER were assayed with UDP-GlcNAc, bilirubin UDP-glucuronyltransferase activity was greater in RER (1272±428) than in SER (893±344), although this difference did not achieve statistical significance ($t=2.2129$; $0.05<p<0.075$).

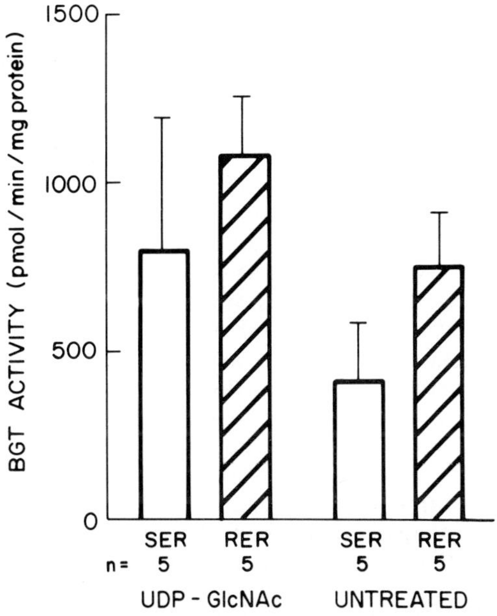

Figure 24.3 Comparison of bilirubin UDP-glucuronyltransferase activity in SER and RER assayed in the presence or absence of UDP-GlcNAc. Comparison of bilirubin UDP-glucuronyltransferase (BGT) activity in SER and RER assayed with or without (i.e. native) UDP-GlcNAc ($n=5$). Enzyme activity in both SER and RER incubated with UDP-GlcNAc was greater than that in native preparations ($p<0.05$ and $p<0.01$, respectively). In native preparations, enzyme activity in RER exceeded that in SER ($p<0.05$). Bilirubin UDP-glucuronyltransferase activities were comparable in SER and RER assayed with UDP-GlcNAc in the incubation mixture. (With permission from Hauser, S.C. *et al.*[31])

DISCUSSION

A variety of important hepatic enzymes are located in more than one subcellular organelle[7–10], but the possibility that bilirubin UDP-glucuronyltransferase activity exists in membranes other than the endoplasmic reticulum has not been systematically explored. Although previous investigators have found bilirubin UDP-glucuronyltransferase in both SER and RER, activity was measured using non-physiologic assay conditions, and the relative distribution of enzyme between SER and RER has remained a source of contention[3–6]. In addition, UDP-glucuronyltransferase activity has been noted in nuclear envelope, but only towards a variety of non-bilirubin substrates[24,25].

Our findings demonstrate that bilirubin UDP-glucuronyltransferase activity is widely distributed among subcellular membranes of the hepatocyte. Despite the sensitivity of the radiochemical enzyme assay, however, activity was not demonstrable in cytosol or plasma membranes (neither sinusoidal nor canalicular-enriched preparations). Although SER and RER account quantitatively for the bulk of hepatic bilirubin conjugating activity (Figure 24.1), bilirubin UDP-glucuronyltransferase in Golgi membranes and nuclear envelope may contribute to the glucuronidation of compartmentalized pools of bilirubin. It appears likely that the same enzyme is present in all membranes, since the pattern of bilirubin diglucuronide and bilirubin monoglucuronide isomer formation was qualitatively similar in all preparations. The presence of bilirubin UDP-glucuronyltransferase activity in multiple subcellular locations, like other enzymes such as glucose-6-phosphatase, may be accounted for by the membrane-flow theory of membrane biogenesis[10,26]. Moreover, this concept is supported by the observations that direct continuity exists between membranes of the RER and nuclear envelope, as well as those of SER and Golgi[27,28].

Evidence obtained using non-bilirubin substrates suggests that UDP-*N*-acetylglucosamine may be a key physiologic regulator of UDP-glucuronyltransferase activity, either by a direct allosteric effect in which the enzyme is made catalytically more efficient[12], or via a postulated membrane permease which enhances access of the cosubstrate, UDP-glucuronic acid, to the active site on the enzyme[11]. When the assay mixture contained UDP-GlcNAc (1 mmol/l) in a concentration similar to that found in the hepatocyte[29], bilirubin UDP-glucuronyltransferase activity in both smooth and rough endoplasmic reticulum exceeded that in native preparations assayed without UDP-GlcNAc (Figure 24.3). These observations support the concept that UDP-GlcNAc is a physiologic activator of bilirubin UDP-glucuronyltransferase at all locations in the hepatocyte, and provide a basis for routinely including this nucleotide–sugar in bilirubin UDP-glucuronyltransferase assays.

The studies, in which digitonin was used to examine the degree of latency of the enzyme in subcellular membranes, indicate that the regulation of bilirubin UDP-glucuronyltransferase activity differs in the various intracellular membranes. Bilirubin UDP-glucuronyltransferase activity in smooth endoplasmic reticulum and in Golgi membranes exhibited considerable latency; thus, the activity in membranes assayed in the presence of UDP-GlcNAc increased two-fold following pretreatment with digitonin (Figure 24.2). In contrast, enzyme activity was not latent in rough endoplasmic reticulum or in nuclear envelope.

The observation that bilirubin UDP-glucuronyltransferase is not latent in nuclear envelope differs from that of other investigators[24,25] who found that activity of the enzyme was latent both in vesicular preparations of nuclear envelope and microsomes, but not in cisternal nuclear envelope. In these studies, however, detergent activated nuclear envelope was compared to native preparations assayed in the absence of UDP-GlcNAc, and bilirubin was not used as substrate. Although it is possible that procedures, such as DNAse digestion, used to prepare nuclear envelope from isolated nuclei, may activate enzyme activity, our finding that vesicular preparations of nuclear envelope and RER do not exhibit latency questions the proposal that latency correlates with vesiculation and is merely an *in vitro* artefact which arises during the isolation of membranes[24].

We conclude from these investigations that bilirubin UDP-glucuronyltransferase in the RER and SER is responsible for the bulk of hepatic bilirubin conjugation, with only minor contributions from Golgi membranes and nuclear envelope. It is possible that the phospholipid microenvironment of bilirubin UDP-glucuronyltransferase in different subcellular membranes may determine whether activity of the enzyme is latent (as in SER and Golgi membranes), either by modulating conformation of the enzyme or by controlling substrate access to its active site. Considering the fact that the rough endoplasmic reticulum comprises approximately 60% of the hepatocyte endoplasmic reticulum[30], and that in contrast to SER, bilirubin UDP-glucuronyltransferase in RER functions at maximal activity in the presence of the presumed physiologic activator, UDP-*N*-acetylglucosamine, it is probable that the RER represents the major site of bilirubin glucuronidation in the hepatocyte.

ACKNOWLEDGEMENTS

These studies were supported by NIH Research Grant AM 30127 and in part by Grant RR 01032 from the General Clinical Research Centers Program of the Division of Research Resources, NIH. We are indebted to Julia Ziurys for considerable technical support, and to Janis Bongiovanni for secretarial assistance.

References

1. Blanckaert, N., Gollan, J. and Schmid, R. (1979). *Proc. Natl. Acad. Sci. USA*, **76,** 2037–41
2. Gordon, E. R. and Goresky, C. A. (1980). *Can. J. Biochem.*, **53,** 1302–10
3. Arias, I. M. (1972). *Semin. Hematol.*, **9,** 55–70
4. Schmid, R. (1972). *N. Engl. J. Med.*, **287,** 703–9
5. White, A. E. (1976). In Bouchier, I. A. D. (ed.) *Bilirubin Metabolism*. pp. 183–7. (Philadelphia: F. A. Davis)
6. Halac, E., DiPiazza, M. and Detwiler, P. (1972). *Biochem. Biophys. Acta*, **279,** 544–53
7. Gunderson, H. M. and Nordlie, R. C. (1973). *Biophys. Res. Commun.*, **52,** 601–7
8. Howell, K. E., Ito, A. and Palade, G. E. (1978). *J. Cell Biol.*, **79,** 581–9
9. Andersson, G. N. and Eriksson, L. C. (1981). *J. Biol. Chem.*, **256,** 9633–9
10. Elhammer, Å, Peterson, E. and Dallner, G. (1983). *Biochim. Biophys. Acta*, **730,** 67–84
11. Berry, C. and Hallinan, T. (1976). *Biochem. Soc. Trans.*, **4,** 650–2

12. Zakim, D. and Vessey, D. A. (1982). In Martonosi, A. N. (ed).) *Membranes and Transport*. Vol. 1, pp. 269–73. (New York: Plenum)
13. Gollan, J., Blanckaert, N. and Hammaker, L. (1981). *Gastroenterology*, **80,** 1334
14. Blanckaert, N. (1980). *Biochem. J.*, **185,** 115–28
15. Ostrow, J. D., Hammaker, L. and Schmid, R. (1961). *J. Clin. Invest.*, **40,** 1442–52
16. Eriksson, L. C., DePierre, J. W. and Dallner, G. (1978). *Pharmac. Ther. A*, **2,** 281–317
17. Hino, Y., Asano, A., Sato, R. and Shimizu, S. (1978). *J. Biochem.*, **83,** 909–23
18. Blobel, G. and Potter, V. R. (1966). *Science*, **154,** 1662–5
19. Kay, R. R., Fraser, D. and Johnston, I. R. (1972). *Eur. J. Biochem.*, **30,** 145–54
20. Song, C. S., Rubins, W., Rifkind, A. B. and Kappas, A. (1969). *J. Cell Biol.*, **41,** 124–32
21. Yousef, I. M, Bloxam, D. L., Phillips, M. J. and Fisher, M. M. (1975). *Can. J. Biochem.*, **53,** 989–97
22. Lowry, O. H., Rosebrough, N. J., Farr, A. L. and Randall, R. J. (1951). *J. Biol. Chem.*, **193,** 265–75
23. Heirweigh, K. P. M., Van De Vijver, M. and Fevery, J. (1972). *Biochem. J.*, **129,** 605–18
24. Wishart, G. J. and Fry, D. J. (1980). *Biochem. J.*, **186,** 687–91
25. Zaleski, J., Bansal, S. K. and Gessner, T. (1982). *Can. J. Biochem.*, **60,** 972–9
26. Sabatini, D. D., Kreibich, G., Morimoti, T. and Adesnik, M. (1982). *J. Cell Biol.*, **92,** 1–22
27. Beaufay, H., Amar-Costesec, A. and de Duve, C. (1981). In Lee, C. P., Schatz, G. and Dallner, G. (eds.). *Mitochondria and Microsomes*. pp. 629–53. (Massachusetts: Addison-Wesley)
28. Franke, W. W., Scheer, U., Krohne, G. and Jarasch, E.-D. (1981). *J. Cell Biol.*, **91,** 39s–50s
29. Zhivkov, V., Tosheva, R. and Zhivkova, Y. (1975). *Comp. Biochem. Physiol.*, **51B,** 421–4
30. Dallner, G., and DePierre, J. W. (1982). In Arias, I., Popper, H., Schachter, D. and Schafritz, D. A. (eds.) *The Liver: Biology and Pathobiology*. Vol. 1, pp. 41–53. (New York: Raven)
31. Hauser, S. C., Ziurys, J. C. and Gollan, J. L. (1984). *J. Biol. Chem.*, **259,** 4527–33

25
The molecular masses and molecular structure of UDP-glucuronyltransferase as determined by radiation-inactivation analysis

W. H. M. PETERS, H. NAUTA AND P. L. M. JANSEN

INTRODUCTION

UDP-glucuronyltransferase consists of a group of enzymes with different substrate specificities, perinatal developmental patterns and induction profiles[1]. Several UDP-glucuronyltransferase isoenzymes have been purified and their subunit molecular weights have been determined[2–5].

With irradiation-inactivation analysis the protein molecular mass of membrane-bound enzymes can be determined *in situ*[6–8]. The minimal molecular mass necessary for enzyme function is determined with this technique. Membrane preparations have to be lyophilized to absolute dryness, and this represents the major limitation of the technique because the enzyme should survive this procedure. In a dry environment, only radiation hits in the enzyme protein molecule itself cause inactivation, and the rate of inactivation as a function of radiation dose is a measure of molecular size. Big enzymes are inactivated more rapidly than small enzymes because big enzymes have a greater chance to receive an inactivating radiation hit per unit time. Exact molecular masses of enzymes can be calculated from the rate of inactivation as a function of cumulative radiation dose. In aqueous environments free radical chain reactions will secondarily inactivate enzymes and the single-hit-one-target theory does not hold any more[6]. Furthermore, heat inactivation should be avoided, and we, therefore, have chosen a radiation dose which does not heat the enzyme preparation. The technique of irradiation-inactivation analysis has been validated by numerous studies on enzymes of known molecular weight[6]. In addition, enzyme structure can be assessed by this method. If enzymes consist of more than one subunit and a particular enzyme reaction is dependent on intactness of all subunits an inactivating radiation hit in one of the several subunits will abolish the activity of that particular enzyme reaction and the molecular mass of the complete oligomeric enzyme is obtained. However, if a particular enzyme reaction is dependent on only a single subunit in an oligomeric enzyme, only hits in that particular subunit will cause inactivation of the enzyme reaction, and the molecular mass of the single subunit is obtained. We have used this technique to study the molecular masses and structure of the UDP-glucuronyltransferase isoenzymes.

METHODS

Microsomes were prepared as described by Cuypers *et al.*[9]. Rat liver microsomes from phenobarbital-treated rats were used. Activation, lyophilization and irradiation of the microsomes were performed as previously described[10]. Enzyme assays and calculation of molecular masses was carried out as described earlier[10,11].

RESULTS AND DISCUSSION

Radiation-inactivation is performed on lyophilized microsomal preparations in the presence of 0.25 mol/l sucrose and 1 mmol/l dithiothreitol. Sucrose serves as a free radical scavenger, and dithiothreitol is present to avoid inactivation due to the possible formation of disulphide (S–S) bridges during lyophilization. The inactivation curves obtained are linear when plotted semilogarithmically, which indicates that the activities measured may reside in single functional units of, for example oligomeric enzymes systems[12], and that the one-hit-single-target theory holds. As endogenous marker enzyme the molecular mass of microsomal β-glucuronidase was determined. A MW of 74 800 was found, which is in excellent agreement with the results of other investigators using similar[13,14] or different techniques[15].

In Figure 25.1 inactivation curves for bilirubin UDP-glucuronyltransferase from human and rat liver microsomes are shown. In both cases, distinct inactivation curves are observed for the conversion of bilirubin (B) to bilirubin monoglucuronide (BMG) and for bilirubin monoglucuronide to bilirubin diglucuronide (BDG). This means that different molecular entities are involved in the formation of BMG and BDG, respectively. Kinetic data also indicated different catalytic units. Formation of BMG is a fast reaction with a low K_M^{UDPGA} (43 μmol/l) and conversion of BMG to BDG is much slower with a high K_M^{UDPGA} (1 mmol/l)[9]. However, in homozygous Gunn rats both glucuronidation steps are absent[16] and, therefore, we postulate that both steps are catalysed by enzymes with one or more common subunits. The present findings and data from earlier work may be combined in the hypothetical model for bilirubin glucuronyltranferase, presented in Figure 25.2. The BDG forming enzyme may be a tetramer, composed of two pairs of identical subunits. BMG may be formed by two identical subunits (1 and 2), which do not necessarily need to

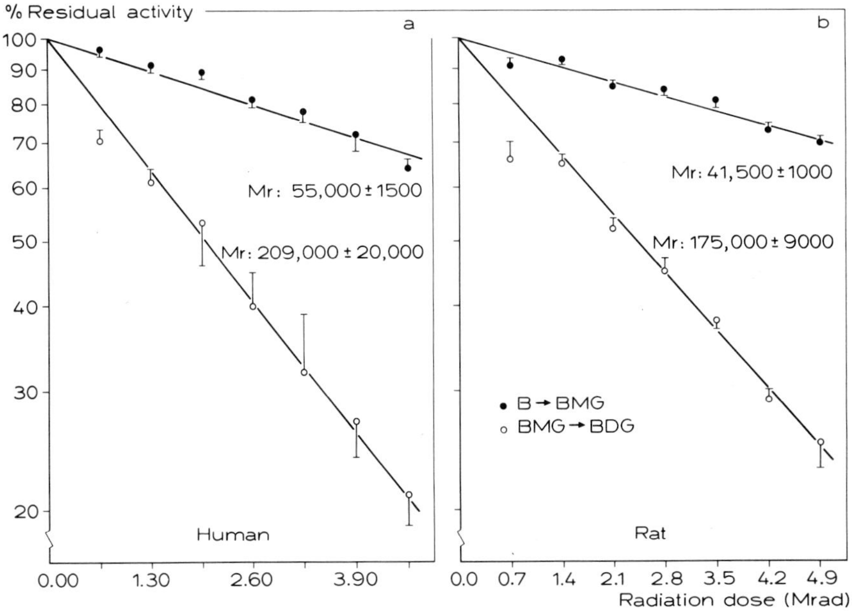

Figure 25.1 Radiation-inactivation of bilirubin UDP-glucuronyltransferase in SDS treated microsomes. BMG (●) and BDG (○) formation is plotted semilogarithmically versus radiation dose. Panel (**A**) shows the data obtained with human microsomes and panel (**B**) the data with Wistar rat microsomes. Values are given ±SE for at least three different microsomal preparations. BMG and BDG formation was determined using high-performance liquid chromatography and with bilirubin as substrate[9]

be combined with each other or with subunits 3 and 4 to be active. Conversion of BMG to BDG is restricted to the tetrameric enzyme. Subunits 3 and 4 are inactive by themselves. In the homozygous Gunn rat a defect in *one* subunit (1 or 2) implicates loss of both BMG and BDG forming activities.

Consistent with theories about mechanisms of enzyme action[17] both subunits within a pair (1 and 2; 3 and 4) are 'out of phase': one is engaged in accepting the substrate, whereas at the same time the other one is releasing the product. At the same time both subunits are in a different conformation. According to this model the enzyme obeys 'half of the sites reactivity', which means that under saturated conditions only half of the substrate binding sites are occupied[17]. These ideas on enzyme action are incorporated in the hypothetical model of Figure 25.2.

In Figure 25.3 the inactivation curves for *p*-nitrophenol (PNP) glucuronidation in Wistar and Gunn rat microsomes are shown. As for the forward reaction, the molecular mass of both enzymes is identical. For the *deconjugation* reactions however, different molecular entities were found: 59 000±7000 and 105 000±9000 for Wistar and Gunn rat, respectively. We earlier postulated that in the deconjugation reaction mainly the UDP/UDPGA binding part of the enzyme is involved and not the complete enzyme[11]. This may explain why in the Wistar rat the reverse reaction is catalysed by an enzyme with a small molecular mass, and the forward reaction by an enzyme approximately twice

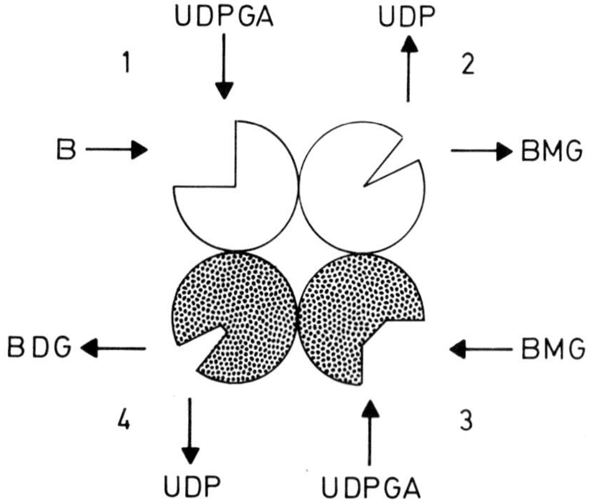

Figure 25.2 Molecular model of bilirubin UDP-glucuronyltransferase. Formation of bilirubin diglucuronide (BDG) is catalysed by a tetrameric enzyme (subunit 1–4) composed of two subunit pairs. Subunit 1 and 3 are identical to subunit 2 and 4, respectively, but are in a different conformation, so that only half of the binding sites are occupied. Formation of monoglucuronide (BMG) is catalysed by a single subunit (subunit 1 or 2)

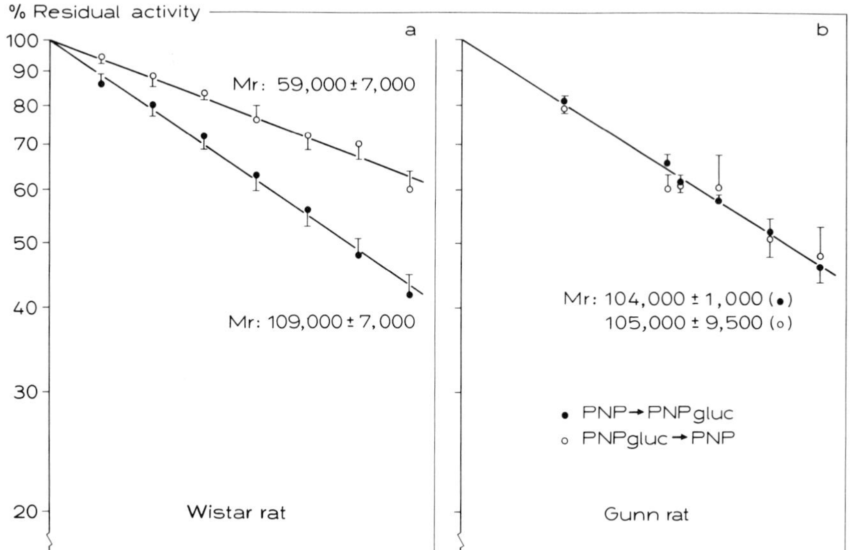

Figure 25.3 Radiation-inactivation of *p*-nitrophenol UDP-glucuronyltransferase. PNP conjugation (●) and PNP-glucuronide deconjugation (○) activity is plotted semilogarithmically versus radiation dose. Panel (**A**) shows the data obtained with Wistar rat microsomes and panel (**B**) with Gunn rat microsomes. Values are means of two different preparations

as big. In contrast, in the Gunn rat enzymes, with equal molecular masses, catalyse both forward and reverse reactions. We suggest the following model. In the Gunn rat not only bilirubin glucuronyltransferase activity is lacking but PNP glucuronyltransferase is also defective[18]. The defect of PNP glucuronyltransferase may be situated in the UDP/UDPGA binding site and comes to expression as decreased affinity of the enzyme for the nucleotide[18]. Whereas in normal functioning UDP-glucuronyltransferase for the reverse reaction to proceed only or mainly the nucleotide binding-site has to be occupied, in the Gunn rat both aglycone-glucuronide *and* nucleotide binding sites have to be occupied for catalysis of the reverse reaction. This might be the reason that in the Gunn rat the molecular mass found for the reverse reaction equals the molecular mass necessary for catalysis of the forward reaction. Whereas in the Wistar rat a part of the enzyme is capable of catalysing the reverse reaction, in the Gunn rat the complete dimeric enzyme is required. Table 25.1 summarizes the UDP-glucuronyltransferase radiation-inactivation data obtained so far[10,11,19], including a number of subunit molecular weights quoted from the literature[3,4,20–23]. Also included is the proposed molecular structure of the different UDP-glucuronyltransferase isoenzymes.

Table 25.1 UDP-Glucuronyltransferase molecular weight determined by radiation-inactivation analysis

Substrate	*Subunit MW* ($\times 10^3$)	*Radiation-inactivation analysis* ($\times 10^3$)	*Proposed structure*
Bilirubin	57 (Burchell[20])[a]	41.5± 1.0 (BMG)[a]	monomer
		175.0± 9.0 (BDG)[a]	tetramer
		55.0± 1.5 (BMG)[b]	monomer
		209.0±20.0 (BDG)[b]	tetramer
p-Nitrophenol	56 (Falany and Tephly[3])[a]	109.0± 6.0 (forward)[a]	dimer
	57 (Burchell[21])[a]	59.0± 7.0 (reverse)[a]	monomer
	59 (Gorski and Kasper[22])[a]	104.0± 1.0 (forward)[c]	dimer
	57 (Burchell[21])[c]	105.0±10.0 (reverse)[c]	dimer
Phenolphthalein	—	159.0±14.0 (forward)[a]	tetramer
		74.0± 8.0 (reverse)[a]	dimer
Testosterone	54 (Matern *et al.*[4])[a]	142.0± 5.0[a]	tetramer
	50 (Falany and Tephly[3])[a]		
Oestrone	57 (Tukey and Tephly[23])[d]	73.5± 9.0	dimer

a = rat, b = human, c = Gunn rat, d = rabbit
Values are presented ±SE for at least three different preparations. Values for the Gunn rat are ±SD for two different preparations

CONCLUSIONS

UDP-glucuronyltransferase consists of a group (homo and/or hetero) oligomeric enzymes with different substrate specificities. BMG formation is catalysed by a monomeric, and BDG formation by a tetrameric isoenzyme. Whether this tetramer is a homo- or hetero-tetramer remains to be elucidated, although kinetic data favour the latter possibility.

The reverse (deconjugation) reactions are catalysed by enzymes with smaller molecular masses than the enzymes catalysing forward (conjugation) reactions, with the exception of the Gunn rat. UDP-glucuronyltransferase isoenzymes probably are oligomeric enzymes consisting of one to four subunits, and only about half the total amount of subunits appears to be required to catalyse reverse reactions.

ACKNOWLEDGEMENT

This study was supported by a grant from FUNGO-ZWO.

References

1. Dutton, G. J. and Burchell, B. (1977). Newer aspects of glucuronidation. *Progr. Drug Metab.*, **2,** 1–70
2. Tukey, R. H., Robinson, R., Holm, B., Falany, C. N. and Tephly, T. R. (1982). A procedure for the rapid separation and purification of UDP-glucuronyltransferase from rabbit liver microsomes. *Drug Metab. Disp.*, **10,** 97–101
3. Falany, C. N. and Tephly, T. R. (1983). Separation, purification and characterization of three iso-enzymes of UDP-glucuronyltransferase from rat liver microsomes. *Arch. Biochem. Biophys.*, **227,** 248–58
4. Matern, H., Matern, S. and Gerok, W. (1982). Isolation and characterization of rat liver microsomal UDP-glucuronyltransferase activity toward chenodeoxycholic acid and testosterone as a single form of enzyme. *J. Biol. Chem.*, **257,** 7422–9
5. Bock, K. W., Josting, D., Lilienblum, W. and Pfeil, H. (1979). Purification of rat liver microsomal UDP-glucuronyltransferase, separation of two enzyme forms inducible by 3-methylcholanthrene or phenobarbital. *Eur. J. Biochem.*, **98,** 19–26
6. Kempner, E. S. and Schlegel, W. (1979). Size determination of enzymes by radiation inactivation. *Anal. Biochem.*, **92,** 2–10
7. Steer, C. J., Kempner, E. S. and Ashwell, G. (1981). Molecular size of the hepatic receptor for asialoglycoproteins determined *in situ* by radiation inactivation. *J. Biol. Chem.*, **256,** 5851–6
8. Lowe, M. E. and Kempner, E. S. (1982). Radiation inactivation of the glycoprotein, invertase. *J. Biol. Chem.*, **257,** 12478–80
9. Cuypers, H. T. M., ter Haar, E. M. and Jansen, P. L. M. (1983). Microsomal conjugation and oxidation of bilirubin. *Biochim. Biophys. Acta*, **758,** 135–43
10. Peters, W. H. M., Jansen, P. L. M. and Nauta, H. (1984). The molecular weights of UDP-glucuronyltransferase determined with radiation-inactivation analysis. A molecular model of bilirubin UDP-glucuronyltransferase. *J. Biol. Chem.* (In press)
11. Peters, W. H. M., Cuypers, H. T. M., Jansen, P. L. M., Nauta, H. and de Abreu, R. A. (1984). UDP-glucuronyltransferase catalyzed conjugation and deconjugation reactions. (Submitted for publication)
12. Verkman, A. S., Skorecki, K. and Ausiello, D. A (1984). Radiation inactivation of oligomeric enzyme systems: theoretical considerations. *Proc. Natl. Acad. Sci. USA*, **81,** 150–4
13. Beauregard, G. and Potier, M. (1982). Radiation inactivation of enzymes at low dose rates: identical molecular weights of rat liver cytosolic and lysosomal neuraminidases. *Anal. Biochem.*, **122,** 379–84
14. Shikita, M. and Hatano-Sato, F. (1973). Functional subunits of liver microsomal cytochrome P-450: molecular weight estimate by radiation inactivation. *FEBS Lett.*, **36,** 187–9
15. Stahl, P. D. and Touster, O. (1971). β-Glucuronidase of rat liver lysosomes: purification, properties, subunits. *Fed. Proc.*, **30,** 1121

16. Blanckaert, N., Gollan, J. and Schmid, R. (1979). Bilirubin diglucuronide synthesis by a UDP-glucuronic acid dependent enzyme system in rat liver microsomes. *Proc. Natl. Acad. Sci. USA*, **76,** 2037–41
17. Levitski, A., Stallcup, W. B. and Koshland, D. E. (1971). Half-of-the-sites reactivity and the conformational states of cytidine triphosphate synthetase. *Biochemistry*, **18,** 3371–8
18. Nakata, D., Zakim, D. and Vessey, D. A. (1976). Defective function of a microsomal UDP-glucuronyltransferase in Gunn rats. *Proc. Natl. Acad. Sci. USA*, **73,** 289–92
19. Peters, W. H. M., ter Haar, E. M., Nauta H. and Jansen, P. L. M. (1983). The molecular weights of UDP-glucuronyltransferase determined by target analysis. *Hepatology*, **3,** 811
20. Burchell, B. (1981). Bilirubin UDP-glucuronyltransferase. *Meth. Enzymol.*, **77,** 188–92
21. Burchell, B. (1978). Substrate specificity and properties of uridine diphosphate glucuronyltransferase purified to apparent homogeneity from phenobarbital-treated rat liver. *Biochem. J.*, **173,** 749–57
22. Gorski, J. P. and Kasper, C. B. (1977). Purification and properties of microsomal UDP-glucuronyltransferase from rat liver. *J. Biol. Chem.*, **252,** 1336–43
23. Tukey, R. H. and Tephly, T. R. (1981). Estrone and 4-nitrophenol UDP-glucuronyltransferases (rabbit liver). *Meth. Enzymol.*, **77,** 177–88

Section 7
Conjugation of Endogenous Compounds:
B. Bile Alcohols, Bile Acids, Lignans

Chairman: A. F. Hofmann

26
The biological utility of bile acid conjugation with glycine or taurine

A. F. HOFMANN, K. R. PALMER, Y.-B. YOON, L. R. HAGEY, D. GURANTZ, S. HUIJGHEBAERT, J. L. CONVERSE, S. CECCHETTI AND E. MICHELOTTI

BIOLOGICAL PERSPECTIVE

In higher vertebrates, bile acids, after their biosynthesis from cholesterol, are efficiently conjugated with glycine or taurine before secretion into bile. The conjugation involves linkage of the carboxylic group of the bile acid side-chain to the amino group of glycine or taurine to form an amide bond. Thus, bile acids are *N*-acyl-glycinates or *N*-acyl-taur(in)ates. The purpose of this article is to review the biological significance of bile acid conjugation with glycine or taurine, emphasizing two aspects. (1) Why has this mode of conjugation evolved for bile acids? To paraphrase, why are bile acids conjugated with glycine or taurine, rather than with glucuronic acid or sulphate, as is observed for most xenobiotics? (2) What would the consequences be for bile acid metabolism if this conjugation with glycine or taurine were not so efficient? Would it matter to the organism if a large fraction of bile acids were secreted into bile in unconjugated form?

PROBLEMS IN NOMENCLATURE

Bile acids are conjugated with glycine or taurine. Glycine (gly) is the simplest amino acid, but taurine (tau) is an amino acid analogue. Taurine belongs to a group of zwitterionic molecules used for osmotic regulation in bacteria, plants and animals[1].

For at least a century, the trivial names for the bile acid conjugates have featured the combining form glyco- or tauro- joined to the name of the bile acid, i.e. glycocholate, taurolithocholate, etc.[2]. (These names were proposed as soon as it was discovered that bile acids were coupled with taurine or glycine;

at this time, however, neither the mode of conjugation nor its influence on physicochemical properties were understood.)

We have argued for some years[3] that it seems preferable to reverse the sequence of the bile acid and its amino acid in the trivial names of the conjugated bile acid, to indicate that the bile acid is linked to the amino acid, rather than vice versa. This recommendation is based on the fact that the ionizing property of a conjugated bile acid is that of its amino acid moiety and not of its bile acid moiety. For example, the name taurocholate suggests that the carboxyl group of cholate is the ionizing group rather than the sulphonic acid group of taurine. In contrast, the name cholyltaurine implies that taurine is still present as a sulphonic acid. There are several advantages to this revised system for trivial names. (1) The non-bile acid expert can grasp immediately from the name that a taurine conjugated bile acid is a strong acid, rather than a weak acid. (2) The structure of bile acid conjugates becomes analogous to that of many peptides such as leucyl-glycine, etc. There has been considerable resistance to the acceptance of this scheme of nomenclature since the older names, such as glycocholate, have been used almost exclusively during the last century, and workers in this field, as in many others, appear to be fond of familiar names and resist the introduction of new names. It has also been stated that a change to a new scheme of nomenclature might confuse scientists in the future.

Regarding fatty acid nomenclature, the Committee on Nomenclature of the International Union of Pure and Applied Chemistry has recommended that the letter 'o' be added to the name of the parent acid, i.e. palmitoic (in place of palmitic). Were this to be done for bile acids, the simplest bile acid would receive the name 'cholanoic acid'. Were this to be applied to the trivial names of bile acid conjugates, one would obtain (adding an 'o' and replacing the 'i' by a 'y'), for example, lithocholoyl-taurine. In general, this has not been done in the bile acid field.

It is also debatable whether the amino acid present in a conjugated bile acid should be referred to as a glycine or a glycinate (and taurine or a taurinate). It seems simplest just to use 'glycine' and 'taurine', since the acidic moiety of these amino acids is fully ionized in most physiological situations, and indeed is ionized even when the substance is isolated in the crystalline form. However, if one crystallized a specific salt, one could justify calling it 'sodium cholyltaurinate', in our judgment. For physiological studies, it seems simplest merely to refer to a conjugated bile acid as, for example, cholylglycine, since the compound will be largely ionized at physiological pH, and the counter ion used to prepare its solution is not relevant.

Relatively few of the C_{24} bile acids have accepted trivial names. Only 20 or 30 bile acids have been named, and in the C_{24} bile acids which predominate in man, only six names are in common usage (cholate, chenodeoxycholate, ursocholate, deoxycholate, ursodeoxycholate, and lithocholate)*. Even these names are cumbersome to use, and in fact, are only partly trivial names. For example, chenodeoxycholate was named 'cheno-cholic acid' when it was isolated from goose bile; 'deoxy' was inserted some decades later, when it was

* In this paper the following abbreviations will be used, as recommended some years ago[4]: cholate (C); chenodeoxycholate (CDC); ursocholate (UC); ursodeoxycholate (UDC); deoxycholate (DC); and lithocholate (LC).

realized that chenodeoxycholic acid had one less oxygen atom than cholic acid. A new name for chenodeoxycholic acid has been proposed by US Pharmacopeial Convention, Inc. a company which assumes responsibility for publishing a dictionary of United States Pharmacopeia (USP) generic names for drugs. These names (United States adopted names) are to be used as generic names for drugs, and thus avoid the problem of trade names in the scientific literature when reporting results with a given drug. For chenodeoxycholic acid, the name 'chenodiol' is now approved. As yet, no generic name has been proposed for ursodeoxycholic acid.

Another problem is what to call the class of bile acids that are conjugated with glycine or taurine. It is now clear that not only sulphation of bile acids, but also glucuronidation of bile acids is a normal biological process. In addition, the work from Norman's laboratory[5] suggests that in cholestasis, bile acids are formed that are doubly conjugated, i.e. the hydroxy group is conjugated with glucuronic acid (by an ether bond) and the carboxy group with glycine or taurine (by an amide bond). In the past, when workers referred to conjugated bile acids, everyone knew that glycine or taurine conjugates were being discussed. Today, having the understanding that bile acids may be conjugated with glycine, taurine, glucuronic acid, or sulphate, we realize that the term 'conjugated bile acid' is ambiguous.

To remedy this situation, our group proposed, several years ago[6], following the original suggestion of Nair *et al.*[7], that bile acids conjugated with glycine or taurine should be referred to as 'amidates'; and the conjugation process with glycine or taurine should be termed 'amidation', analogous to sulphation or glucuronidation.

Time will tell whether these proposals have merit. In this paper, we will use the revised name for bile acid conjugates, e.g. cholyltaurine; we will refer to both glycine and taurine as amino acids; and we will refer to bile acids conjugated with these amino acids as amidates.

ENZYMOLOGY AND PHYSIOLOGY

Bile acid amidation occurs only in the liver and is mediated by two enzymes. The first enzyme is a cholanoyl-Coenzyme A ligase, which forms the Coenzyme A (CoA) thioester of the bile acid[8,9]. This activation is reversible, so that CoA derivatives are rapidly formed and hydrolysed (for review, *see* Ref. 9). The enzyme is present in the microsomes, and there has been considerable progress in its characterization[8].

The second enzyme is a cholanoyl-CoA amino acid transferase which transfers the bile acid moiety of the CoA bile acid thioester to glycine or taurine[10], forming the amidated bile acid and releasing CoA. The enzyme is present in the cytosol and has been purified[10,11]. This step, in contrast to the CoA ligase step, is irreversible. In some species, β-alanine may also serve as an acceptor. No other amino acids have been shown to act as acceptors, although extensive studies of taurine analogues have not been performed. There appears to be striking specificity in the structural requirements for the bile acid: nor-cholyl CoA[12], and presumably other nor-bile acid CoA thioesters (*see* below), show no reaction with the enzyme. In some species of mammals (for example the dog and cat), and in birds, reptiles, fish, amphibians, and reptiles, the amidation enzymes use taurine exclusively[13]. In the dog, if taurine becomes deficient, amidation does not occur; and unconjugated bile acids are secreted into bile[14]. In rodents and man, the rate of amidation with taurine has been shown to be linearly proportional to the concentration of taurine in the hepatocyte; but if taurine becomes deficient, amidation proceeds with glycine[13]. Thus, in these species, the mode of conjugation, i.e. the proportion of bile acids amidated with glycine or taurine, is influenced by the level of hepatic taurine. It is believed that the *total* rate of amidation, however, is not influenced by taurine availability (for review, *see* Refs. 9, 15, 16).

There are two sources of hepatocyte taurine. Taurine may be actively transported into the cell or synthesized (from cysteine-sulphinic acid via cysteine) (for review, *see* Ref. 17). In the rat, which has been studied in some detail, taurine is actively transported into the hepatocyte[18], and indeed, it seems probable that the same occurs in all species. Taurine, at least in the rat, is used exclusively for bile acid conjugation; accordingly, the hepatocyte concentration of taurine depends on the relative rates of transport into the cell (plus the rate of endogenous taurine synthesis) in relation to the rate of usage for bile acid conjugation. In man and cat, taurine cannot be synthesized, but is derived solely from dietary sources[19–21].

The current experimental evidence suggests that taurine availability [from transport and synthesis (in those species capable of *de novo* synthesis)] often lags behind the amidation rate; accordingly, taurine is said to be rate-limiting for bile acid conjugation[21]. The rate of taurine transport into the cell presumably depends on its concentration in sinusoidal plasma and the usual enzymatic kinetic parameters for its transport. Taurine is well absorbed from the diet, and addition of taurine to the diet enhances the concentration of taurine in the hepatocyte and the rate of bile acid amidation with taurine[16,20,21]. Thus, the working hypothesis is that in man, taurine availability does not influence the rate of total amidation, but only influences the proportion of bile acids conjugated with taurine.

The efficiency of bile acid conjugation has usually been assumed to be quite high as older analyses, using paper chromatography, indicated that unconjugated bile acids were not present in bile[22]. In our own studies in the hamster, we consistently found a small fraction (3–8%) of unconjugated cholate in bile, and if a radioactive unconjugated dihydroxy bile acid was given intravenously, a small fraction (2–5%) appeared in bile in unconjugated form[23]. The availability of improved analytical methods, such as high pressure liquid chromatography (HPLC) coupled with enzyme-based detectors[24], should permit the proportion of unconjugated bile acids in bile to be measured with accuracy in the future*. As will be proposed later in this chapter, if dihydroxy

* When using HPLC to separate bile acids, it is customary to quantitate the eluted peaks by measuring the amide bond absorbance at 200 nm. The unconjugated bile acids, lacking an amide bond, have much less absorbance at this wave length. An enzyme detector has been described by Okuyama *et al.*[24]. The detector is based on a coil containing immobilized 3-hydroxy-steroid dehydrogenase. The detector is reported to give an identical response to all bile acids with an unsubstituted 3-hydroxyl group, whether amidated or unconjugated.

bile acids are secreted into bile in unconjugated form, they are likely to be reabsorbed during their passage down the biliary tree. Accordingly, the previous hypothesis that bile acid amidation is nearly 100% efficient is likely to require modification for two reasons: first, the analytical methods were not sufficiently sensitive to detect small proportions of unconjugated bile acids; second, as will be proposed later in this essay, appreciable amounts of unconjugated bile acids are likely to be secreted into bile but reabsorbed in the biliary tree.

Bile acid amidates are actively transported out of the liver into bile by a canalicular transport system. The direction of transport for the common bile acid amidates is unidirectional; there is extremely little reflux of bile acid conjugates back into sinusoidal plasma (for review of data, *see* Ref. 25). (There is one exception to this generalization; both sulpholithocholylglycine and sulpholithocholyltaurine, sulphated amidates, show appreciable reflux from the hepatocyte into sinusoidal plasma in man[26].

PHYSICAL PROPERTIES OF BILE ACIDS AND THE EFFECT OF AMIDATION

Bile acids are amphipathic substances somewhat analogous to ionic detergents. One side of the molecule is hydrophobic, and the other side, which possesses the hydroxyl substituents, is hydrophilic. In solution, bile acids self-associate to form multimers or micelles. For a given bile acid, this association occurs over a relatively narrow concentration range called the critical micellar concentration (CMC), above which the molecules are present as micelles in equilibrium with monomers (whose concentration is approximately equal to that of the CMC). The common bile acids have CMC values ranging from 2 to 10 mmol/l[27]. It is possible to modify bile acid structure chemically so that the hydrophobic area of the bile acid molecule is diminished, for example by changing a hydroxyl group to an oxo (keto) group or from an α-configuration to a β-configuration. Such bile acids have considerably higher CMC values, and indeed, if both sides of the molecules are rendered hydrophilic, there is no micellar association whatsoever. *Thus it would appear that during biological evolution, the structure of the natural bile acids has been selected to give molecules that aggregate at relatively low aqueous concentrations.*

Bile acids do not occur in body fluids in simple micelles, but rather in the form of mixed micelles composed of bile acids and other lipids. The formation of mixed micelles occurs at a bile acid concentration well below its CMC. The biological 'purpose' of such a formation of mixed micelles is the transport of lipid molecules out of and into the organism: the micelles in bile transport cholesterol out of the organism; the micelles in intestinal content transport lipolysis products and fat soluble vitamins into the organism[28,29].

The CMC of bile acids is also influenced by the length of the side-chain. The natural C_{24} bile acids have a C_5 side-chain. If bile acids are prepared with a shorter side-chain, for example C_{23} bile acids, the CMC is considerably higher. Indeed, the logarithm of the CMC values rises linearly as the side-chain is shortened[27] from C_5 to C_4 to C_3. (The bile acids with one less methylene group in the side-chain are referred to as nor-bile acids; those with two less carbon atoms, as bis-nor bile acids.) It would be predicted that elongating the side-chain of bile acids, for example as with a C_{25} bile acid (termed a homo-bile acid), would further diminish the CMC value.

Amidation of bile acids with glycine or taurine elongates the length of the side-chain of bile acids, and, *a priori*, it would be predicted that an amidated bile acid would have considerably lower CMC values than its corresponding unconjugated precursor. In fact, this is not the case. In a study comparing the CMC values of unconjugated bile acids with those of their corresponding glycine and taurine amidates, it was found that amidation with glycine or taurine had no consistent effect on the CMC values[27]. Apparently the effect of elongation of the side-chain (which would tend to lower the CMC value) was fully counterbalanced by the effect of the polarity of the amide bond. This study thus indicated that amidation of the natural bile acids with glycine or taurine does not alter their amphipathic properties.

Amidation with glycine or taurine does, however, profoundly affect not only the physical, but also the physiological properties. Bile acid amidates are stronger acids than unconjugated bile acids. The natural bile acids, as any substituted isopentanoic acid, have a pK_a of about 5 [30]. This value is obtained at concentrations where they are dispersed as single ions; when present in micelles the pK_a (of the molecules in micellar state) is about 1 pK_a unit higher[31]. Glycine amidated bile acids have a pK_a of about 2.6; and taurine conjugated bile acids, <1. (The pK_a value of the bile acid amidates is also about 1 pK_a unit higher when they are present in micellar form.) A major change in physical properties caused by amidation is a greater solubility at acidic pH: solutions of glycine conjugated bile acids are generally stable above pH 5–6; and taurine conjugates are resistant to precipitation even under extremely acidic conditions[32,33]. A second change is resistance to heavy metal precipitation: taurine conjugated bile acids are quite soluble in the presence of high concentrations of calcium and other polyvalent metal ions.

Because of the lower pK_a values, the bile acid amidates remain charged at the pH present in bile (pH 7–8), and largely charged at the pH present in small intestinal content (pH 5.5–7.5).

INFLUENCE OF BILE ACID AMIDATION ON ENTEROHEPATIC CYCLING

The bile acid amidates which enter canalicular bile have a pK_a value of 2.6 or <1, and are fully ionized at the pH of canalicular bile which is probably about 7. Bile acids, whether conjugated or unconjugated, are too large to pass through the tight junctions connecting the epithelial cells of the biliary tract[34]; and their charge prevents dissolution in the lipid membrane of these cells. Accordingly, the current view is that none of the bile acid amidate molecules entering the biliary tract will be absorbed in the bile ducts, but all will reach the small intestine. *Thus, amidation of bile acids prevents their reabsorption in the biliary tree.*

The situation changes in the upper small intestine. Duodenal and upper jejunal pH fluctuates between 5.5 and 6.5, since acidic gastric contents which empty into the duodenal bulb are not always immediately neutralized by intestinal and pancreatic bicarbonate secretion[35]. As a consequence, a small fraction of the glycine conjugated bile acids are now present in protonated form.

Extensive studies of the rules of passive absorption of drugs and lipids have clearly shown that the rate of passive membrane permeation is directly proportional to hydrophobicity (measured operationally as the octanol/water distribution ratio)[36]. (The octanol/water distribution ratio is determined by the free energy of moving each part of a molecule from an aqueous environment to a non-aqueous environment; a major factor decreasing partition into octanol is the presence of polar groups which form hydrogen bonds with water molecules[37].) In general, charged molecules which are too large to traverse the aqueous pores are considered to have little or no passive absorption from the small intestine.

In jejunal content, during digestion, the concentration of bile acids is about 10 mmol/l. Using the Henderson–Hasselbalch equation, it can be calculated that the percentage of the glycine amidates that would be present in protonated form at pH 5.5 would be about 0.3%. Thus, the concentration of bile acids present in protonated form would be 0.03 mmol/l. Those bile acids whose steroid moiety is not too hydrophilic can be absorbed passively by dissolution (of the non-ionized molecule) in the lipid membrane of the enterocyte.

The influence of the chemical structure of the steroid moiety of bile acids on small intestinal membrane resistance to passive bile acid absorption has been defined by measuring the absorption rate of unconjugated bile acids using the perfused jejunum in the rat[38] or man[39]. Experimentally, it is found that dihydroxy bile acids with two α-OH groups are absorbed so rapidly that diffusion through the unstirred water layer becomes rate limiting[38]. Trihydroxy bile acids are well absorbed, but more slowly. The effect of the amide bond on membrane resistance, for a given state of ionization, is approximately equal to that of a hydroxy substituent. Thus, for a given degree of ionization, chenodeoxycholylglycine (with two α-OH groups) should be absorbed at about the same rate as cholate.

Although there is a lack of direct experimental evidence, a number of lines of indirect evidence suggest that glycine conjugated dihydroxy (and monohydroxy) bile acids are passively absorbed to some extent from the relatively acidic upper small intestinal content (for summary, see Ref. 40). (Some bile acid precipitation is also likely to occur[41].) *Thus bile acid amidation with glycine permits limited absorption of the most hydrophobic bile acids in the upper small intestine, but prevents absorption of the more polar bile acids. Taurine amidates are not appreciably absorbed.*

In the distal ileum, both taurine and glycine amidates are actively absorbed by an active transport system[28,29,42]. The anatomical localization of the site for active bile acid transport to the distal ileum results in bile acids being available throughout the entire small intestine to facilitate fat absorption. The initial uptake step involves a sodium coupled transport system[43], and it is likely that there may be a second carrier mediated transport system on the basolateral cell membranes of the terminal ileocytes[44].

INFLUENCE OF BILE ACID AMIDATION ON INTESTINAL BIOTRANSFORMATION

The amide bond of the glycine and taurine amidates of bile acids is resistant to hydrolysis by either pancreatic or enterocyte brush border peptidases. On the other hand, the amide bond of the natural bile acids is readily cleaved by bacterial enzymes which are known collectively as cholylglycine hydrolases[7].

Bacterial deconjugation of bile acids (which will be termed de-amidation) begins in the distal small intestine. De-amidation proceeds more slowly than active intestinal absorption, so that in healthy man, most bile acids are absorbed in the form of the intact amidate from the small intestine[16,25,28,29,45].

During enterohepatic cycling of bile acids, however, there is always some de-amidation of bile-acids with absorption of the liberated unconjugated bile acid moiety. This is absorbed in part and efficiently re-amidated in the liver. Thus, during the normal enterohepatic cycling of bile acids, there is continuous de-amidation and re-amidation of bile acids. The experimental evidence for this de-amidation and re-amidation is indirect, but convincing. If doubly-labelled bile acid amidates are prepared, for example [^{3}H]-cholyl-glycine-1-[^{14}C], the turnover of the glycine moiety is several fold more rapid than that of the steroid moiety[41]. The rate of deconjugation is readily assessed by the appearance of $^{14}CO_2$ in breath derived by bacterial and tissue catabolism of liberated glycine[28,45].

BIOLOGICAL BASIS FOR CONJUGATION WITH GLYCINE OR TAURINE

It seems curious that bile acids are conjugated exclusively with glycine or taurine, despite the great variety of amino acids potentially available for bile acid conjugation in the hepatocyte. It was known, as shown over a half century ago by von Beznak[46], working in the Verzar laboratory , that bile acid amidates were not cleaved by pancreatic trypsin. This idea was generalized to the widely accepted view that bile acids are resistant to all pancreatic enzymes. Additional evidence for this viewpoint was the finding that no de-amidation of bile acids was detectable in germ-free mice[47].

We wondered whether bile acids amidated with other amino acids would be equally resistant to pancreatic peptidases. To test this, we synthesized the choloyl amidates of a variety of the common α-amino bile acids. We found these were readily cleaved by human pancreatic juice, presumably by its carboxypeptidases. The only amino acid conjugate of cholic acid that was resistant to de-amidation by pancreatice juice was the aspartate conjugate[48].

Thus, bile acid amidation with glycine or taurine results in the formation of useful detergent molecules which are resistant to digestive enzymes. If bile acids were amidated with other amino acids in the liver, such amidates would be hydrolysed during digestion.

BIOLOGICAL BASIS FOR LACK OF CONJUGATION WITH GLUCURONATE OR SULPHATE*

A related question is why the naturally-occurring bile acids are not conjugated with glucuronate or sulphate. We do not know, but a few speculations may be useful.

Conjugation with glucuronate

If the natural bile acids were conjugated with glucuronate rather than with glycine or taurine, i.e. if the carboxyl group of the side-chain were esterified to the 1-hydroxyl group of glucuronate, the resulting O-acyl conjugates would probably have satisfactory detergent properties. The nature of the polar group in a detergent does not have an important effect on its CMC[49]. Such bile acid ester glucuronides could be actively transported into bile, since they could take advantage of the favourable electrical gradient, and an active transport system for bilirubin glucuronates is considered to be present. However, it seems possible that such bile acid ester glucuronides would be hydrolysed in the intestine by digestive enzymes. As they have not been synthesized, their susceptibility to pancreatic enzymes is not known. Huijghebaert[50] found that the 3-ether glucuronide of cholate was cleaved by the intestinal contents.

It is also to be noted that one naturally-occurring bile acid, hyodeoxycholic acid, is glucuronidated in the 6-position when given orally to man; the glucuronide is rapidly eliminated in bile and urine[51], so that the compound does not undergo an enterohepatic circulation and does not accumulate in bile when administered chronically[52].

Conjugation with sulphate

Bile acids can be sulphated only on the hydroxyl groups and, in cholestasis, such sulphated bile acids are formed at a greatly increased rate. The bile acid sulphates reflux from the hepatocyte and are rapidly secreted in urine[53,54].

Sulphation on a hydroxyl group should markedly change the physicochemical properties of bile acids, since the resulting conjugate now has two charges, one on the nucleus and one on the side-chain. The physicochemical properties of bile acid sulphates have not been defined.

In lower vertebrates, such as the shark, C_{27} bile alcohols are the major detergents in bile; after biosynthesis from cholesterol, they are sulphated on the terminal hydroxyl group of the side-chain to form an ester or 'ethereal' sulphate[55]. Thus, in these species, the bile salts arc bile alcohol sulphates, in contrast to the higher vertebrates where the bile salts are bile acid amidates[22]. The metabolism of such bile alcohol sulphates in man has not been defined.

Finally, it should be noted that the magnitude of bile acid amidation with glycine can be considerable (3–10 mmol/day)[45], because of the large flux of

* Although it is customary to refer to conjugation with glucuronic acid, we have used the term 'glucuronate' since glucuronic acid will invariably be ionized, even when present in the cell as UDP-glucuronate.

unconjugated bile acids which return from the intestine. The availability of sulphate may be rate limiting in sulphate conjugation[56,57] whereas there is an unlimited supply of glycine. Thus conjugation with glycine not only results in products that are resistant to hydrolysis in the small intestine, but it is also a process that uses a substance for conjugation which is present in an inexhaustible amount.

BIOLOGICAL CONSEQUENCES OF DEFICIENT AMIDATION: STUDIES WITH NOR-BILE ACIDS

To gain further insight in the biological significance of bile acid conjugation, it would be useful to have an animal model with a genetic deficiency in bile acid conjugation. Such a model exists for bilirubin metabolism. The Gunn rat lacks the ability to conjugate bilirubin with glucuronate, and this animal has been widely used to gain insight into the biological significance of bilirubin conjugation[58].

An animal model in which the liver is incapable of conjugating bile acids has not as yet been identified.

An alternative approach is to synthesize a bile acid whose side-chain is modified in such a manner as to preclude hepatic amidation. Lindstedt and Tryding reported in 1957 that nor-cholate (nor-C) was secreted in unconjugated form in the rat[59]. This observation was subsequently confirmed by Vessey *et al.*[60] and by O'Maille *et al.* in this laboratory[61]. Nor-C was secreted predominantly in unconjugated form. It induced the formation of a relatively large volume of bile. The choleretic properties of nor-C were considered to be explained by its relatively high CMC value[27].

Czuba and Vessey[12], as noted above, provided a biochemical explanation for these pharmacological observations. They prepared the CoA derivative of nor-C and showed that it did not react with the amino acid transferase. This observation, together with their earlier observation that the formation of CoA derivatives of bile acids is a rapidly reversible process, suggested that even if a nor-bile acid were converted to its CoA derivative in the hepatocyte, the CoA derivative should rapidly revert to the acid. (It is not known whether nor-bile acids are converted efficiently to the CoA derivative when they enter the hepatocyte.) At any rate, the view, until quite recently, has been that any nor-bile acid entering the liver cell would be secreted into bile in unconjugated form.

Our interest in nor-bile acids arose from quite different considerations. Chenodeoxycholic acid (CDC) and ursodeoxycholic acid (UDC) are now widely used for gallstone dissolution. A major problem in the therapeutic use of these bile acids is that the optimal dose for gallstone dissolution is relatively large – usually above 0.6 g/day[62,63]. This large dose is required, despite the excellent bioavailability of the administered bile acid, and is explained by relatively poor intestinal conservation of the amidates which are formed in the liver[40].

We reasoned that greater intestinal conservation would occur if a derivative of UDC or CDC could be prepared which would be secreted in bile largely in non-amidated form. We speculated that such a compound would undergo much more passive absorption in the small intestine, and its biological halflife would be much greater. Accordingly, smaller doses would be required for gallstone dissolution.

To this end, we synthesized nor-CDC and administered it intravenously to the hamster, an animal whose response to infused bile acid has been characterized extensively in our laboratory[23]. To our astonishment, we found that the response in the hamster differed strikingly from that observed for any other bile acid, in three ways: (1) nor-CDC induced a striking choleresis; (2) nor-CDC (and/or its metabolites) was recovered in bile more slowly than CDC; and (3) nor-CDC was incompletely amidated, but was biotransformed to unusual metabolites. After some thought, we surmised that nor-CDC was secreted into bile, but reabsorbed in the biliary ductules; we reasoned further that after absorption into the cholangiocytes, the nor-CDC would pass out of the cholangiocytes into the plasma of periductular capillary plexus which surrounds the biliary ductules, be transported to the hepatic sinusoid, and be resecreted into bile. Since that time, a large number of experiments have been carried out not only in the hamster, but also in the rat. The experiments have been extended to include a systematic comparison of nor-CDC and nor-UDC with CDC and UDC, as well as their respective conjugates. The overall aim of these experiments has been to test the hypothesis that nor-CDC and nor-UDC undergo such a novel enterohepatic circulation, and that such an uncommon hepatic transport pathway results in additional effects on bile flow and on hepatic biotransformaton of these dihydroxy bile acids.

Only the major findings of our work will be reported here, since they have been published in abstract form only[64–67], and additional experiments must be conducted to firmly establish the multiple speculations advanced below. Rather than present experimental results in chronological form, we will attempt to propose general principles that should apply to the metabolism and enterohepatic circulation of nor-bile acids (or for that matter any bile acid undergoing such a novel circulation). We will then show briefly that the experimental results are not in conflict with the principles that are corollaries of the hypothesis.

PRINCIPLES THAT SHOULD APPLY TO 'NON-AMIDATABLE' BILE ACIDS

If bile acids entered the hepatocyte and could not be amidated with glycine or taurine, a number of potential fates could be envisioned. First, they could undergo no biotransformation and either accumulate in the hepatocyte, be secreted into bile, or reflux from the cell into sinusoidal plasma and be secreted in urine. Second, they could be conjugated with glucuronate or sulphate (or both), and these conjugates could undergo any of the three possible transport schemes already mentioned.

If nor-bile acids were secreted into bile, they should remain in bile or be reabsorbed back through the canalicular membrane as they passed down the canaliculi, or, after they passed through the canals of Herring, or back through the epithelium of the bile ductules (cholangiocytes) according to the rules of passive absorption. In general, as noted, lipophilic substances will be absorbed in direct relationship to their hydrophobicity, or in inverse relationship to their hydrophilicity[36,68]. Charged molecules cannot be absorbed passively, once their size exceeds that of the paracellular aqueous pores. Only the uncharged form can be absorbed. Thus, passive absorption is pH dependent, just as the distribution ratio of any weak acid is pH dependent[36,69]. At a sufficiently alkaline pH, there will be little partition into the non-aqueous phase.

These considerations predict that unless the pH of bile was extremely alkaline, unconjugated nor-dihydroxy bile acids would be absorbed passively into the membrane of the canaliculus or the cholangiocyte. Presumably the nor-bile acid is secreted in ionized form from the hepatocyte and uses the canalicular active transport system; its reabsorption is in the uncharged form, so that a proton must be donated by an acid in the ductular bile. The obvious donor is carbonic acid. Thus absorption of a bile acid in protonated form is responsible for the formation of one bicarbonate anion. The passive absorption should be slowed, unless there is an active proton pump in the canalicular or cholangiocyte membrane.

We reasoned that the absorbed bile acid should dissolve in the lipid membrane of the canaliculus or the lipid membrane of the cholangiocyte and would be removed from solution. In so doing, it would lose its osmotic activity. The osmotic activity that it did possess would now have been transferred to the bicarbonate ion which was generated by the bile acid molecule accepting a proton from carbonic acid. The net result would be that bile acids moved intracellularly, yet left their initial osmotic effect in the canalicular or ductular lumen by generating a bicarbonate anion. The proposed scheme is identical to that proposed for short chain fatty acid absorption from the distal large intestine[70].

The cholangiocyte is drained by a periductular capillary plexus that originates from the hepatic arterioles and drains into the sinusoids[71]. Thus, bile acid molecules which enter the cholangiocyte would (somehow) pass through the cell and into the plasma of the periductular capillary plexus. They would return via this capillary blood flow to the liver and be extracted by the hepatocyte, to re-enter the liver cell. In the liver cell, they would be again secreted into bile, and thus cycle repeatedly between ductular bile and the hepatocyte.

Absorption of substances from the biliary ductules has been discussed for several decades. Guzelian and Boyer[72] showed, in a classic study, that glucose was absorbed from the biliary ductules, and proposed the term bilio-hepatic circulation. We suggest the name 'cholehepatic shunt' pathway. The choice of this term is based on the following considerations. (1) The name is etymologically correct, as both chole and hepato are of Greek origin. (2) The name is harmonious with the usual term 'enterohepatic' which is applied to the circulation of bile acids from the intestine to the liver. (3) The term shunt indicates a short cut from the usual route. (The term 'cholehepatic shunt' was suggested by Dr E. W. Moore.)

CONSEQUENCES OF A CHOLEHEPATIC SHUNT PATHWAY OF DIHYDROXY BILE ACIDS

Effect on bile flow

The bile acid dependent component of bile flow is considered to result from the osmotic activity of actively secreted bile anions into the canaliculus which pulls a flux of water and accompanying electrolytes through the tight junctions. Thus the bile acid dependent flow is directly proportonal to the number of osmotically active particles secreted into the canaliculus. If bile acid anions do not associate (or if this association does not change over the course of the experiment), there should be a linear relationship between canalicular bile acid secretion and bile flow. This slope of the curve relating bile flow to bile acid secretion has not been named, but it may be useful to propose the term 'apparent specific choleretic activity', which has the units of μl (bile)/μmole (bile acid). The apparent specific choleretic activity of conjugated synthetic bile acids with relatively high CMC values (>20 mmol/l) is higher (12–15 μl/μmol) than that of the natural conjugated bile acids (7–12 μl/μmol) that have low CMC values[23,73–76], presumably because these synthetic bile acids do not aggregate after secretion into bile.

Thus each time a nor-bile acid is secreted into the canaliculus, it should generate an osmotic flow of water and electrolyte. Yet, as noted above, when a nor-bile acid is absorbed in non-ionized form, its osmotic power is transferred stoichiometrically to luminal bicarbonate. The bile acid output measured in hepatic bile is the small amount of bile acid that has escaped ductular reabsorption. Accordingly, there should be a spectacular apparent specific choleretic activity of nor-bile acids, not because they possess any remarkable choleretic properties, but because most of the bile acid secretion through the canaliculus, which is responsible for canalicular bile formation, has not been recovered in hepatic bile. The magnitude of the canalicular secretion cannot be estimated from biliary recovery, just as, for the enterohepatic circulation, the amount of bile acid secretion into the intestine cannot be estimated by measuring faecal bile acids.

Effect on bile acid biotransformation

If nor-dihydroxy bile acids are not amidated with glycine or taurine, they remain in relatively non-polar form within the hepatocyte. Accordingly, it would be predicted that they would partition into the microsomes and might undergo biotransformation. It might be speculated that biotransformations which usually take place to a limited extent might be greatly increased; or novel biotransformations might occur. For bile acids, one considers additional hydroxylations of the nucleus or side-chain, oxidation of the nucleus, shortening of the side-chain, or conjugation of the nucleus, with sulphate, or conjugation of the nucleus with glucuronate (in an ether linkage), or conjugation of the side-chain with glucuronate (in ester linkage). The fate of the non-conjugated derivatives could be subsequent glucuronidation, sulphation, or amidation; no additional biotransformation would be anticipated for the conjugates.

The biotransformation products might be secreted in bile, or might reflux from the cell and be secreted in urine. If they were secreted into bile, their fate would depend on their polarity and charge. To the extent that polarity was increased or they were charged, they would escape ductular reabsorption and be secreted into hepatic bile. Thus the nor-bile acids would continue to recycle until all of the molecules had been converted to sufficiently polar derivatives that they could escape the vast lipid surface of the epithelium of the canaliculi and the cholangiocytes.

EXPERIMENTAL RESULTS

Hepatic uptake, transport, and biliary recovery of nor-dihydroxy bile acids

Nor-CDC and nor-UDC were rapidly extracted from the perfusate of the isolated perfused hamster liver. The mechanism of this uptake was not defined, but is presumably by passive lipophilic absorption (passive non-ionic diffusion). This belief is based on: (1) the finding that dihydroxy bile acids are absorbed rapidly and passively by isolated hepatocytes[77,78], and (2) the finding that nor-CDC and nor-UDC are rapidly and passively absorbed from the perfused rat jejunum[38].

Nor-CDC and nor-UDC were rapidly secreted into bile, but the time course of biliary secretion was much slower than that of the corresponding C_{24} homologue. Biliary secretion persisted for 6 h after the infusion was discontinued. Eventually more than 80% of infused nor-CDC or nor-UDC was recovered, based on measurement of biliary radioactivity. No appreciable urinary excretion occurred.

To test whether nor-UDC was transported into bile by the canalicular transport system, ursocholoyl-taurine (UCT) was infused at a supra-maximal rate (24 μmol kg^{-1} min^{-1}). This dose exceeded the maximal canalicular transport rate, yet the anaesthetized animals showed no ill-effects; apparently, this bile acid is devoid of hepatotoxicity, in contrast to many other bile acids[79]. During the infusion of UCT at a saturating dose, an infusion of nor-UDC was superimposed. The biliary secretion of UCT fell, and that of nor-UDC increased; thus competition of the two bile acids for the canalicular transport system appears to occur. (This experimental design was based on a similar experiment by O'Maille[76].)

Thus, together, these results suggest that nor-CDC and nor-UDC are rapidly extracted by the liver, rapidly secreted into bile by the canalicular transport system, and subsequently reabsorbed in part by the cholangiocytes.

Hepatic biotransformation

Nor-CDC and nor-UDC showed an uncommon pattern of hepatic biotransformation as compared to that of their corresponding C_{24} homologues. When radioactive CDC or UDC were given to bile fistula animals or the isolated perfused liver, the predominant form of biliary radioactivity was in the form of the glycine and taurine amidates. A small percentage ($<5\%$) escaped amidation. In addition, there was formation of two metabolites, one tentatively identified as the 3-oxo-derivative; the other, as an ester glucuronate.

In contrast, when nor-CDC and nor-UDC were administered, biliary radioactivity had an extremely complex pattern. Considerably more radioactivity (30–40%) was present in an 'unconjugated' fraction, the majority of which was the unaltered nor-bile acid. In addition, there was evidence of oxidation at the 3-position to form the 3-oxo compound, as well as formation of the ester glucuronates. The conjugated fraction was also quite complex. There appeared to be no formation of glycine amidates, only trace formation of taurine amidates, but extensive formation of glucuronides.

Thus, the nor-bile acids have deficient amidation, greatly increased type I biotransformations of the nucleus and side-chain (oxidation and hydroxylation), and a novel pattern of conjugation–glucuronidation.

Effect of nor-CDC and nor-UDC on bile flow

In early experiments, bile acid output was determined by the 3-hydroxysteroid dehydrogenase (HSD) end-point enzymatic method[80]. When bile flow was plotted against bile acid output, a spectacular choleresis appeared to be induced by nor-CDC and nor-UDC. For nor-CDC, the apparent specific choleretic activity was 200 μl/μmol, at least an order of magnitude higher than any previously reported values. This remarkable value did not astonish us, because we speculated that there was a great deal of ductular reabsorption of bile acids, so that the biliary secretion rate of bile acids was far greater than was determined enzymatically.

Some time later, we became aware that novel biotransformations of the nor-bile acids generated compounds which were not measured using the HSD method. Obviously, 3-oxo bile acids and 3-glucuronides do not react with the enzyme. Accordingly, we prepared 2,4-^{3}H and ^{14}C-labelled nor-CDC and nor-UDC, so that true biliary recovery could be determined. When bile flow was plotted against output of radioactivity, the apparent specific choleretic activity of these nor-bile acids became lower – 30–100 μl/μmol. This value is still higher than all previous values, and is considered to be caused by cholehepatic shunting.

In the hamster, the specific choleretic activity of UC derivatives is about 15 μl/μmol[23], and as these bile acids have quite a high CMC value (30–40 mmol/l)[27], this figure is likely to reflect the osmotic activity of bile acid monomers in this species. As the CMC values of the nor-bile acids are also somewhat above those of the natural bile acids, it may be possible to estimate, at least approximately, the amount of canalicular secretion and ductular reabsorption of the nor-bile acids. A precise calculation will be impossible because of the complexity of hepatic biotransformation. On the other hand, in unpublished experiments with N. Marassi, we have found that nor-DC also induces an anomalously large choleresis, and its only biotransformation pattern is nor-C, whose specific choleretic activity is easily measurable. Thus, in time, it may be possible to make a semi-quantitative estimate of transcanalicular and transductular flux of at least this bile acid with some confidence.

REPRISE: SIGNIFICANCE OF BILE ACID AMIDATION WITH GLYCINE OR TAURINE

In this essay, we have shown that hepatic amidation of bile acids with glycine or taurine results in the formation of amphipathic molecules that are not reabsorbed from the biliary tree and not degraded by digestive enzymes. By preparing derivatives that cannot be amidated, we have shown (or at least presented evidence consistent with the hypothesis) that such derivatives undergo a cholehepatic shunt pathway, causing a disproportionate choleresis, and leading to a novel pattern of hepatic biotransformation, presumably because of greater exposure to intracellular enzymes. (The remote possibility that nor-bile acids are more susceptible than the natural bile acids to biotransformation by tissue enzymes has not as yet been excluded.) *Thus, hepatic amidation with glycine or taurine appears to have a third benefit: it decreases hepatic biotransformation.*

We speculate that these observations on unnatural bile acids apply to natural bile acids. The natural unconjugated dihydroxy bile acids, when infused into the hamster, also cause a disproportionate choleresis, if compared to their corresponding amidates[23]. If these bile acids are incompletely amidated and undergo a cholehepatic shunt pathway, then their greater specific choleretic activity can be explained. Erlinger and his colleagues have shown that infusions of UDC can cause a remarkable choleresis[81], and further that this bile acid is conjugated with difficulty[82]. Again, were this bile acid to circulate via the cholehepatic shunt pathway, its anomalous choleretic properties would have an explanation.

Finally, we also speculate that drugs which are weak acids, and which are conjugated incompletely in the liver, and are secreted into bile in unconjugated form may also undergo such a cholehepatic shunt pathway. This could explain the choleretic activity of a number of polycyclic weak acids[83].

All of our experimental results do not exclude a specific effect of the nor-bile acids and/or their metabolite products on ion pumping by the hepatocyte. However, at the moment, we have been unable to design an experiment which would permit us to quantitate the magnitude of such an effect on the hepatocyte alone.

ACKNOWLEDGEMENTS

The Biliary Disease Research Laboratory is supported in part by NIH Grants AM 21506 and AM 32130 and a grant-in-aid from the Falk Foundation.

References

1. Yancey, P. H., Clark, M. E., Hand, S. C., Bowlus, R. D. and Somero, G. N. (1982). Living with water stress: Evolution of osmolyte systems. *Science*, **217,** 1214–22
2. Sobotka, H. (1937). *Physiological Chemistry of the Bile*, p. 202. (Baltimore: Williams and Wilkins)
3. Hofmann, A. F. (1972). Metabolism of the steroid and amino acid moieties of glycine and taurine conjugated bile acids in man. In Back, P. and Gerok, W. (eds.). *Bile Acids in Human Disease*, pp. 79–85. (Stuttgart: F. K. Schattauer Verlag)

4. Haslewood, G. A. D., Danielsson, H., Sjovall, J., Hofmann, A. F., Dowling, R. H. and Low-Beer, T. (1976). Recommendations on bile salt nomenclature. In Taylor, W. (ed.). *The Hepatobiliary System*, pp. 639–41. (New York: Plenum Press)
5. Hedenborg, G., Norlander, A., Norman, A. and Sundblad, R. (1982). Conjugation and excretion of ^{14}C-chenodeoxycholic acid during total extrahepatic cholestasis. *Scand. J. Clin. Lab. Invest.*, **42,** 557–61
6. Raedsch, R., Hofmann, A. F. and Tserng, K-Y. (1979). Separation of individual sulfated bile acid conjugates as calcium complexes using reversed-phase partition thin-layer chromatography. *J. Lipid Res.*, **20,** 796–800
7. Nair, P. P., Gordon, M. and Reback, J. (1967). The enzymatic cleavage of the carbon-nitrogen bond in 3α,7α,12α-trihydroxy-5β-cholan-24-oylglycine. *J. Biol. Chem.*, **242,** 7–11
8. Killenberg, P. G. (1978). Measurement and subcellular distribution of choloyl-CoA synthetase and bile acid-CoA : amino acid *N*-acyltransferase activities in rat liver. *J. Lipid Res.*, **19,** 24–31
9. Schersten, T. (1971). Bile acid conjugation. In Fishman, W. H. (ed.). *Metabolic Conjugation and Metabolic Hydrolysis*, Vol. 2. pp. 75–121. (New York: Academic Press)
10. Killenberg, P. G. and Jordan, J. T. (1978). Purification and characterization of bile acid-CoA : amino acid *N*-acyltransferase from rat liver. *J. Biol. Chem.*, **253,** 1005–10
11. Vessey, D. A. (1979). The co-purification and common identity of cholyl CoA:glycine- and cholyl CoA:taurine-*N*-acyltransferase activities from bovine liver. *J. Biol. Chem.*, **254,** 2059–63
12. Czuba, B. and Vessey, D. A. (1982). The effect of bile acid structure on the activity of bile acid-CoA : glycine/taurine-*N*-acyltransferase. *J. Biol. Chem.*, **257,** 8761–5
13. Vessey, D. A. (1978). The biochemical basis for the conjugation of bile acids with either glycine or taurine. *Biochem. J.*, **174,** 621–6
14. O'Maille, E. R. L., Richards, T. G. and Short, A. H. (1967). The influence of conjugation of cholic acid on its uptake and secretion: hepatic extraction of taurocholate and cholate in the dog. *J. Physiol.*, **189,** 337–50
15. Garbutt, J. T., Lack. L. and Tyor, M. P. (1971). Physiological basis of alterations in the relative conjugation of bile acids with glycine and taurine. *Am. J. Clin. Nutr.*, **24,** 218–28
16. Hepner, G. W., Sturman, J. A., Hofmann, A. F. and Thomas, P. J. (1973). Metabolism of steroid and amino acid moieties of conjugated bile acids in man. III. Cholyl taurine (taurocholic acid). *J. Clin. Invest.*, **52,** 433–40
17. Sturman, J. A. (1978). Biology of taurine in nutrition and development. In Draper, H. H. (ed.). *Advances in Nutritional Research*, Vol. 3. pp. 231–99. (New York: Plenum)
18. Hardison, W. G. M. and Weiner, R. G. (1980). Taurine transport by rat hepatocytes in primary culture. *Biochem. Biophys. Acta (Biomembranes)*, **598,** 145
19. Jacobsen, J. G. and Smith, L. H. (1968). Biochemistry and physiology of taurine and taurine derivatives. *Physiol. Rev.*, **48,** 424–511
20. Sturman, J. A., Hepner, G. W., Hofmann, A. F. and Thomas, P. J. (1975). Metabolism of ^{35}S taurine in man. *J. Nutr.*, **105,** 1206–14
21. Hardison, W. G. M. (1978). Hepatic taurine concentration in dietary taurine as regulators of bile acid conjugation with taurine. *Gastroenterology*, **75,** 71–5
22. Haslewood, G. A. D. (1967). Bile salt evolution. *J. Lipid Res.*, **8,** 535–50
23. Gurantz, D. and Hofmann, A. F. (1984). Influence of bile acid structure on bile flow and biliary lipid secretion in the hamster. *Am. J. Physiol.* (In press)
24. Okuyama, S., Kokubun, N., Higashidate, S., Uemura, D. and Hirata, Y. (1979). A new analytical method of individual bile acids using high performance liquid chromatography and immobilized 3-hydroxysteroid dehydrogenase in column form. *Chem. Lett.*, 1443–6
25. Hofmann, A. F., Molino, G., Milanese, M. and Belforte, G. (1983). Description and simulation of a physiological pharmacokinetic model for the metabolism and enterohepatic circulation of bile acids in man. Cholic acid in healthy man. *J. Clin. Invest.*, **71,** 1003–22
26. Cowen, A. E., Korman, M. G., Hofmann, A. F. and Thomas, P. J. (1975). Metabolism of lithocholate in man. III. Plasma disappearance of radioactivity after intravenous injection of labeled lithocholate and its derivatives. *Gastroenterology*, **69,** 77–82
27. Roda, A., Hofmann, A. F. and Mysels, K. J. (1983). The influence of bile salt structure on self-association in aqueous solutions. *J. Biol. Chem.*, **258,** 6362–70

28. Hofmann, A. F. (1977). The enterohepatic circulation of bile acids in man. *Clin. Gastroenterol.*, **6,** 3–24
29. Carey, M. C. (1982). The enterohepatic circulation. In Arias, I. M., Popper, H., Schachter, D. and Shafritz, D. A. (eds.). *The Liver*, pp. 429–65. (New York: Raven Press)
30. Fini, A., Roda, A. and De Maria, P. (1982). Chemical properties of bile acids. II. pK_a values in water and aqueous methanol of some hydroxy bile acids. *Eur. J. Med. Chem.*, **17,** 467–70
31. Ekwall, P., Rosendahl, T. and Lofman, N. (1957). Studies on bile acid salt solutions. I. The dissociation constants of the cholic and deoxycholic acids. *Acta Chem. Scand.*, **11,** 590–8
32. Hofmann, A. F. and Small, D. M. (1967). Detergent properties of bile salts: Correlation with physical function. *Ann. Rev. Med.*, **18,** 333–76
33. Small, D. M. (1971). The physical chemistry of the cholanic acids. In Nair, P. P. and Kritchevsky, D. (eds.). *The Bile Acids: Chemistry, Physiology and Metabolism*, pp. 249–356. (New York: Plenum Publishing)
34. Higuchi, W. I., Ho, N. F. H., Park, J. Y. and Komiya, I. (1981). Rate limiting steps and factors in drug absorption. In Prescott, L. F. and Nimmo, W. S. (eds.). *Drug Absorption*, p. 35. (New York: Adis Press)
35. McCloy, R. F., Greenberg, R. G. and Baron, J. H. (1984). Duodenal pH in health and duodenal ulcer disease: effect of a meal, Coca-Cola, smoking, and cimetidine. *Gut*, **25,** 386–92
36. Jackson, M. J. (1981). Absorption and secretion of weak bile electrolytes in the gastrointestinal tract. In Johnson, L. R. (ed.). *Physiology of the Gastrointestinal Tract*. pp. 1243–70. (New York: Raven Press)
37. Flynn, G. L. (1971). Structural approach to partitioning: Estimation of steroid partition coefficients based upon molecular constitution. *J. Pharm. Sci.*, **60,** 345–53
38. Dupas, J-L., Moreau, M. and Hofmann, A. F. (1983). Polymeric dyes are ideal non-absorbable reference markers for intestinal absorption studies. *Gastroenterology*, **84,** 1142 (abstract)
39. Hislop, I. G., Hofmann, A. F. and Schoenfield, L. J. (1967). Determinants of the rate and site of bile acid absorption in man. *J. Clin. Invest.*, **46,** 1070 (abstract)
40. Hofmann, A. F. (1983). Pharmacology of chenodeoxycholic and ursodeoxycholic acid in man. In Paumgartner, G., Stiehl, A. and Gerok, W. (eds.). *Bile Acids and Cholesterol in Health and Disease*, pp. 301–36. (Lancaster: MTP Press)
41. Zentler-Munro, P. L., Fine, D. R., Fitzpatrick, W. J. F. and Northfield, T. C. (1984). Effect of intrajejunal acidity on lipid digestion and aqueous solubilisation of bile acids and lipids in health, using a new simple method of lipase inactivation. *Gut*, **25,** 491–9
42. Weiner, I. M. and Lack, L. (1968). Bile salt absorption: enterohepatic circulation. In Code, C. F. (ed.). *Handbook of Physiology: Alimentary Canal*, pp. 1439–55. (Washington, DC: American Physiological Society)
43. Luke, H., Stange, G., Kinne, R. and Murer, H. (1978). Taurocholate sodium co-transport by brush border membrane vesicles isolated from rat ileum. *Biochem. J.*, **174,** 951–8
44. Simon, F. R., Molitoris, B. A. and Sutherland, E. (1984). Taurocholate (TC) receptors in rat ileum: identification and differences between brush border (BB) and basolateral membrane (BLM) binding. *Gastroenterology*, **86,** 1253 (abstract)
45. Hepner, G. W., Hofmann, A. F. and Thomas, P. J. (1972). Metabolism of steroid and amino acid moieties of conjugated bile acids in man. II. Glycine-conjugated dihydroxy bile acids. *J. Clin. Invest.*, **51,** 1898–1905
46. von Beznak, A. (1929). Die Wirkung von Trypsin auf die gapaarten Gallensaeuren. *Biochem. Z.*, **210,** 261–4
47. Gustafsson, B. E. and Norman, A. (1962). Comparison of bile acids in intestinal contents of germ-free and conventional rats. *Proc. Soc. Exptl. Biol. Med.*, **110,** 387
48. Huijghebaert, S. and Hofmann, A. F. (1984). A biological explanation for the specificity of amino acids used for bile acid conjugation. Abstract for presentation at *VIII Bile Acid Meeting*, September, Berne, Switzerland.
49. Shinoda, K., Nakagawa, T., Tamamushi, B-I. and Isemura, T. (1963). *Colloidal Surfactants. Some Physicochemical Properties.* (New York and London: Academic Press)
50. Huijghebaert, S. (1983). Intestinale Microbiele Galzuur-Sulfatase-Aktiviteit Pharm. Sci. D. *Doctoral Thesis*. University of Leuven (Belgium)

51. Sacquet, E., Parquet, M., Riottot, M., Raizman, A., Jarrige, P., Huguet, C. and Infante, R. (1983). Intestinal absorption, excretion, and biotransformation of hyodeoxycholic acid in man. *J. Lipid Res.*, **24,** 604–13
52. Thistle, J. L. and Schoenfield, L. J. (1971). Induced alterations in composition of bile of persons having cholelithiasis. *Gastroenterology*, **61,** 488–96
53. Stiehl, A. (1977). Disturbances of bile acid metabolism in cholestasis. *Clin. Gastroenterol.*, **6,** 45–67
54. van Berge Henegouwen, G. P., Brandt, K-H., Eyssen, H. and Parmentier, G. (1976). Sulfated and unsulfated bile acids in serum bile and urine of patients with cholestasis. *Gut*, **17,** 861–9
55. Hoshita, T. and Kazuno, T. (1968). Chemistry and metabolism of bile alcohols and higher bile acids. In Paoletti, R. and Kritchevsky, D. (eds.). *Advances in Lipid Research*, pp. 207–54. (New York: Academic Press)
56. Levy, G., Galinsky, R. E. and Lin, J. H. (1982). Pharmacokinetic consequences and toxicity implications of endogenous substrate depletion. *Drug Metab. Rev.*, **13,** 1009–20
57. Krijgsheld, K. R., Scholtens, E. and Mulder, G. J. (1982). The dependence of the rate of sulphate conjugation on the plasma concentration of inorganic sulphate in the rat *in vivo. Biochem. Pharmacol.*, **31,** 3997–4000
58. Blankaert, N. and Schmid, R. (1982). Physiology and pathophysiology of bilirubin metabolism. In Zakim, D. and Boyer, T. D. (eds.). *Hepatology*, pp. 246–96. (Philadelphia: W. B. Saunders)
59. Lindstedt, S. and Tryding, N. (1957). On the metabolism of bishomocholic, homocholic, and norcholic acid in the rat. *Ark. Kemie*, **11,** 137–44
60. Vessey, D. A., Whitney, J. and Gollan, J. L. (1983). The role of conjugation reactions in enhancing biliary secretion of bile acids. *Biochem. J.*, **214,** 923–7
61. O'Maille, E. R. L., Kozmary, S. V., Hofmann, A. F. and Gurantz, D. (1984). Differing effects of norcholate and cholate on bile flow and biliary lipid secretion in the rat. *Am. J. Physiol.*, **246,** G67–G71
62. Stiehl, A. (1981). Effects of chenodeoxycholic acid and ursodeoxycholic acid on bile acid and biliary lipid metabolism in patients with radiolucent gallstones. Correlation with efficacy and toxicity. In Paumgartner, G., Stiehl, A. and Gerok, W. (eds.). *Bile Acids and Lipids*. pp. 309–17. (Lancaster: MTP Press)
63. Erlinger, S., Le Go, A. and Husson, J. M. (1984). Franco–Belgian study of ursodeoxycholic acid in the medical dissolution of gallstones: A double-blind randomized dose-response study and comparison with chenodeoxycholic acid. *Hepatology*, **4,** 308–14
64. Palmer, K. R., Gurantz, D., Hofmann, A. F. and Ljungwe, E. B. (1983). Novel choleretic properties of nor-chenodeoxycholate. *Hepatology*, **3,** 816 (abstract)
65. Palmer, K. R., Hofmann, A. F., Gurantz, D., Ljungwe, E. B. and Michelotti, E. L. (1984). The singular conjugation pattern of nor-chenodeoxycholate, a bile acid with a shortened side chain. *Gastroenterology*, **86,** 1335 (abstract)
66. Yoon, Y. B., Hagey, L. R., Gurantz, D., Cecchetti, S. and Hofmann, A. F. (1984). The unusual physiological properties of nor-ursodeoxycholate. *Hepatology*. (In press) (abstract)
67. Hagey, L. R., Yoon, Y. B., Gurantz, D., Michelotti, E. and Hofmann, A. F. (1984). Unique hepatic biotransformation of nor-ursodeoxycholate: a clue to the biological significance of bile acid conjugation. *Hepatology*. (In press) (abstract)
68. Diamond, J. M. and Wright, E. M. (1969). Biological membranes: the physical basis of ion and non-electrolyte selectivity. *Ann. Rev. Physiol.*, **31,** 581–646
69. Golumbic, C., Orchin, M. and Weller, S. (1949). Partition studies on phenols. Relation between partition coefficient and ionization constant. *J. Am. Chem. Soc.*, **71,** 2624–7
70. Von Engelhardt, W. and Rechkemmer, G. (1984). Colonic transport of short-chain fatty acids and the importance of the microclimate. In Skadhauge, E. and Heintze, K. (eds.). *Intestinal Absorption and Secretion*, pp. 93–101. (Lancaster: MTP Press)
71. Rappaport, A. M. (1980). Hepatic blood flow: morphologic aspects and physiologic regulation. In Javitt, N. B. (ed.). *Liver and Biliary Tract, Physiology I. International Review of Physiology*, Vol. 24, pp. 1–63. (Baltimore: University Park Press)
72. Guzelian, P. and Boyer, J. L. (1974). Glucose reabsorption from bile – evidence for a biliohepatic circulation. *J. Clin. Invest.*, **53,** 526–35
73. Sewell, R., Hoffman, N. E., Smallwood, R. and Cockbain, S. (1980). Bile acid structure

and bile formation: a comparison of hydroxy and keto bile acids. *Am. J. Physiol.*, **239,** G10–G17

74. Danzinger, R. G., Nakagaki, M., Hofmann, A. F. and Ljungwe, E. B. (1984). Differing effects of hydroxy-7-oxotaurine conjugated bile acids on bile flow in the dog. *Am. J. Physiol.*, **246,** G166–G172
75. Cummings, S. A. and Hofmann, A. F. (1984). Physiological determinants of biliary calcium secretion in the dog. *Gastroenterology*, **87,** 664–73
76. O'Maille, E. R. L. and Richards, T. G. (1976). The secretory characteristics of dehydrocholate in the dog: Comparison with the neutral bile salts. *J. Physiol.*, **261,** 333–57
77. Van Dyke, R. W., Stephens, J. E. and Scharschmidt, B. F. (1982). Bile acid transport in cultured rat hepatocytes. *Am. J. Physiol.*, **243,** G484–92
78. Bartholomew, T. C. and Billing, B. H. (1983). The effect of 3-sulphation and taurine conjugation on the uptake of chenodeoxycholic acid by rat hepatocytes. *Biochim. Biophys. Acta*, **754,** 101–9
79. Hardison, W. G. M., Hatoff, D. E., Miyai, K. and Weiner, R. G. (1981). The nature of bile acid maximum secretory rate in the rat. *Am. J. Physiol., Gastrointestinal and Liver Physiology*, **4,** G337–44
80. Turley, S. D. and Dietschy, J. M. (1978). Reevaluation of the 3α-hydroxy-steroid dehydrogenase assay for total bile acids in bile. *J. Lipid Res.*, **19,** 924–8
81. Dumont, M., Erlinger, S. and Uchman, S. (1980). Hypercholeresis induced by ursodeoxycholic acid and 7-ketolithocholic acid in the rat. Possible role of bicarbonate transport. *Gastroenterology*, **79,** 82–9
82. Zouboulis-Vafiadis, I., Dumont, M. and Erlinger, S. (1982). Conjugation is rate limiting in hepatic transport of ursodeoxycholate in the rat. *Am. J. Physiol.*, **243,** G208–13
83. Cook, D. L., Bianchi, R. G. and Hambourge, W. E. (1950). Studies on five long-acting choleretics. *J. Pharmacol. Exp. Ther.*, **100,** 421–8

27
Direct analysis of bile alcohol glucuronides in urine of patients with cerebrotendinous xanthomatosis

B. EGESTAD, P. PETTERSSON, S. SKREDE AND J. SJÖVALL

INTRODUCTION

Patients with cerebrotendinous xanthomatosis (CTX) excrete large amounts of bile alcohols in urine[1,2]. The behaviour on ion exchangers and hydrolysis by β-glucuronidase indicate that the main part of these compounds is conjugated with glucuronic acid. In order to obtain direct evidence for the nature of the conjugates we have analysed extracts of urine with fast atom bombardment (FAB) mass spectrometry[3]. It also appeared likely that this method would provide a rapid means for the diagnosis of CTX, as has been shown for inborn errors of steroid hormone biosynthesis[4].

The results reported in this paper show that bile alcohol glucuronides are readily detected by FAB mass spectrometry of extracts of urine from CTX patients, and that the method provides a rapid and unambiguous diagnosis of the disease.

MATERIALS AND METHODS

Samples of urine from a patient with CTX (A. F., 42 years old, female, clinical data described previously[5]) and a healthy niece (daughter of a sister of A. F. – I. J. who also suffers from CTX) were studied. The samples were kept at −20°C until analysed. One ml of urine was extracted with a Sep-Pak C_{18} cartridge, and 80 μg of sodium taurocholate were added as internal standard to the methanol eluate. The solvent was evaporated, the residue was dissolved in 0.5 ml 70% (v/v) aqueous methanol and 0.5 ml of glycerol was added. About 2 μl of the thoroughly mixed solution was placed on the probe tip for FAB mass spectrometry. A VG 7070E (VG Analytical Ltd, Manchester, England) double focussing instrument equipped with a FAB source and Ion Tech atom gun was used. Argon was used as the bombarding gas and spectra of positive and negative ions were recorded.

RESULTS AND DISCUSSION

The urine extracts, with added sodium taurocholate, gave intense spectra both in the positive and negative mode of operation. In agreement with the results of studies of conjugated steroids[3] and bile acids[6], the spectra of positive ions were more complex than those of the negative ones. This is due to the formation of positive ions with different numbers of cations (sodium, potassium) for each acid present in the sample. Thus, the negative ion spectra were much simpler and more useful for analysis of urine samples. These spectra were dominated by quasimolecular ions with a mass corresponding to $[M-H]^-$ (where M signifies the undissociated acid).

With the amounts of urine extract analysed, samples from the healthy subject only gave ions originating from the added taurocholate in the high mass region (Figure 27.1). Samples from the CTX patient gave a series of ions corresponding to $[M-1]^-$ of bile alcohol glucuronides (Figure 27.1). The peaks at m/z 611, 627, 643 and 659 correspond to glucuronides of C_{27} bile alcohols with 4, 5, 6 and 7 hydroxyl groups, respectively. The occurrence of such bile alcohols in urine has been shown by gas chromatographic–mass spectrometric analyses of their trimethylsilyl ethers after hydrolysis[1,2] (and unpublished results). If it is assumed that all bile alcohol glucuronides give the same yield of quasimolecular ions, the relative amounts of tetrols, pentols, hexols and heptols can be calculated from the respective ion clusters to be about 15, 55, 25 and 5%, respectively. Although the accuracy of this type of quantitation is probably low, the result is in reasonable agreement with that obtained by gas chromatographic analysis after hydrolysis.

In addition to the peaks due to C_{27} bile alcohol glucuronides, a small peak (larger than that of an isotope peak) is observed at m/z 613. This corresponds to $[M-H]^-$ of a C_{26}-pentol glucuronide known to be present in urine of healthy subjects and patients with cholestasis[1]. This compound, or an isomer, is also found in urine from CTX patients[1] (unpublished). The concentration in urine from healthy subjects is too low to permit detection with the amounts analysed in this study.

Because of the high and typical excretion of bile alcohols in urine of patients with CTX, very little sample is required to obtain FAB spectra of the glucuronides. The amount put on the probe to obtain the spectra shown in Figure 27.1 corresponds to $2\,\mu l$ of urine and $0.16\,\mu g$ of taurocholate. Thus, it would be possible to put urine directly in glycerol on the probe, but a Sep-Pak extraction was performed to decrease the concentration of cations and to minimize contamination of the ion source. If the yield of quasimolecular ions of taurocholate and bile alcohol glucuronides were the same (which is unlikely to be the case, taurocholate probably producing a more intense spectrum), the concentration of bile alcohol glucuronides is calculated to be about $200\,\mu g/ml$.

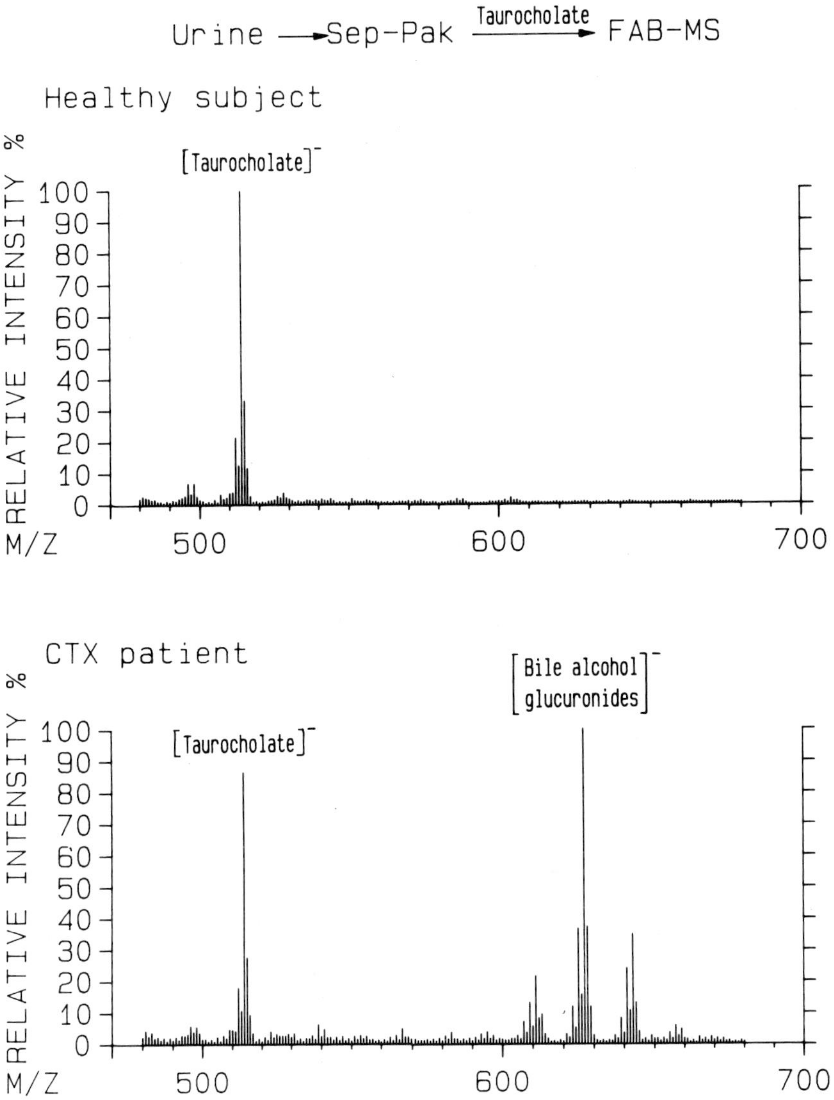

Figure 27.1 High mass region of the negative ion spectra obtained with extracts of urine from a healthy subject (top) and a patient with CTX (bottom). Sodium taurocholate (m/z 514, $[M-H]^-$) was added as internal standard

The value measured by gas chromatography after hydrolysis was about 300 μg/ml (700 μmol/day)[1].

The FAB mass spectra strongly support the identification of the bile alcohol conjugates in urine as glucuronides. This is in agreement with previous indirect evidence[1,2], and with the identification of bile alcohol glucuronides in bile of patients with CTX[7].

There is no other known disease with high excretion of bile alcohol glucuronides in urine. Thus, FAB mass spectrometry can give an unambiguous diagnosis of CTX in less than half an hour after the collection of a urine sample. The method should be further examined with a view to direct analysis of the amniotic fluid for the prenatal diagnosis of cerebrotendinous xanthomatosis. In the normal fetus, bile acid conjugates have been found in the gall bladder at least as early as a gestational age of 22 weeks[8].

ACKNOWLEDGEMENTS

This work was supported by grants from the Swedish Medical Research Council (grant no. 03X-219) and the Council for Planning and Coordination of Research (grant for purchase of the VG 7070E).

References

1. Karlaganis, G., Karlaganis, V. and Sjövall, J. (1983). Bile alcohol glucuronides in urine: Secondary metabolites of intermediates in the formation of bile acids from cholesterol? In Paumgartner, G., Stiehl, A. and Gerok, W. (eds.) *Bile Acids and Cholesterol in Health and Disease*. pp. 119–27. (Lancaster: MTP Press)
2. Wolthers, B. G., Volmer, M., van der Molen, J., Koopman, B. J., de Jager, A. E. J. and Waterreus, R. J. (1983). Diagnosis of cerebrotendinous xanthomatosis (CTX) and effect of chenodeoxycholic acid therapy by analysis of urine using capillary gas chromatography. *Clin. Chim. Acta*, **131,** 53–65
3. Shackleton, C. H. L. and Straub, K. M. (1982). Direct analysis of steroid conjugates: The use of secondary ion mass spectrometry. *Steroids*, **40,** 35–51
4. Shackleton, C. H. L. (1983). Inborn errors of steroid biosynthesis: Detection by a new mass spectrometric method. *Clin. Chem.*, **29,** 246–9
5. Oftebro, H., Björkhem, I., Skrede, S., Schreiner, A. and Pedersen, J. I. (1980). Cerebrotendinous xanthomatosis: a defect in mitochondrial 26–hydroxylation required for normal biosynthesis of cholic acid. *J. Clin. Invest.*, **65,** 1418–30
6. Whitney, J. O., Lewis, S., Straub, K. M., Thaler, M. M. and Burlingame, A. L. (1981). Analysis of conjugated bile salts in human duodenal bile using fast atom bombardment and field desorption mass spectrometry. *Koenshu-Iyo Masu Kenkyukai*, **6,** 33–44
7. Hoshita, T., Yasuhara, M., Une, M., Kibe, A., Itoga, E., Kito, S. and Kuramoto, T. (1980). Occurrence of bile alcohol glucuronides in bile of patients with cerebrotendinous xanthomatosis. *J. Lipid Res.*, **21,** 1015–21
8. Bongiovanni, A. M. (1965). Bile acid content of gall bladder of infants, children and adults. *J. Clin. Endocrinol. Metab.*, **25,** 678–85

28
Glucuronidation of bile alcohols in liver disease

G. KARLAGANIS AND P.-Y. ZAUGG

INTRODUCTION

Hepatic glucuronidation of relatively insoluble exogenous and endogenous compounds is important in promoting their excretion. The non-steroidal anti-inflammatory drug zomepirac, which undergoes hepatic 'ester' glucuronidation in excess of 90%, has been investigated as a model compound for studying glucuronidation in patients with cirrhosis of the liver. It was found that in cirrhotics the apparent oral clearance of zomepirac was significantly reduced, in parallel with galactose elimination capacity, suggesting that the functioning liver cell mass is the major determinant of the rate of zomepirac disposition. Presumably, therefore, ester-glucuronidation may be abnormal in liver disease[1]. In contrast, however, other investigators have shown that ether-glucuronidation of oxazepam, lorazepam and morphine proceed normally even in the presence of severe hepatic impairment[2–4]. In order to determine whether glucuronidation of endogenous substrates is affected in hepatic disease, we measured unconjugated and glucuronidated bile alcohols in urine from 12 female patients with primary biliary cirrhosis (PBC) and from six age and sex matched healthy volunteers.

Bile alcohols have the bile acid type of nuclear structure and a sterol side-chain containing one or several hydroxyl groups. They can probably be regarded as intermediates and side-products from the normal pathways in bile acid biosynthesis[5]. The major urinary bile alcohol in man has been found to be 27-nor-5β-cholestane-3α,7α,12α,24,25-pentol (C_{26} pentol)[6–9], which was also measured in this study in its unconjugated and glucuronidated form (Figure 28.1)

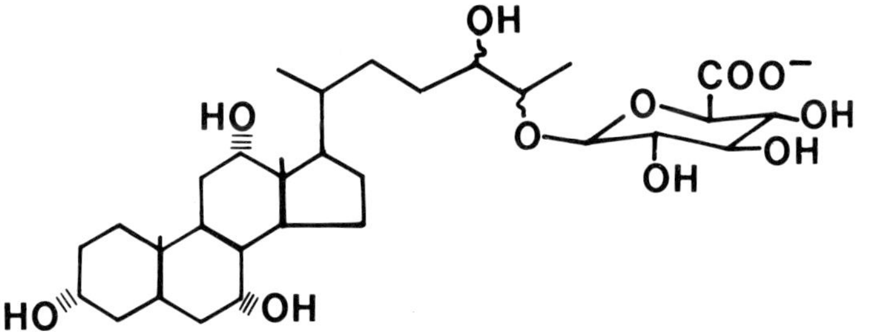

Figure 28.1 Structure of the major urinary bile alcohol 27-nor-5β-cholestane-3α,7α,12α,24,25-pentol glucuronide (C_{26} pentol glucuronide). The position of the glucuronyl moiety is based on data derived from mass spectra of the intact glucuronide[6], but needs to be confirmed by microchemical reactions

MATERIALS AND METHODS

Subjects

Twelve female patients with primary biliary cirrhosis (stage II–IV), aged 43–76 years (mean age 58), and six healthy female volunteers, aged 45–60 years (mean age 63), were studied. Diagnosis was based on typical clinical and laboratory findings, including positive antimitochondrial antibodies with titres over 1 : 100 and elevated IgM levels in plasma over 3.8 g/l. To assess functional impairment of the liver, galactose elimination capacity was measured[10] and aminopyrine breath test was performed[11,12]. The diagnosis was confirmed by percutaneous biopsy.

Collection of samples

Twenty-four hour urine samples were collected and kept refrigerated at −20°C until analysis. After overnight fasting, 10 ml of blood was taken (in the morning of the same day of urine collection).

Analysis of bile alcohols

Fifty ml of filtered urine was submitted to analysis of bile alcohols, as previously described by Karlaganis *et al.*[13]. Briefly, [^{14}C]testosterone glucuronide (kind gift of Prof S. Matern, Freiburg, FRG) was added for estimation of recoveries. Bile alcohols were extracted using Sep-Pak C_{18} cartridges. The extract was filtered over a column of SP-Sephadex C25 in H^+ form. The unconjugated (free) bile alcohol fraction and the bile alcohol glucuronide fraction were isolated by ion-exchange chromatography on Lipidex-DEAP. Bile alcohol glucuronides were hydrolysed at 37°C for 20 h with β-glucuronidase from *Helix pomatia* intestinal juice. Hydrolysed steroids were extracted with Sep-Pak C_{18} cartridges and further purified by filtration through Lipidex-DEAP. Twenty-five nmol of coprostanol were added as internal standard to both the unconjugated and the glucuronide fraction for analysis by computerized combined capillary gas chromatography–mass spectrometry (GC–MS). Bile alcohols were converted to trimethylsilyl (TMS) ethers and dissolved in 50 μl of hexane.

GC–MS was carried out using an automated Finnigan 1020 instrument equipped with a persilanized glass capillary column coated[14] with OV-73. Operational conditions were as follows: temperature of injector and GC–MS interface both 250°C; splitless injection was performed. The column temperature was increased from 70 to 260°C by 20°C/min. Helium was used as the carrier gas. The energy of bombarding electrons was 32 eV. Repetitive magnetic scanning was carried out over the mass range of 34–800 atomic mass units. Peak areas of mass chromatograms were quantified by the data system of the GC–MS for m/z 321 (C_{26} pentol) and for m/z 370 (internal standard coprostanol), and the ratio of the two was calculated. Cholic acid methyl ester trimethylsilyl ether (m/z 253) was used as the external standard for calibration. Percentage ionizations of m/z 321 (C_{26} pentol) and of m/z 253 (cholic acid) compared to total ionization were taken from the corresponding mass spectra, and the results were corrected for this difference of percentage ionization between C_{26} pentol and the external standard[15], as well as for losses during sample preparation from the recovery of [^{14}C]testosterone.

RESULTS

A representative mass chromatogram of TMS derivatives of bile alcohols of the glucuronide fraction of urine from a patient with PBC is depicted in Figure 28.2. The large peak in the upper tracing at scan 515 shows the major isomer of the C_{26} pentol, which was measured in this study. The peak at scan 481 corresponds to a minor isomer of the C_{26} pentol and the peak at scan 579 to 5β-cholestane-3α,7α,12α,24,25-pentol. As expected, only a few bile alcohols are seen in this mass chromatogram (Figure 28.2), compared to the gas chromatogram with the whole bile alcohol profile[6,8]. The area of the internal standard (coprostanol) was taken from the lower tracing (m/z 370, scan 251).

In normal volunteers the excretion of the major urinary bile alcohol, 27-nor-5β-cholestane-3α,7α,12α,24,25-pentol (C_{26} pentol) in the glucuronide fraction was $0.6 \pm$ SD 0.3 μmol/24 h (Figure 28.3), and none could be detected in the unconjugated fraction. In patients with PBC, the urinary excretion of C_{26} pentol glucuronide was significantly increased (mean $\pm$ SD $= 5.2 \pm 3.5$ μmol/24 h; $p < 0.01$). In the same group of patients the excretion of C_{26} pentol in the unconjugated fraction was only 0.09 ± 0.07 μmol/24 h. Hence, in PBC 98% of the C_{26} pentol was excreted as glucuronide, and only 2% in its unconjugated form. In six urine samples from patients with PBC, the sulphate fraction was also eluted from the DEAP-Lipidex column[16], and solvolysis was performed[16]. However, the concentration of C_{26} pentol sulphate in urine was below the detection limit.

DISCUSSION

In a previous study, the intact C_{26} pentol glucuronide (Figure 28.1) was analysed by GC–MS as the methyl ester TMS ether derivative[6]. The mass spectrum showed fragment ions corresponding to loss of the glucuronyl moiety,

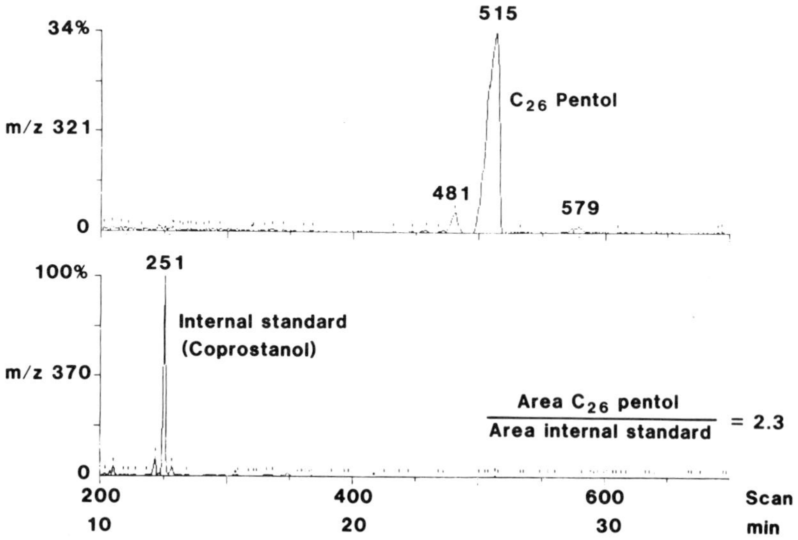

Figure 28.2 Mass chromatograms of the trimethylsilyl ethers of bile alcohols from the glucuronide fraction of urine from a patient with primary biliary cirrhosis

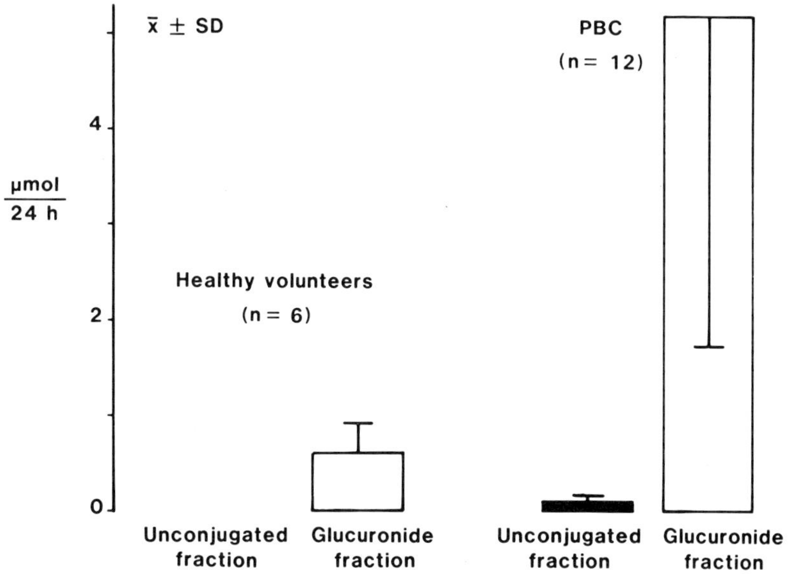

Figure 28.3 Excretion of unconjugated and glucuronidated C_{26} pentol in urine of patients with primary biliary cirrhosis and of healthy volunteers

and peaks typical for the glucuronide and the C_{26} pentol derivative. The mass spectrum indicated that C_{25} might be the site of conjugation[6].

The present investigation presents no data on the biliary excretion of bile alcohols, and no information about the total overall production of bile alcohol glucuronides is available. However, in urine from patients with PBC 98% of the C_{26} pentol was excreted as glucuronide, and only 2% in its unconjugated form. Recently, Hoshita and co-workers reported the excretion of C_{26} pentol in urine from healthy adults[9]. They found, similarly, 95% in the glucuronide and 5% in the unconjugated fraction. In PBC the urinary excretion of the C_{26} pentol was several fold increased compared to healthy controls, but still almost all was excreted as the glucuronide. Therefore, in PBC glucuronidation seems to be maintained in proportion to bile alcohol production, and glucuronidation seems not to be specifically affected by this disease. In addition to these events in the liver, it is possible that extrahepatic glucuronidation (e.g. by the kidneys) might play an important role.

Glucuronidation of xeno- and endobiotics in patients with liver disease is dependent on the kind of substrate: urinary excretion of bile salt glucuronides (ether glucuronides) in patients with intra- and extrahepatic cholestasis was found to be increased compared to healthy subjects[17]. Ether-glucuronidation of oxazepam[2], lorazepam[3] and morphine[4] have been reported to proceed normally despite advanced liver disease. In contrast, ester-glucuronidation of zomepirac in patients with cirrhosis of different aetiology may be significantly reduced. These different observations could be explained by activation or inactivation of the enzyme UDP-glucuronyltransferase[18], depending on the kind of substrate. In addition, adaptive changes of glucuronidation in patients with advanced liver disease (e.g. extrahepatic glucuronidation) have to be taken into consideration.

ACKNOWLEDGEMENTS

This investigation was supported by the Swiss National Science Foundation and the Sandoz Stiftung. The authors would like to thank Prof S. E. Bradley and Prof R. Preisig for fruitful discussions. The technical assistance of Mr Th. Weber and the secretarial help of Miss R. Steiner are gratefully acknowledged.

References

1. Witassek, F., Bircher, J., Huguenin, P. and Preisig, R. (1983). Abnormal glucuronidation of zomepirac in patients with cirrhosis of the liver. *Hepatology*, **3,** 415–22
2. Shull, H. J., Wilkinson, G. R., Johnson, R. and Schenker, S. (1976). Normal disposition of oxazepam in acute viral hepatitis and cirrhosis. *Ann. Intern. Med.*, **84,** 420–5
3. Kraus, J. W., Desmond, M. B., Marshall, J. P., Johnson, R. F., Schenker, S. and Wilkinson, G. R. (1978). Effects of aging and liver disease on disposition of lorazepam. *Clin. Pharmacol. Ther.*, **24,** 411–9
4. Patwardhan, R. V., Johnson, R. F., Hoyumpa, A. Jr., Sheehan, J. J., Desmond, P. V., Wilkinson, G. R., Branch, R. A. and Schenker, S. (1981). Normal metabolism of morphine in cirrhosis. *Gastroenterology*, **81,** 1006–11
5. Karlaganis, G. and Sjövall, J. (1984). Formation and metabolism of bile alcohols in man. *Hepatology*, **4,** 966–73
6. Karlaganis, G., Almé, B., Karlaganis, V. and Sjövall, J. (1981). Bile alcohol glucuronides in urine. Identification of 27-nor-5β-cholestane-3α.7α,12α,24ξ,25ξ-pentol in man. *J. Steroid Biochem.*, **14,** 341-5
7. Karlaganis, G., Bremmelgaard, A., Karlaganis, V. and Sjövall, J. (1983). Precursor of 27-nor-5β-cholestane-3α,7α,12α,24,25-pentol in man. *J. Steroid Biochem.*, **18,** 725–9

8. Karlaganis, G., Karlaganis, V. and Sjövall, J. (1984). Identification of 27-nor-5β-cholestane-3α,7α,12α,24,25,26-hexol and partial characterization of the bile alcohol profile in urine from man. *J. Lipid Res*, **25,** 693–702

9. Kuwabara, M., Ushiroguchi, T., Kihira, K., Kuramoto, T. and Hoshita, T. (1984). Identification of bile alcohols in urine from healthy humans. *J. Lipid Res.*, **25,** 361–8

10. Bircher, J., Blankart, R., Halpern, A., Häcki, W., Laissue, J. and Preisig, R. (1973). Criteria for assessment of functional impairment in patients with cirrhosis of the liver. *Eur. J. Clin. Invest.*, **3,** 72–85

11. Hepner, G. W. and Vessell, E. S. (1975). Quantitative assessment of hepatic function by breath analysis after oral adminstration of ^{14}C-aminopyrine. *Ann. Intern. Med.*, **83,** 632–8

12. Bircher, J., Küpfer, A., Gikalov, I. and Preisig, R. (1976). Aminopyrine demethylation measured by breath analysis in cirrhosis. *Clin. Pharmacol. Ther.*, **20,** 484–92

13. Karlaganis, G., Nemeth, A., Hammarskjöld, B., Strandvik, B. and Sjövall, J. (1982). Urinary excretion of bile alcohols in normal children and patients with α_1-antitrypsin deficiency during development of liver disease. *Eur. J. Clin. Invest.*, **12,** 399–405

14. Grob, K., Grob, G., Blum, W. and Walther, W. (1982). Preparation of inert glass capillary columns for gas chromatography. *J. Chromatogr.*, **244,** 197–208

15. Axelson, M., Cronholm, T., Curstedt, T., Reimendal, R. and Sjövall, J. (1974). Quantitative analysis of unlabelled and polydeuterated compounds by gas chromatography–mass spectrometry. *Chromatographia*, **7,** 502–9

16. Setchell, K. D. R., Almé, B., Axelson, M. and Sjövall, J. (1976). The multicomponent analysis of conjugates of neutral steroids in urine by lipophilic ion exchange chromatography and computerised gas chromatography–mass spectrometry. *J. Steroid Biochem.*, **7,** 615–29

17. Fröhling, W. and Stiehl, A. (1976). Bile salt glucuronides: identification and quantitative analysis in the urine of patients with cholestasis. *Eur. J. Clin. Invest.*, **6,** 67–74

18. Dutton, G. J. (1980). *Glucuronidation of Drugs and Other Compounds.* 1st Edn. (Boca Raton, Florida: CRC Press)

29
Glucuronide conjugation of bile acids in cholestasis

G. HEDENBORG AND A. NORMAN

It is well known that bile acids in bile occur conjugated with either glycine or taurine. The introduction of isotope-labelled bile acids demonstrated that the bile acids are excreted in bile only in a conjugated form. In 1967 Palmer was able to demonstrate the presence of sulphate esters of lithocholate in bile[1]. Later, sulphate esters of primary and secondary bile acids were identified. During cholestasis the main excretion of bile acids occurs via the urine as sulphate esters, which have been revealed by means of the HPLC technique to be mainly 3-sulphates of the glycine- or taurine-conjugates[2].

Back *et al.*[3], in 1974, reported that β-glucuronidase treatment of a polar bile acid fraction obtained from urine of jaundiced patients yielded additional amounts of bile acids. The occurrence of bile acid glucuronides was later established by isolation and identification of chenodeoxycholic acid-3β-D-glucuronide after enzymatic hydrolysis of bile acids with cholylglycine hydrolase[4]. Fröhling and Stiehl[5] synthesized, enzymatically, glucuronides of the common bile acids and developed methods for quantitation of these in urine. They found that most of the patients with liver disease excreted glucuronides, indicating that glucuronidation of bile acids represents a metabolic pathway in patients with cholestasis.

Glucuronic acid conjugates of deuterium-labelled deoxycholic and lithocholic acids have been synthesized via the Koenigs–Knorr condensation reaction[6]. These conjugates were used as internal standards in an accurate microassay for the determination of serum bile acid glucuronides by mass fragmentography. A defined amount of deuterium-labelled glucuronides was added to serum, and after enzymatic cleavage of the amide bonds, bile acids were group-separated into unconjugated, glucuronidated and sulphated bile acids by column chromatography using piperidinohydroxypropyl Sephadex LH-20[7].

Bile acid glucuronides obtained from serum or urine can be separated prior to enzymatic hydrolysis by chromatography on diethylaminohydroxypropyl Sephadex LH-20[8–10]. The main part of the glucuronides containing C or CDC were eluted after the taurine conjugates, but prior to the sulphates. Individual glucuronides could be separated by TLC, and by means of splitting the glucuronides of C and CDC by treatment with *Helix pomatia*, it was found that these were present as double conjugates of either glycine or taurine conjugates. The released bile acid glucuronides could be separated by capillary GLC, and were tentatively identified by GC–MS[10].

Available methods have made it possible to study the occurrence of glucuronides in man both in normal conditions of health as well as with liver disease. Determination by mass spectrometry has shown that the glucuronides comprise 8% of total fasting serum bile acids[6]. Using capillary GLC determinations after group separation on DEAP-LH-20, 10% of CDC were found as glucuronides[11]. In healthy subjects, only trace amounts of C and CDC glucuronides are present in bile and urine. The serum glucuronides were found to be present as double conjugates of glycine or taurine conjugates, and no postprandial increase was observed[11]. This indicates that these glucuronides do not follow the same hepatic excretion or intestinal absorption as the amidated bile acids. Individual bile acid conjugates are glucuronidated to varying extents, and the proportion of glucuronides of CDC and DC is higher than that of C in serum[6]. Glucuronides of unconjugated 6-hydroxylated bile acids have been found in a patient with malabsorption[12].

During liver disease, the concentration of glucuronides in serum increases[7] as well as in the urinary excretion[5]. However, the percentage of glucuronides in total bile acids was about 5%, which is rather lower than in normal subjects. In patients with liver cirrhosis, glucuronidation of bile acids was diminished, as indicated by a decrease of glucuronidated serum bile acids, expressed as per cent of total bile acids[7]. In cases of cholestasis, glucuronides of bile acids have been reported to be 16%[5] or 10%[2] of excreted urinary bile acids. Glucuronidation has been shown to increase the renal clearance of bile acids[13].

To compare glucuronidation with other conjugations of bile acids in cholestasis, [24-^{14}C]chenodeoxycholic acid was given to patients with total obstruction 2 days prior to establishing an external biliary drainage, and the isotope excretion in urine and bile followed[2]; 51–75% of administered isotope were excreted. All labelled compounds were excreted as conjugates, 21–59% as glycine and taurine conjugates, 16–30% as sulphates and 0.1–2.4% as glucuronides. Both sulphates and glucuronides were found to be double conjugates, and no glucuronides of unconjugated CDC were isolated. The results indicate that in patients with extrahepatic cholestasis the glucuronidation is a minor pathway compared to sulphation.

References

1. Palmer, R. H. and Bolt, M. G. (1971). Bile acid sulfates. I. Synthesis of lithocholic acid sulfates and their identification in human bile. *J. Lipid Res.*, **12,** 671–9
2. Hedenborg, G., Norlander, A. and Norman, A. (1985). Conjugation, metabolism and excretion of [24-^{14}C]chenodeoxycholic acid in patients with extrahepatic cholestasis before and after biliary drainage. – Analysis of conjugated bile acids by HPLC. *Scand. J. Clin. Lab. Invest.* (In press)
3. Back, P., Spaczynski, K. and Gerok, W. (1974). Bile-salt glucuronides in urine. *Hoppe-Seyler's Z. Physiol. Chem.*, **335,** 749–52

4. Back, P. (1976). Bile acid glucuronides, II. Isolation and identification of a chenodeoxycholic acid glucuronide from human plasma in intrahepatic cholestasis. *Hoppe-Seyler's Z. Physiol. Chem.*, **357,** 213–7
5. Fröhling, W. and Stiehl, A. (1976). Bile salt glucuronides: Identification and quantitative analysis in the urine of patients with cholestasis. *Eur. J. Clin. Invest.*, **6,** 67–74
6. Takikawa, H., Otsuka, H., Beppu, T., Seyama, Y. and Yamakawa, T. (1982). Quantitative determination of bile acid glucuronides in serum by mass fragmentography. *J. Biochem.*, **92,** 985–98
7. Takikawa, H., Otsuka, H., Beppu, T., Seyama, Y. and Yamakawa, T. (1983). Serum concentrations of bile acid glucuronides in hepatobiliary diseases. *Digestion*, **27,** 189–95
8. Almé, B. and Sjövall, J. (1980). Analysis of bile acid glucuronides in urine: identification of $3\alpha,6\alpha,12\alpha$-trihydroxy-5β-cholanoic acid. *J. Steroid. Biochem.*, **13,** 907–16
9. Stiehl, A., Raedsch, R., Rudolph, G., Czygan, P. and Walker, S. (1982). Analysis of bile acid glucuronides in urine: group separation on a lipophilic anion exchanger. *Clin. Chim. Acta*, **123,** 275–85
10. Hedenborg, G. and Norman, A. (1984). The nature of urinary bile acid conjugates in patients with extrahepatic cholestasis. *Scand. J. Clin. Lab. Invest*, **44.** (In press)
11. Hedenborg, G. and Norman, A. (1985). Fasting and postprandial serum bile acid concentration with special reference to variations in the conjugate profile. *Scand. J. Clin. Lab. Invest.*. (In press)
12. Almé, B., Nordén, Å. and Sjövall, J. (1978). Glucuronides of unconjugated 6-hydroxylated bile acids in urine of a patient with malabsorption. *Clin. Chim. Acta*, **86,** 251–9
13. Back, P. and Gerok, W. (1977). Differences in renal excretion between glyco-tauroconjugates, sulfoconjugates and glucuronoconjugates of bile acid in cholestasis. In *Bile Acid Metabolism in Health and Disease*. Falk Symposium 24 (Lancaster: MTP Press)

30
Characterization of bile acid glucuronidation in microsomes of the liver, kidney and intestinal mucosa of man

S. MATERN, H. MATERN AND W. GEROK

INTRODUCTION

Bile acid glucuronides were first described by Back *et al.* in 1974[1], and have been shown to be present in serum[2] and urine[3,4] of healthy man, as well as in biological material of patients with hepatobiliary disease[1-3]. However, little is known about the enzyme catalysing the glucuronidation of bile acids in man[5-7]. The present paper characterizes the bile acid UDP-glucuronosyltransferase in microsomes of the liver, kidney and intestinal mucosa of healthy man, and shows a decreased hepatic bile acid glucuronidation in patients with liver cirrhosis compared to healthy subjects.

MATERIALS AND METHODS

Specimens of human liver were obtained either at laparotomy or laparoscopy, or after percutaneous needle biopsy. Classification of liver disease was made on the basis of histological findings of liver biopsy specimens and clinical assessments of the patients. Intestinal biopsy specimens were obtained from patients who had undergone either gastrectomy due to gastric cancer, or intestinal resection, due either to Crohn's disease or carcinoma of the colon. Kidney samples were obtained from nephrectomy due to kidney cancer. Only macroscopic apparently normal intestinal or renal tissue was used. The liver and renal tissue were immediately frozen at −20°C. Gut segments were washed with ice-cold saline and stepwise frozen at −70°C as described by Hoensch *et al.*[8]. The bile acid UDP-glucuronosyltransferase activity was found to be stable for at least 4 weeks under these conditions.

Human liver, kidney or intestinal homogenates and microsomes were prepared as described previously[5,9]. For the determination of UDP-glucuronosyltransferase activity toward bile acids about 100 μg of hepatic, renal or intestinal microsomal protein were incubated for 30 min at 37°C in a reaction mixture containing 9 mmol/l UDP-glucuronic acid, 5 mmol/l $MgCl_2$, 5 mmol/l saccharolactone, 0.1 mol/l imidazole/HCl (ph 6.7) containing one of the following labelled bile acids: 0.5 mmol/l [^{14}C]chenodeoxycholic acid (0.8 μCi/μmol) or 0.2 mmol/l [^{14}C]deoxycholic acid (2 μCi/μmol) or 0.05 mmol/l [^{14}C]lithocholic acid (8 μCi/μmol) or 0.1 mmol/l [^{3}H]glycolithocholic acid (3.5 μCi/μmol) or 0.5 mmol/l [^{3}H]ursodeoxycholic acid (0.7 μCi/μmol). Details of the assays and identificiation of bile acid glucuronides are described in previous reports[9,10]. Determination of UDP-glucuronosyltransferase activity toward chenodeoxycholic acid using human liver homogenate as enzyme source was performed as described previously[5].

Bilirubin was estimated by the method of Michaëlsson *et al.*[11]. DNA was determined according to Burton[12] using calf thymus DNA as standard. Protein was estimated by the method of Lowry *et al.*[13] from the trichloroacetic acid-precipitable material using crystalline bovine serum albumin as standard.

Values are expressed as means ± standard deviations. Means of groups were compared by impaired Student's *t*-test; $p < 0.05$ was considered statistically significant. Linear regression analysis was performed by the least squares method[14].

RESULTS AND DISCUSSION

Microsomal bile acid UDP-glucuronosyltransferase activity in liver, kidney and intestinal mucosa of healthy man

Kinetic parameters

Kinetic parameters of microsomal hepatic and extrahepatic UDP-glucuronosyltransferase activities toward the bile acids lithocholic acid, chenodeoxycholic acid, deoxycholic acid and ursodeoxycholic acid are shown in Table 30.1. Kinetic parameters for glycolithocholic acid were only determined with liver microsomes as the enzyme source, since in the presence of glycolithocholic acid as substrate the reaction rate with renal or duodenal microsomes was too low to perform correct determinations of enzyme activity (less than 0.01 nmol min^{-1} mg of protein^{-1}). For all bile acids estimated as the variable substrates of UDP-glucuronosyltransferase from microsomes of liver, kidney and duodenal mucosa, initial rate data yielded straight lines when graphed as double reciprocal plots according to Lineweaver–Burk.

It may be seen in Table 30.1 that the apparent K_m values for various bile acids as substrates indicate a similar affinity of the individual bile acids to the enzymes from liver, kidney or small intestine. However, among the individual bile acids marked differences in the affinities to the respective enzymes were observed independent of the enzyme source. The monohydroxylated bile acid lithocholic acid exhibited about a 4–15-fold higher affinity to the enzymes from liver, kidney or small intestinal mucosa compared to the dihydroxylated bile

Table 30.1 Kinetic parameters of microsomal UDP-glucuronosyltransferase activities toward bile acids in different organs of man

Bile acid substrates		*Liver*		*Kidney*		*Duodenum*	
		K_m (mmol/l)	V_{max}	K_m (mmol/l)	V_{max}	K_m (mmol/l)	V_{max}
Lithocholic acid	(3α-ol)	0.019	0.54	0.017	0.27	0.015	0.18
Glycolithocholic acid	(3α-ol)	0.11	0.083	—	—	—	—
Chenodeoxycholic acid	(3α,7α-ol)	0.083	0.23	0.081	0.11	0.10	0.11
Deoxycholic acid	(3α,12α-ol)	0.11	0.24	0.17	0.11	0.11	0.08
Ursodeoxycholic acid	(3α,7β-ol)	0.29	0.42	0.26	0.25	0.21	0.23

The kinetic parameters were calculated from double reciprocal plots of the initial rates of enzyme activities as a function of varying concentrations of the individual bile acids, while the concentration of UDP-glucuronic acid was kept constant at 9 mmol/l. The bile acid concentrations in the assay mixtures varied between 0.002 mmol/l and 0.05 mmol/l for lithocholic and glycolithocholic acids, between 0.01 mmol/l and 0.5 mmol/l for chenodeoxycholic and ursodeoxycholic acids and between 0.01 mmol/l and 0.2 mmol/l for deoxycholic acid. The assay mixtures contained 100 μg of microsomal protein from normal liver, kidney or duodenal mucosa and 0.7 mg of Triton X-100 per mg of protein. The position and configuration of hydroxyl groups in the bile acid skeleton are given in parentheses. V_{max}, nmol of bile acid conjugated min^{-1} mg of microsomal $protein^{-1}$

acids chenodeoxycholic acid, deoxycholic acid or ursodeoxycholic acid. Among the dihydroxylated bile acids the highest K_m value was obtained for ursodeoxycholic acid (Table 30.1). Since ursodeoxycholic acid is more hydrophilic than chenodeoxycholic or deoxycholic acids, these results suggest that the affinity of bile acids to hepatic, renal and intestinal UDP-glucuronosyltransferase appears to increase with an increasing hydrophobicity of bile acids. Furthermore, conjugation of bile acids with amino acids appears to decrease the affinity of bile acids to UDP-glucuronosyltransferase, since in the presence of glycolithocholic acid a 6-fold lower affinity to hepatic microsomal UDP-glucuronosyltransferase was observed compared to unconjugated lithocholic acid (Table 30.1).

In contrast to the K_m values, the V_{max} values for individual bile acids exhibited organ specific differences (Table 30.1). The V_{max} values for individual bile acids showed that microsomal UDP-glucuronosyltransferase activity toward bile acids in liver is about twice that found in kidney, and about two to three times that observed in duodenal mucosa. Among the individual bile acids, the reaction rate with chenodeoxycholic acid approximately equalled the reaction rate with deoxycholic acid, and both rates were about half to one-third the reaction rates observed in the presence of ursodeoxycholic or lithocholic acids when either microsomes from liver, kidney or duodenal mucosa were used as enzyme source (Table 30.1).

In order to investigate whether or not UDP-glucuronosyltransferase activity toward bile acids is equally distributed throughout the whole human intestine, different segments of intestinal mucosa were assayed for UDP-glucuronosyltransferase activity toward chenodeoxycholic acid. As shown in Table 30.2, the relative glucuronidation rates with chenodeoxycholic acid in different segments of human intestinal mucosa indicate a decrease in the activity of

Table 30.2 UDP-glucuronosyltransferase activity toward chenodeoxycholic acid from microsomes of different segments of human intestinal mucosa

Gut segment	*No. of patients*	*Enzyme activity* (nmol min^{-1} mg of $protein^{-1}$)
Duodenum	9	0.10 ± 0.02
Jejunum	4	0.085 ± 0.02
Ileum	6	0.06 ± 0.02
Colon	5	0.03 ± 0.01

UDP-glucuronosyltransferase toward bile acids when going from the oral end of the small intestine to the colon, where it was 30% of the duodenal level. Since a similar decrease of the mixed function mono-oxygenase system was observed from the duodenum to ileum of rats[15], enzymes involved in the biotransformation of foreign or endogenous compounds appear to be concentrated in the upper small intestine. However, the biological significance of the bile acid UDP-glucuronosyltransferase activity in human intestine has to be determined.

Effect of divalent metal ions

The effect of divalent metal ions on the activity of hepatic and extrahepatic microsomal UDP-glucuronosyltransferase toward chenodeoxycholic acid is shown in Table 30.3. Addition of magnesium, manganese or calcium had no significant effect on the rates of chenodeoxycholic acid glucuronidation in renal and small intestinal microsomes, whereas one of these divalent metal ions was required to achieve maximal activity of chenodeoxycholic acid glucuronidation in hepatic microsomes (Table 30.3). Lack of stimulation of enzyme activity by magnesium, manganese or calcium in intestinal or renal microsomes cannot be explained by the presence of these ions which may not have been removed by washing of the microsomes, since conjugating activity toward chenodeoxycholic acid in renal or small intestinal microsomes was about the same in the presence and absence of EDTA, as well as in the presence and absence of magnesium, manganese or calcium (Table 30.3). Marked differences between chenodeoxycholic acid glucuronidation in hepatic, renal and small intestinal microsomes were observed with regard to their response to other divalent metal ions such as Co^{2+}, Ni^{2+} or Fe^{2+} which either were without effect or were inhibitory to the enzyme activities depending on the enzyme source (Table 30.3). Whether or not these differences between hepatic, renal and small intestinal microsomes, with regard to the effect of divalent metal ions on enzyme activities, indicate the existence of different organ specific UDP-glucuronosyltransferase activities toward bile acids can only be clarified when the purified enzymes become available[16].

Table 30.3 Effect of divalent metal ions on hepatic and extrahepatic UDP-glucuronosyltransferase activity toward chenodeoxycholic acid

Addition to assay	*Enzyme activity in microsomes of*		
	liver	*duodenal mucosa* (% of control)*	*kidney*
None	100	100	100
10 mmol/l EDTA	97	109	98
5 mmol/l Mg^{2+}	138	108	100
5 mmol/l Mn^{2+}	134	90	91
5 mmol/l Ca^{2+}	135	88	89
5 mmol/l Ba^{2+}	101	104	89
5 mmol/l Co^{2+}	35	89	64
5 mmol/l Ni^{2+}	44	101	74
5 mmol/l Zn^{2+}	6	40	14
5 mmol/l Fe^{2+}	13	64	92
5 mmol/l Pb^{2+}	16	38	30

* Control: enzyme activity without addition of EDTA and metal ions

Bile acid UDP-glucuronosyltransferase activity in liver disease

Since, with the exception of the enzyme(s) catalysing the glucuronidation of bilirubin[17], the knowledge about UDP-glucuronosyltransferase activities toward endogenous compounds in human liver disease is scanty, studies were carried out on UDP-glucuronosyltransferase activity toward the bile acid chenodeoxycholic acid in liver biopsy specimens from patients with a variety of liver diseases, such as fatty liver, fatty liver hepatitis, liver fibrosis, granulomatous hepatitis or liver cirrhosis (Figure 30.1). Whereas patients with normal liver exhibited a mean value of UDP-glucuronosyltransferase activity toward chenodeoxycholic acid of $201 \pm 77.6\,\text{nmol}\,h^{-1}\,mg^{-1}$ of DNA (0.063 ± 0.024 $\text{nmol}\,min^{-1}\,mg$ of $protein^{-1}$), the mean value of bile acid UDP-glucuronosyltransferase activity was significantly reduced in patients with liver cirrhosis to about half the mean value observed in normal liver samples (Figure 30.1). The reduced bile acid UDP-glucuronosyltransferase activity in liver biopsy specimens of patients with liver cirrhosis is in agreement with diminished serum bile acid concentrations found in patients with liver cirrhosis, amounting to 0.8–1.8% of the total serum bile acids, whereas in healthy subjects 8.6% of the total serum bile acids were glucuronidated[18]. The decreased hepatic bile acid UDP-glucuronosyltransferase activity observed in patients with liver cirrhosis (Figure 30.1) may be explained by the reduced amounts of hepatocytes per mg of DNA. However, the diminished bile acid UDP-glucuronosyltransferase activity observed in liver biopsy specimens of patients with liver cirrhosis may also be explained by an inhibitory effect of bilirubin on bile acid UDP-glucuronosyltransferase activity, since it has been shown that bilirubin competitively inhibits the glucuronidation of bile acids in human liver microsomes[5,6]. Furthermore, an inverse correlation was observed between the concentrations of total serum bilirubin and hepatic bile acid UDP-glucuronosyltransferase activity (Figure 30.2) when the values of total serum bilirubin were plotted against the corresponding values of UDP-glucuronosyltransferase activity to-

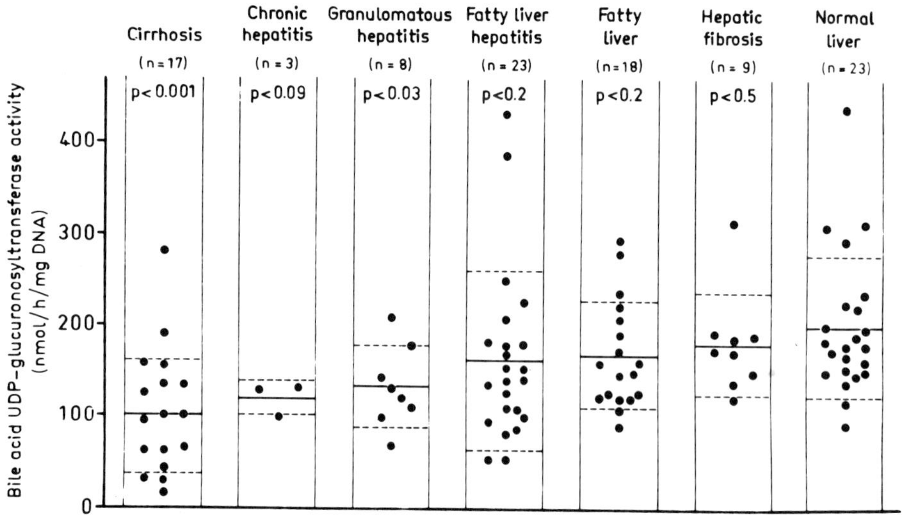

Figure 30.1 UDP-glucuronosyltransferase activity toward chenodeoxycholic acid in liver biopsy specimens from patients with normal liver and various liver disease. Enzyme activity and DNA were determined from 10 g/100 ml liver homogenates (wet weight) prepared with 0.25 mol/l sucrose containing 5 mmol/l Tris/HCl, pH 7.4. Horizontal lines represent means ± SD. p-Values < 0.05 were considered significant when compared with the normal liver. n, number of liver biopsy specimens.

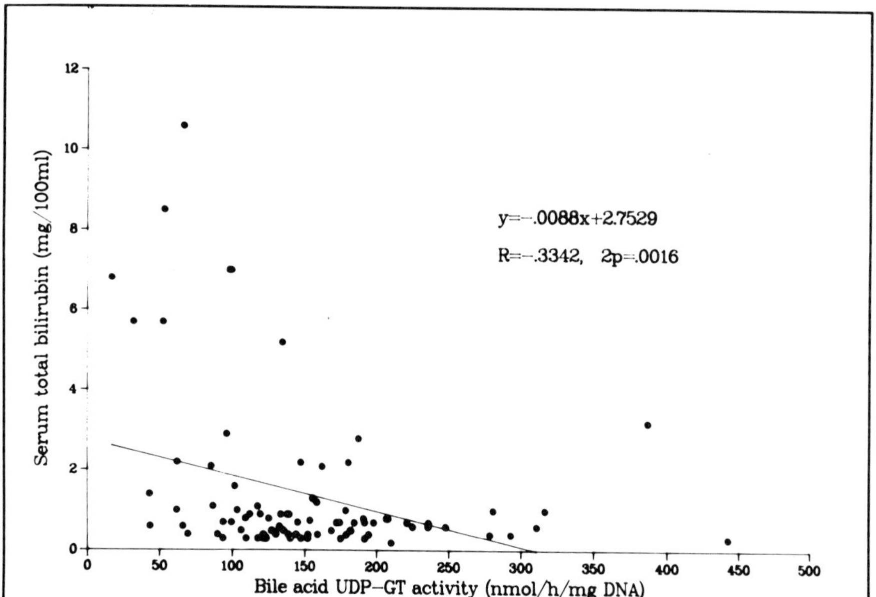

Figure 30.2 Correlation of human hepatic UDP-glucuronosyltransferase (UDP-GT) activity toward chenodeoxycholic acid with total serum bilirubin concentrations. Enzyme activities were obtained from liver biopsy specimens of patients with and without liver disease (values of Figure 30.1)

ward chenodeoxycholic acid measured in human liver biopsy specimens shown in Figure 30.1. Whether or not the observed inverse correlation between total serum bilirubin and bile acid UDP-glucuronosyltransferase activity may be due to bilirubin acting as a competitive inhibitor of chenodeoxycholic acid glucuronidation as previously observed in *in vitro* studies[5,6] or due to an unspecific inhibitory effect of bilirubin on bile acid UDP-glucuronosyltransferase because of its toxicity[19] can only be clarified when the purified UDP-glucuronosyltransferase(s) becomes available from human liver.

ACKNOWLEDGEMENTS

This work was supported by the Deutsche Forschungsgemeinschaft (SFB 154-84). H.M. is the recipient of a Heisenberg award from the Deutsche Forschungsgemeinschaft.

References

1. Back, P., Spaczynski, K. and Gerok. W. (1974). Bile salt glucuronides in urine. *Hoppe-Seyler's Z. Physiol. Chem.*, **355,** 749-52
2. Takikawa, H., Otsuka, H., Beppu, T., Seyama, Y. and Yamakawa, T. (1982). Quantitative determination of bile acid glucuronides in serum by mass fragmentography. *J. Biochem.*, **92,** 985–98
3. Almé, B. and Sjövall, J. (1980). Analysis of bile acid glucuronides in urine. Identification of 3α,6α,12α-trihydroxy-5β-cholanoic acid. *J. Steroid Biochem.*, **13,** 907–16
4. Saquet, E., Parquet, M., Riottot, M., Raizman, A., Jarrige, P., Huguet, C. and Infante, R. (1983). Intestinal absorption, excretion and biotransformation of hyodeoxycholic acid in man. *J. Lipid Res.*, **24,** 604–13
5. Matern, H., Matern, S., Schelzig, C. and Gerok, W. (1980). Bile acid UDP-glucuronyltransferase from human liver. Properties and studies on aglycone substrate specificity. *FEBS Lett.*, **118,** 251–4
6. Matern, H., Matern, S. and Gerok, W. (1981). Characterization of bile acid UDP-glucuronyltransferase from human liver. In Paumgartner, G., Stiehl, A. and Gerok, W. (eds.). *Bile Acids and Lipids*, pp. 111–6. (Lancaster: MTP Press)
7. Matern, S., Matern, H. and Gerok, W. (1983). Detoxification and protection. In Bianchi, L., Gerok, W., Landmann, L., Sickinger, K. and Stalder, G. A. (eds.). *Liver in Metabolic Diseases*, pp. 325–39. (Lancaster: MTP Press)
8. Hoensch, H. P., Hutt, R. and Hartmann, F. (1979). Biotransformation of xenobiotics in human intestinal mucosa. *Environ. Health Perspect.*, **33,** 71–8
9. Matern, H., Matern, S. and Gerok, W. (1983). A rapid and sensitive method for the assay of UDP-glucuronosyltransferase activity toward bile acids. *Anal. Biochem.*, **133,** 417–24
10. Matern, S., Matern, H., Farthmann, E. H. and Gerok, W. (1984). Hepatic and extrahepatic glucuronidation of bile acids in man. Characterization of bile acid uridine 5′-diphosphate-glucuronosyltransferase in hepatic, renal, and intestinal microsomes. *J. Clin. Invest.*, **74,** 402–10
11. Michaëlsson, M., Nosslin, B. and Sjölin, S. (1965). Plasma bilirubin determination in newborn infant: methodological study with special reference to influence of hemolysis. *Pediatrics*, **35,** 925–31
12. Burton, K. (1968). Determination of DNA concentration with diphenylamine. In Grossman, L. and Moldave, K. (eds.). *Methods in Enzymology*, **12B,** pp. 163–5. (New York: Academic Press)
13. Lowry, O. H., Rosebrough, N. J., Farr, A. L. and Randall, R. J. (1951). Protein measurement with the folin phenol reagent. *J. Biol. Chem.*, **193,** 265-75

14. Sachs, L. (1982). *Statistische Methoden.* 5th Edn. (Berlin, Heidelberg, New York: Springer)
15. Hoensch, H., Woo, C. H., Raffin, S. B. and Schmid, R. (1976). Oxidative metabolism of foreign compounds in rat small intestine: cellular localization and dependence on dietary iron. *Gastroenterology*, **70,** 1063–70
16. Arias, I. M. (1968). On specificity of glucuronyltransferase(s). In Beck, K. (ed.). *Ikterus*, pp. 15–6. (Stuttgart, New York: Schattauer)
17. Black, M. and Billing, B. H. (1969). Hepatic bilirubin UDP-glucuronyltransferase activity in liver disease and Gilbert's syndrome. *N. Engl. J. Med.*, **280,** 1266–71
18. Takikawa, H., Otsuka, H., Beppu, T., Seyama, Y. and Yamakawa, T. (1983). Serum concentrations of bile acid glucuronides in hepatobiliary diseases. *Digestion*, **27,** 189–95
19. Charbonnier, A. (1968). On the toxicity of bilirubin. In Beck, K. (ed.). *Ikterus*, pp. 93–7. (Stuttgart, New York: Schattauer)

31
Hepatic conjugation of enterolactone and enterodiol: the first mammalian lignans

K. D. R. SETCHELL

Enterolactone (2,3-bis(3-hydroxybenzyl)butyrolactone) and enterodiol (2,3-bis(3-hydroxybenzyl)butane-1,4-diol) are the trivial names that were adopted for the first and quantitatively two most important lignans to be identified in biological fluids of man and several animal species[1-4], and their structures are illustrated in Figure 31.1. Lignans are, by definition, compounds having a 2,3-dibenzylbutane skeleton[5], and are widely distributed as minor constituents in many plants[6-8]. These two lignans differ significantly in chemical structure from all known plant lignans[3], which excludes their direct dietary origin.

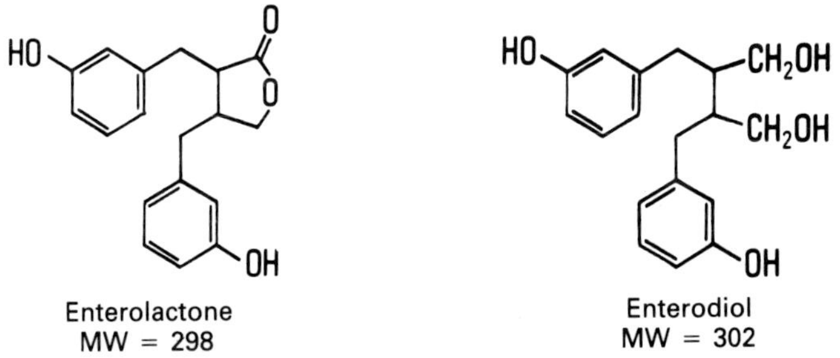

Figure 31.1 Structures of enterolactone and enterodiol

Both lignans were identified following their persistent occurrence in the gas chromatographic profiles of urinary steroids[9], and after the serendipitous observation of a cyclicity in their quantitative excretion during the menstrual cycle of the vervet monkey[10] and man[1,2,11], in which maximum excretion occurred during thc luteal phase, suggesting that their production and/or excretion was controlled in some way by hormonal status. Studies in rats have demonstrated that gonadotrophins play a role in the controlling mechanism[12].

Quantitatively, the urinary excretion of these lignans[13] is comparable to many of the neutral steroids, and well in excess of the phenolic oestrogens. Enterolactone and enterodiol have also been identified in blood[4,14], bile[15] and semen[14], and in common with many endogenous compounds an efficient enterohepatic circulation was observed[15].

In view of the close similarity in physicochemical properties and physiological characteristics of the lignans to oestrogenic steroids, synthesis by the ovaries was initially considered[4], but excluded when experiments comparing urinary lignan excretion in conventional and germ-free rats fed identical diets, confirmed their bacterial production[15]. These findings were supported by data demonstrating a complete suppression of lignan excretion in man after oral antibiotic administration[4] and also from *in vitro* studies of faecal flora[16].

Unequivocal evidence that these novel lignans were not of a direct dietary origin was obtained when the normal pelleted diet of rats was switched to a semi-synthetic diet, and lignan excretion showed a pronounced decrease to undetectable levels[17]. When the normal diet was re-introduced, lignan excretion was re-established. In our search for a precursor of these lignans, a variety of foodstuffs of plant origin were added to the semi-synthetic diet and lignan production assessed from urinary excretion[17]. Many of the grains tested contained precursors, but linseeds in particular were found to be rich in a precursor identified as a complex plant lignan, secoisolariciresinol-diglycoside[17]. This compound, after hydrolysis, demethylation and oxidation[17], reactions which have been shown to occur *in vitro* with faecal flora[16], is converted in the gastrointestinal tract to enterodiol. Further bacterial oxidization of enterodiol results in the production of enterolactone.

Following the absorption of lignans from the gastrointestinal tract they are transported via the portal venous system[15] to the liver where efficient conjugation to glucuronic acid is presumed to occur[13]. The more water soluble conjugate is then excreted via the kidneys and by the biliary route where it is present primarily as the mono-glucuronide conjugate in the urine and bile. The finding of high concentrations of enterolactone-glucuronide in the portal blood[14], suggests that this intact conjugate may be re-absorbed from the gastrointestinal tract but, if so, the mechanism and site of absorption are at present unknown.

Experiments were carried out which establish *in vitro* conjugation of enterolactone and enterodiol to glucuronic acid by hepatic microsomes. Solubilized rat liver microsomes were prepared from adult Sprague-Dawley rats, and using uridine diphosphoglucuronic acid as the glucuronyl donor, various concentrations of synthetically prepared enterolactone and enterodiol[18-20] were incubated. The conversion of free lignans to glucuronide conjugates was measured by gas liquid chromatography–mass spectrometry[21] and high performance liquid chromatography.

At constant substrate concentration (50 μg each lignan incubated per tube) both lignans were rapidly converted to their respective glucuronide conjugates (Figure 31.2). Varying substrate concentrations over the range 0.08–1 mmol/l and incubating for 20 minutes, the K_m value for the conjugation of enterolactone was found to be 0.296 mmol/l. In separate experiments using rabbit liver microsomes the K_m values for the conjugation of enterolactone and enterodiol were found to be 0.30 mmol/l and 0.23 mmol/l, respectively[22].

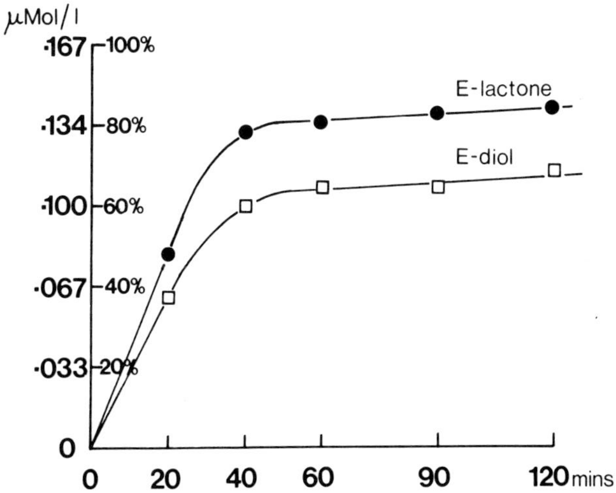

Figure 31.2 Time course for the *in vitro* conjugation of enterolactone and enterodiol to glucuronic acid by solubilized rat liver microsomes

While these experiments clearly indicate the capacity of solubilized rat liver microsomes to conjugate enterolactone and enterodiol to glucuronic acid, it remains to be established whether conjugation similarly takes place during transport across the intestinal mucosa. The high levels of conjugated lignans in portal venous blood[15] may be explained by uridine diphosphoglucuronyltransferase activity of intestinal microsomes, which is known to be active upon other aromatic compounds[23,24].

Interest in the potential physiological importance of these compounds has gained impetus following speculation of a possible beneficial role in diseases, such as breast cancer[25,26] and colon cancer[4], stimulated from the finding that vegetarians excrete significantly increased quantities of lignans compared with non-vegetarians[25,27], and the known lower incidence of these diseases in such populations. Preliminary studies have recently indicated that both lignans are inhibitory upon hepatic cholesterol-7α-hydroxylase and acyl coenzyme A : cholesterol acyltransferase enzymes *in vitro*[28] and, if such effects are confirmed, *in vivo*, lignans may alter bile acid metabolism and could prove to be of importance in many common diseases. Conjugation of these compounds to glucuronic acid may, therefore, influence the effective biological activity of enterolactone and enterodiol.

References

1. Setchell, K. D. R., Lawson, A. M., Mitchell, F. L., Adlercreutz, H., Kirk, D. N. and Axelson, M. (1980). Lignans in man and animal species. *Nature*, **287**, 740–2
2. Stitch, S. R., Toumba, J. K., Groen, M. B., Funke, C. W., Leemhuis, J., Vink, J. and Woods, G. F. (1980). Excretion, isolation and structure of a new phenolic constituent of female urine. *Nature*, **287**, 738–40
3. Setchell, K. D. R., Lawson, A. M., Conway, E., Taylor, N. F., Kirk, D. N., Cooley, G., Farrant, R. D., Wynn, S. and Axelson, M. (1981). The definitive identification of

the lignans *trans*-2,3-bis(3-hydroxybenzyl)-γ-butyrolactone and 2,3-*bis*(3-hydroxybenzyl)-butane-1,4-diol in human and animal urine. *Biochem. J.*, **197**, 447–58
4. Setchell, K. D. R., Lawson, A. M., Borriello, S. P., Harkness, R., Gordon, H., Morgan, D. M. L., Kirk, D. N., Anderson, L. C., Adlercreutz, H. and Axelson, M. (1981). Lignan formation in man – microbial involvement and possible roles in relation to cancer. *Lancet*, **2**, 4–8
5. Haworth, R. D. and Slinger, F. H. (1940). The constituents of natural phenolic resins. Part XVII. A synthesis of 1-matairesinol. *J. Chem. Soc.*, 1098–1101
6. Rao, C. B. S. (1978). *The Chemistry of Lignans*. (Andhra: University Press, Waltair, India)
7. Hartwell, J. L. (1976). Types of anticancer agents isolated from plants. *Cancer Treat. Reps.*, **60**, 1031–67
8. Barclay, A. S. and Perdue, R. E. Jr. (1976). Distribution of anticancer activity in higher plants. *Cancer Treat. Reps.*, **60**, 1081–113
9. Setchell, K. D. R., Lawson, A. M., Borriello, S. P., Aldercreutz, H. and Axelson, M. (1981). Formation of lignans by intestinal microflora. In Malt, R. A. and Williamson, R. C. N. (eds.). *Colonic Carcinogenesis*, pp. 93–9. (Lancaster: MTP Press)
10. Setchell, K. D. R., Bull, R. and Adlercreutz, H. (1980). Steroid excretion during the reproductive cycle and in pregnancy of the vervet monkey (*Ceropithecus aethiopus pygerythrus*). *J. Steroid Biochem.*, **12**, 375–84
11. Setchell, K. D. R., Lawson, A. M., Axelson, M. and Adlercreutz, H. (1979). The excretion of two new phenolic compounds during the menstrual cycle and in pregnancy. In Adlercreutz, H., Bullbrook, R. D., Van der Molen, H. J., Vermeulen, A. and Sciarra, F. (eds.). *Endocrinological Cancer Ovarian Function and Disease*, pp. 207–15. (Amsterdam: Excerpta Medica)
12. Coert, A., Vonk Noordegraaf, C. A., Groen, M. B. and Van der Vies, J. (1982). The dietary origin of the urinary HPMF. *Experientia*, **38**, 904–5
13. Axelson, M. and Setchell, K. D. R. (1980). Conjugation of lignans in human urine. *FEBS Letts.*, **122**, 49–53
14. Dehennin, L., Reiffsteck, A., Jondef, M. and Thibler, M. (1982). Identification and quantitative estimation of a lignan in human and bovine semen. *J. Reprod. Fert.*, **66**, 305–9
15. Axelson, M. and Setchell, K. D. R. (1981). Excretion of lignans in rats – evidence for an intestinal bacterial source for this new group of compounds. *FEBS Letts.*, **123**, 337–42
16. Borriello, S. P., Setchell, K. D. R., Axelson, M. and Lawson, A. M. (1984). Production and metabolism of lignans by the human fecal flora. *J. Appl. Bacteriol.* (In press)
17. Axelson, M., Sjövall, J., Gustafsson, B. E. and Setchell, K. D. R. (1982). Origin of lignans in mammals and identification of a precursor from plants. *Nature*, **298**, 659–60
18. Cooley, G., Farrant, R. D., Kirk, D. N., Patel, S., Wynn, S., Buckingham, M. J., Hawkes, G. E., Hursthouse, M. B., Galas, A. M. R., Lawson, A. M. and Setchell, K. D. R. (1984). Structural analysis of the urinary lignan 2,3-bis(3-hydroxybenzyl)butan-4-olide (enterolactone). A 400 MHz nuclear magnetic resonance study for the solution state and X-ray study for the crystal state. *J. Chem. Soc. Perk. Trans.*, **II**, 489-97
19. Cooley, G., Farrant, R. D., Kirk, D. N. and Wynn, S. (1981). Chemical synthesis of the first lignans to be found in humans and animals. *Tetrahedron Letts.*, **22**, 349–50
20. Kirk, D. N., McLaughlin, L. M., Lawson, A. M., Setchell, K. D. R. and Patel, S. K. (1984). Synthesis of [^{2}H]-labelled urinary lignans enterolactone and enterodiol. *J. Chem. Soc. Perk. Trans.*, **I.** (In press)
21. Setchell, K. D. R., Lawson, A. M., McLaughlin, L. M., Patel, S., Kirk, D. N. and Axelson, M. (1983). Measurement of enterolactone and enterodiol, the first mammalian lignans, using stable isotope dilution and gas chromatography mass spectrometry. *Biomed. Mass Spectrom.*, **10**, 227–35
22. Brunner, G., Tegtmeier, F., Kirk, D. N. and Setchell, K. D. R. (1984). Enzymatic synthesis and purification of lignan glucuronides. *FEBS Letts.* (Submitted for publication)
23. Schwenk, M. (1984). Glucuronide conjugation in isolated cells from intestine, liver and kidney. In Matern, S., Bock, K. W. and Gerok, W. (eds.). *Proceedings of Falk Symposium No. 40, Advances in Glucuronide Conjugation*, pp. 163–73. (Lancaster: MTP Press).
24. Koster, A. S. (1984). Intestinal glucorinidation. *In vivo* and *in vitro* model systems. In Matern, S., Bock, K. W. and Gerok, W. (eds.). *Proceedings of Falk Symposium No. 40, Advances in Glucuronide Conjugation*, pp. 175–93. (Lancaster: MTP Press).

25. Adlercreutz, H., Fotsis, T., Heikkinen, R., Dwyer, J. T., Woods, M., Goldin, B. R. and Gorbach, S. L. (1982). Excretion of the lignans enterolactone and enterodiol and of equol in omnivorous and vegetarian post-menopausal women and in women with breast cancer. *Lancet*, **2,** 1295–9
26. Adlercreutz, H. (1984). Does fiber-rich food containing lignan precursors protect against both colon and breast cancer? An extension of the fiber hypothesis. *Gastroenterology*, **86,** 761–6
27. Adlercreutz, H., Fotsis, T., Heikkinen, R., Dwyer, J. T., Goldin, B. R., Gorbach, S. L., Lawson, A. M. and Setchell, K. D. R. (1981). Diet and urinary excretion of lignans in female subjects. *Med. Biol.*, **59,** 259–61
28. Sanghvi, A., Dixen, W. F., Seltman, H., Warty, V., Rizk, M., Kritchevsky, D. and Setchell, K. D. R. (1984). Inhibition of rat liver cholesterol 7α-hydroxylase and acyl CoA: cholesterol acyl transferase activities by enterodiol and enterolactone. In *Proceedings of the 8th International Symposium on Drugs Affecting Lipid Metabolism.* (New York: Plenum Press). (In press)

Section 8
Conjugation Reactions in Preneoplastic Liver

Chairman: K. W. Bock

32
Aspects of drug metabolism in hepatocyte nodules in rats

L. C. ERIKSSON

INTRODUCTION

During the process of chemical carcinogenesis in the rat, liver foci of altered cells and hepatocyte nodules appear[1-3]. After 8–12 months hepatocellular carcinomas develop in these livers. In certain cases hepatomas have been seen to develop within hepatocyte nodules[4-8]. Many researchers, therefore, consider these nodules to be preneoplastic lesions in the liver. Although their status as obligate precursors for hepatocellular carcinomas remains to be proven, a material continuity beween the nodule and the malignant liver tumour has been shown. The process starts by the induction of alterations in a few cells of the liver. These cells, referred to as initiated cells, are brought to proliferate and expand into focal lesions and hepatocellular nodules. This selective expansion, obviously necessary for the progress of the cancer development, is referred to as selection or promotion, although the term promotion means more than just proliferation. There are several experimental models available for the production of liver carcinomas which have been very useful in the search for the mechanisms of cancer induction by chemicals[9]. Some use one chemical to perform the initiation and another for the selection or promotion of the process, while others consist of longterm feeding of only one chemical carcinogen. The promotion regimens vary considerably in duration, but are always terminated long before the malignant liver tumour appears, i.e. the longest part of the process is self-generating once the promotion has been performed.

The general hypothesis of the multistep procedure of chemical carcinogenesis states that every step will generate a new cell population, with phenotypic properties favouring the survival and growth of the cells and also the next step in the carcinogenic process. This hypothesis is nicely illustrated in the models where nodules are generated by intermittent feeding of either 2-acetylaminofluorene or ethionine or by initiation with diethylnitrosamine, and the subsequent brief promotion with 2-acetylaminofluorene in combination with a mitogenic stimulus, such as partial hepatectomy. These nodules are resistant to the cytotoxic effect of carbon tetrachloride and dimethylnitrosamine[10], and to the mitoinhibitory effect of 2-acetylaminofluorene[11]. The capability of the initiated cells to grow in the presence of 2-acetylaminofluorene is regarded to be the key to clonal proliferation and the development of hepatocyte nodules in these models. Therefore, the biochemical investigation of the nature of this resistance seems to be important in the understanding of the mechanisms of chemical carcinogenesis.

The resistant hepatocyte model

In the resistant hepatocyte model described by Solt and Farber[12], initiation is performed with diethylnitrosamine. After 2 weeks the initiated cells are selected by dietary treatment of the animals with 2-acetylaminofluorene, which effectively inhibits mitoses and proliferation of liver cells. Only cells resistant to the mitoinhibitory effect of the drug will be able to respond to mitogenic stimuli, e.g. partial hepatectomy, and go through several cell divisions to develop into focal lesions and hepatocyte nodules. The differential inhibition of cell division is the prerequisite for nodular development in this model. Work performed by Hayes[13] has shown that if phenobarbital or 3-methylcholanthrene is administered together with 2-acetylaminofluorene during selection in this model no nodules develop, but the entire liver will respond to partial hepatectomy with cell proliferation. That is, phenobarbital or methylcholanthrene treatment will render the surrounding cells resistant to the mitoinhibitory effect of 2-acetylaminofluorene. These experiments focus our minds on altered drug metabolism being the mechanism for the resistance phenomenon, as these drugs are known to be potent inducers of drug metabolizing enzymes.

In this presentation data will be presented from work performed on drug metabolism in hepatocyte nodules and normal liver tissue, and the implications of the specific phenotype of the nodules on their resistance to cytotoxic drugs will be discussed. Data are presented from work on nodules produced by intermittent chronic exposure of 2-acetylaminofluorene[14] and by the resistant hepatocyte model[12].

UPTAKE OF 2-ACETYLAMINOFLUORENE

From a theoretical point of view there may be many differences between normal and nodular cells which may explain their different sensitivity to 2-acetylaminofluorene. Figure 32.1 illustrates some of those that have been investigated in the resistant hepatocyte model and in the model of intermittent feeding of 2-acetylaminofluorene. The drug is transported to the liver and to the nodules in the portal blood. It has been shown, with the use of microspheres, that hepatocyte nodules are preferentially perfused by arterial blood, and to a lesser extent by blood from the portal vein[15,41]. This would create a situation where the nodules have escaped from the toxic blood flow in the portal vein carrying drugs reabsorbed from the gut. This effect is seen in large nodules, and is not evident for small and intermediate sized lesions. In addition, even

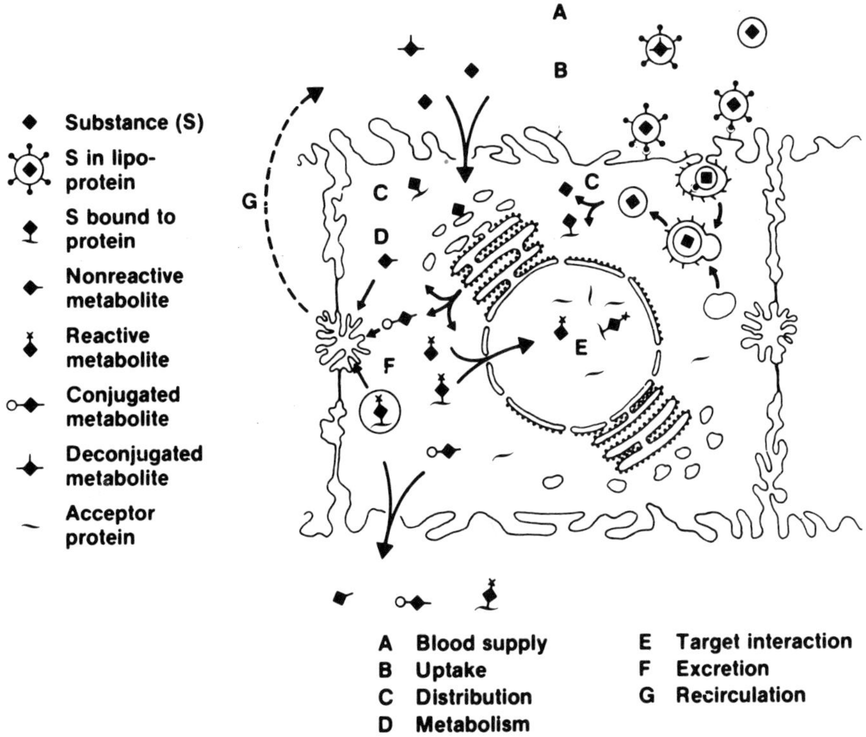

Figure 32.1 Schematic presentation of a liver parenchymal cell and the theoretical alternatives for drug uptake, distribution, metabolism and elimination

if the drug is injected directly in the portal vein equilibration will have taken place in the blood after only 2–3 minutes[16].

The mechanisms of uptake of 2-acetylaminofluorene are not known in detail, but from *in vivo* and *in vitro* experiments[16] there seems to be no evidence for receptor-mediated or carrier-mediated uptake processes in the liver for 2-acetylaminofluorene. When a tracer amount of radioactive 2-acetylaminofluorene was injected into the mesenteric vein of a normal rat, the drug was very quickly taken up by the liver cells with kinetic parameters indicating partition between sites of affinity in the blood and in the cells. The parent compound seemed to move freely across the cell membrane facing the sinusoids. As will be discussed later, this was not true for passage of the compound across the bile canalicular membrane.

INTRACELLULAR DISTRIBUTION

The initial intracellular distribution of 2-acetylaminofluorene was very specific, Figure 32.2. Most of the drug was non-covalently associated to the membranes recovered in the microsomal fraction within the first few minutes, only very little could be found associated to other cell compartments such as mitochondria. The elimination from the cell was also very fast during the initial minutes. This fast rate of elimination was partly due to the fact that the parent compound moved from the cell to free sites in the blood, and partly due to the metabolism, redistribution and elimination of metabolites.

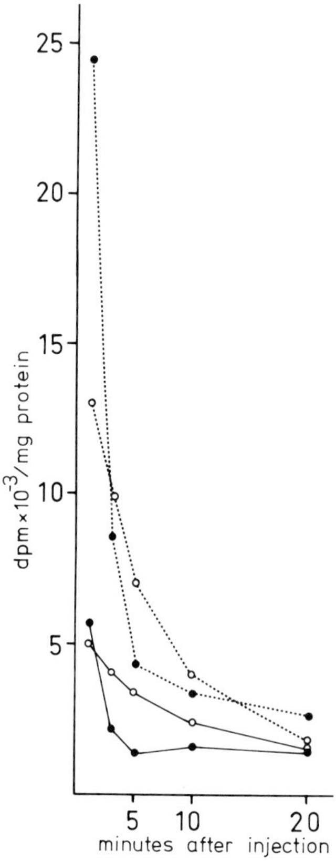

Figure 32.2 Intracellular distribution of radioactivity after intramesenteric injection of [9-^{14}C]2-acetylaminofluorene in normal and nodular liver tissue. The substance was dissolved in rat serum and injected (0.23 mg/kg body weight) into a branch of the superior mesenteric vein. After the time points indicated the livers were perfused with ice-cold 0.25 mol/l sucrose. Tissue was harvested and fractions prepared as described in Ref. 14
Normal microsomes: ●......● Normal mitochondria: ●——● Nodular microsomes: ○......○ Nodular mitochondria: ○——○

The amount of covalently bound tracer increased with time in all liver cell fractions investigated. In this case, there was no specificity in the binding pattern as was seen for the initial non-covalent binding. Eventually all fractions contained the same amount of radioactive tracer, expressed per mg of protein. Two hours after the tracer injection, 70% was covalently and the rest non-covalently bound as judged by TCA precipitation. The rate of covalent binding differed between different subfractions. The microsomal membranes reached the maximal amount of covalent binding after 10 minutes, while the mitochondria and cytosol proteins did not reach this relative level of binding until 90 minutes and 2 hours respectively. In nodular tissue uptake was also very fast, and the initial uptake seemed to be as high as that in the normal liver. This was supported by the finding that the initial amount of radioactivity associated with mitochondrial membranes was as high in nodular tissue as it was in normal liver cells. The specific binding to microsomal membranes was much lower in nodules than in normal liver. Nodular cells, therefore, retained less of the drug in the intracellular compartment. In nodules the elimination rate was also considerably lower than the rate in normal liver, as was the formation of covalent binding to cellular macromolecules. Eventually the amount of 2-acetylaminofluorene derivatives covalently bound to macromolecules in the nodular cells amounted to around one-fifth of that found in normal liver.

The specific affinity of the endoplasmic reticulum for 2-acetylaminofluorene seemed to be correlated to the amount of cytochrome P-450 in the membranes. This statement is based on comparisons between the high binding to normal membranes, the low binding to nodular membranes low in cytochrome P-450, and the very high binding to membranes in rats treated with 3-methylcholanthrene where cytochrome levels were dramatically increased.

DRUG METABOLIZING ENZYMES IN HEPATOCYTE NODULES

It has been reported from many laboratories, using a series of different experimental models for chemical carcinogenesis, that the amount of cytochrome P-450 measured with differential spectroscopy is very low in microsomes prepared from hepatocyte nodules[14,17-24]. Different enzymatic reactions catalysed by cytochrome P-450 have also been reported to be markedly reduced, the most extensive characterization being made by Åström *et al.*[23], Table 32.1.

Table 32.1 Relative levels of cytochrome P-450 and cytochrome P-450 catalysed activities in microsomes from hepatocyte nodules. Normal activity = 1

Cytochrome P-450	0.25
Aminopyrine N-demethylase	0.24
Benzo(a)pyrene mono-oxygenase	0.06
Ethoxyresorufin *O*-deethylase	0.12
Ethoxycoumarin *O*-deethylase	0.45
2-AAF 1-hydroxylase	0.02
2-AAF 3-hydroxylase	0.24
2-AAF 5-hydroxylase	0.63
2-AAF 7-hydroxylase	0.06
2-AAF 9-hydroxylase	0.05
2-AAF N-hydroxylase	0.04

Data from Ref. 23

All mono-oxygenase reactions analysed showed a reduced specific activity in hepatocyte nodules, but the degrees of reduction were different. Some activities retained half or more than half of the control activity, e.g. ethoxycoumarin *O*-deethylase and 2-acetylaminofluorene 5-hydroxylase, while other activities were only 5% of control activity, e.g. benzo(a)pyrene mono-oxygenase, 2-acetylaminofluorene 1-hydroxylase and 2-acetylaminofluorene *N*-hydroxylase. These variations point out a certain specificity in the reduction of these enzyme activities, making an unspecific alteration in the cells less probable as the mechanism for the reported phenotypic differences between normal and nodular cells. The consequences of the reduced mono-oxygenase activities in the cells during 2-acetylaminofluorene promotion are slow formation of ring hydroxylated compounds of the drug for excretion and a slow rate of formation of *N*-hydroxylated compounds, regarded as precursors for reactive species of the parent compound.

Enzymes participating in the second phase of drug metabolism, Table 32.2, were all markedly increased in activities and amounts in hepatocyte nodules compared to normal tissue. The activity of UDP-glucuronosyltransferase in the microsomal fraction of liver nodules was five times the normal activity, when 1-naphthol[23,25,26] or 4-methylumbelliferone[25] were used as substrates (UDP-glucuronosyltransferase I), while the activities using 4-hydroxybiphenyl, morphine, chloramphenicol, bilirubin or oestrone were not changed or changed to only a limited extent[25] (Figure 32.3).

Table 32.2 Relative levels of various drug metabolizing enzyme activities, glutathione and γ-glutamyltransferase in hepatocyte nodules produced by intermittent feeding of 2-acetylaminofluorene. Normal activities and amounts = 1

UDP-glucuronosyltransferase I (microsome)*	4.9
Glutathione S-transferase (cytosol)†	4.7
DT-diaphorase (cytosol)‡	13.1
Epoxide hydrolase (microsome)‡	5.0
Glutathione (cytosol)‖	3.0
γ-Glutamyltransferase (homogenate)†	3.5

* Data from Ref. 25
† Data from Ref. 14
‡ Data from Ref. 23
‖ Data from Ref. 24

Immunoprecipitation techniques and immunohistochemical investigations confirmed that there was an increased amount of the glucuronosyltransferase I protein in cells in hepatocyte nodules[25–27].

The cytosolic forms of glutathione S-transferase using 1-chloro-2,4-dinitrobenzene as substrate were also markedly increased[14,23,24], which was not true for the forms associated with the endoplasmic reticulum membrane[14]. Recently Sato *et al.*[28] showed that in hepatocyte nodules a placental form of glutathione S-transferase, usually not measurable in normal liver, was tremendously increased in the nodules. Work recently performed by Pickett *et al.*[29] using hepatocyte nodules from the resistant hepatocyte model also established that the mRNA levels for Ya/Yc subunits as well as Yb subunits of glutathione S-transferase were 3 and 5 times the levels found in normal liver, respectively.

DT-Diaphorase activity determined in cytosols from hepatocyte nodules exceeded the activity in normal rat liver cytosol 12 times[23,24,30]. This was also found to be the case using histochemical techniques[30]. The work of Pickett *et al.*[29] confirmed that the mRNA for cytosolic DT-diaphorase was elevated 5–7-fold in nodules over the levels in normal rat liver.

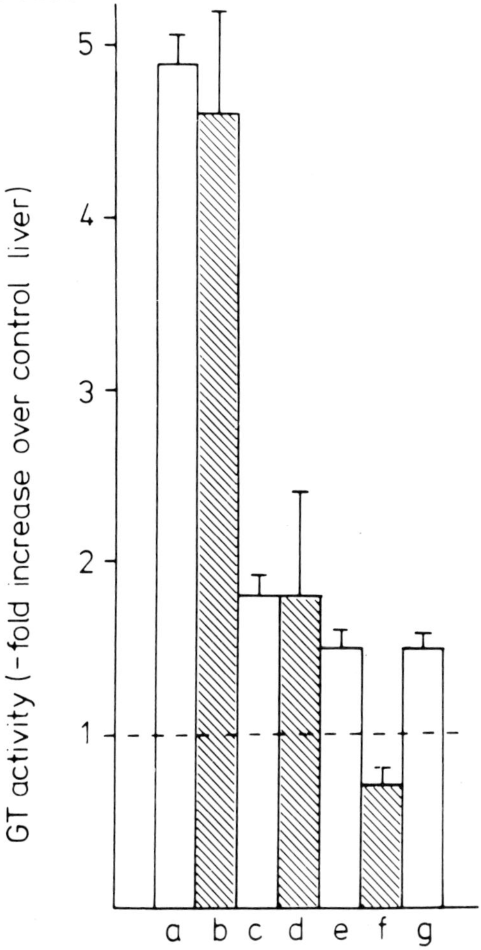

Figure 32.3 The activity of UDP-glucuronosyltransferase in hepatocyte nodules using different substrates. Normal activity = 1. a = 1-naphthol, b = 4-methylumbelliferone, c = 4-hydroxybiphenyl, d = morphine, e = chloramphenicol, f = bilirubin, g = oestrone. Data from Ref. 25

Microsomal epoxide hydrolase was reported by Levin[31] to be elevated in hepatocyte nodules produced by intermittent feeding of 2-acetylaminofluorene. This was later reported by other authors[23,32,33]. Oesch[33] showed that in contrast to the membrane bound form the cytosolic form of the epoxide hydrolase was not altered in hepatocyte nodules.

The activity of sulphotransferase in cytosol of hepatocyte nodules has been reported by King *et al.*[34] to be reduced using histochemical methods. Ringer *et al.*[35] reported decreased activity of this enzyme in liver cytosols from rats fed carcinogens.

Other characteristic phenotypic properties of nodular cells related to drug metabolism are the high levels of glutathione found in the cytosol[24] and the very high activity of γ-glutamyl transferase in membranes[14,24,25,36] and cytosol[14,24] from nodular cells as well as in serum of nodule-bearing rats[14,24].

EXCRETION OF 2-ACETYLAMINOFLUORENE DERIVATIVES

With the background of the specific pattern of drug-metabolizing enzymes presented above we have investigated not only the *in vivo* uptake and binding[16] of 2-acetylaminofluorene in hepatocyte nodules and in normal rat liver tissue, but also the *in vivo* metabolism[37] as well as the excretion of metabolites of the drug in bile and urine[38]. The rate of elimination of metabolites and the accumulated excretion of metabolites over a prolonged period of time give valuable information of how liver cells deal with a given dose of a foreign compound. These experiments were performed using normal rats and rats treated with 2-acetylaminofluorene to generate hepatocyte nodules that from a practical point of view replaced almost the entire liver. Experiments shown in Figure 32.2 illustrate how nodules initially retained less of the injected compound, and that the rate of elimination from the nodules of 2-acetylaminofluorene was lower than from normal liver. Table 32.3 shows that 180 minutes

Table 32.3 Accumulated excretion of 2-AAF metabolites from normal and nodule-bearing rats 180 min after injection. Data are the mean ± SD of four experiments

	% Given dose			
	Total	*Ether extractable*	*Glucuronides*	*Other*
Normal rat	82 ± 8	4.7	8.7	57
Nodule-bearing rats	60 ± 6	5.1	24.0	25

[9-^{14}C]2-AAF, [9-^{14}C]2-acetylaminofluorene, was dissolved in rat serum and injected (0.23 mg/kg body weight) in a branch of the superior mesenteric vein. Bile was collected from a bile cannula in 100 μl fractions. Urine was collected by puncture of the bladder 180 min after injection. Nodule-bearing rats were produced by intermittent feeding of 2-acetylaminofluorene. Metabolites were separated by fractionated ether extraction. *Ether extractable metabolites* (ring-hydroxylated compounds) are radioactivity extractable with ether from bile and urine. *Glucuronides* are radioactivity extractable after β-glucuronidase treatment. *Other metabolites* are remaining radioactivity

after the intramesenteric injection of a tracer dose of 2-acetylaminofluorene (0.23 mg/kg body weight) 82% of the given dose had been excreted from a normal rat, while only 60% of the dose was excreted from nodule-bearing rats in bile and urine together. Five per cent of the excreted dose was excreted as ring-hydroxylated compounds which can be extracted from urine and bile with ether. From normal rats, 9% of the dose was excreted as glucuronidated compounds, extractable after treatment with β-glucuronidase. Nodule-bearing rats excreted as much as 24% of the given dose as glucuronidated compounds, leaving 25% as yet uncharacterized derivatives, probably sulphate and glutathione conjugated metabolites. The corresponding value for normal rats was 57%. No free 2-acetylaminofluorene was excreted in bile or urine.

Table 32.4 shows how the excreted derivatives were divided between bile and urine. Normal rats excreted most of the dose (65%) via the bile, only 18% being found in the urine. On the other hand, nodule-bearing rats excreted less in the bile and most of the excreted compounds were found in the urine (38% of given dose). Evidently the vast majority of the formed glucuronic acid conjugates were excreted in the urine (90%).

Table 32.4 Accumulated excretion of 2-AAF metabolites in bile and urine from normal and nodule-bearing rats 180 min after injection. Data are the mean ± SD of four experiments

	Bile (% given dose)				Urine (% given dose)			
	Total	*Ether extract.*	*Glucuronides*	*Other*	*Total*	*Ether extract.*	*Glucuronides*	*Other*
Normal rats	65 ± 7	4.6	6.5	48	18 ± 6	0.1	2.2	8.5
Nodule-bearing rats	22 ± 5	4.1	2.0	13	38 ± 5	1.0	22	12

Experiments were performed as given in legend Table 32.3

Most of the detected *N*-hydroxy-2-acetylaminofluorene was excreted conjugated with glucuronic acid. Table 32.5 shows that the excretion of glucuronic acid esters of *N*-hydroxy-2-acetylaminofluorene was the same in bile from normal and nodule-bearing rats, but that the urine from nodule-bearing rats contained 14-fold the amount in urine from normal rats, at 180 minutes after injection of the tracer dose of 2-acetylaminofluorene. Taking urine and bile products together three times as many *N*-hydroxy compounds were excreted from nodule-bearing rats as were excreted from normal rats. On the other hand, 1.9% of the given dose of 2-acetylaminofluorene was recovered as compound covalently bound to macromolecules in the liver cells from normal rats, while only 0.3% of the dose was bound to macromolecules in the hepatocyte nodules. The data led us to conclude that the formation of *N*-hydroxy-2-acetylaminofluorene over a 3 hour period was equal in normal liver and in the livers replaced by hepatocyte nodules. Thus, in spite of the fact that the rate of *N*-hydroxylation was faster in normal liver, the substrate was available for a longer period of time in the nodule-bearing rats, which compensated for the slow rate of metabolism. In the case of nodular tissue the conjugation with glucuronic acid was more efficient, and the abundant glucuronosyltransferase enzyme trapped the formed *N*-hydroxyl compounds, which consequently were excreted instead of being further processed and bound to intracellular macromolecules. Of course, some of these conjugates may be already sulphated derivatives of the drug.

Table 32.5 Total amounts of glucuronic acid esters of *N*-OH-2-AAF eliminated in bile and urine of normal and nodule-bearing rats, and amount of compound bound to macromolecules 180 min after injection

	N-OH-2-AAF-glucuronide nmoles excreted at 180 min			*% Given dose excreted as N-OH-compound*	*% Given dose bound to macromols. in liver*
	Bile	*Urine*	*Total*		
Normal rat	1.38	0.29	1.67	0.8	1.9
Nodule-bearing rats	1.38	3.82	5.20	2.2	0.3

Experiments were performed as given in legend Table 32.3. *N*-OH-2-AAF was isolated from the fraction of glucuronides from bile and urine by HPLC chromatography using a modification of the technique discribed by Ryzewski and Malejka-Giganti (1982)[40]

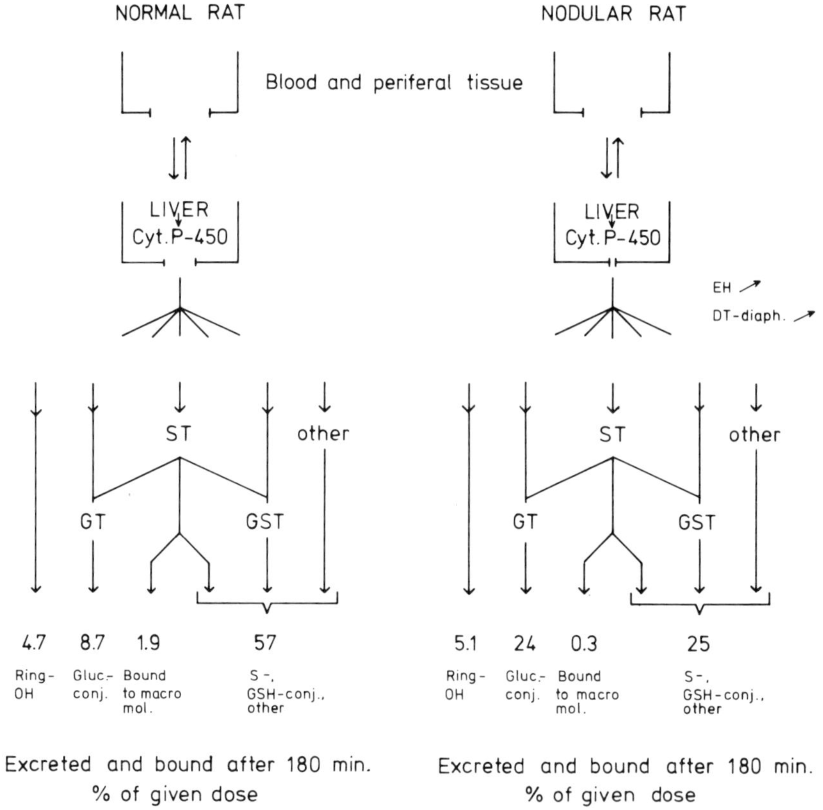

Figure 32.4 Schematic presentation of the flow of 2-acetylaminofluorene and its metabolites through the livers of normal and nodule-bearing rats

In summary, Figure 32.4 illustrates the flow of 2-acetylaminofluorene and its metabolites through the livers of normal and nodule-bearing rats. There seemed to be no hindrance for the uptake of 2-acetylaminofluorene to nodular tissue, but in nodules less drug was non-covalently attracted to cytochrome P-450 and the rate of metabolism was also slower in nodule cells than in normal liver cells. In the normal rat liver the formation of hydroxylated compounds was fast, and a lot of products were formed within a short period of time. These formed substances were substrates for the phase II enzymes in the different cell compartments. The affinities of these enzymes for the available substrates and the capacities of the enzymes to catalyse the reactions determined the formation of products for excretion or binding to intracellular structures. In the situation of excess substrate, high capacity enzymes are favoured on behalf of high affinity, low capacity enzymes. As can be seen from Figure 32.4, in the normal rat, 4.7% of the given dose was excreted as ring-hydroxylated compounds, 9% as glucuronic acid esters, 57% as other compounds while 1.9% of the dose was bound to macromolecules in the cell.

In the nodular rat the situation was different. Hydroxylated compounds were formed relatively slowly, but were produced over a prolonged period of time.

The phase II enzymes present in different relative amounts in nodules were exposed to low amounts of substrate, which should favour the enzymes with the highest affinity even if the capacity of these enzymes was low. In this case a large amount of the drug was glucuronidated and excreted in the urine resulting in a low amount of binding to cellular macromolecules. In our view, the specific phenotype of the nodular cells renders them resistant to cytotoxic drugs by a decreased rate of activation in combination with an efficient conjugation capacity where the formation of glucuronic acid conjugates seems to play an important role.

There are still many obscure processes in the mechanisms of resistance of hepatocyte nodules to cytotoxic drugs. Currently work is being performed to try to show the importance of sulphotransferase for the formation of reactive species of *N*-hydroxy-2-acetylaminofluorene, and how that enzyme is altered in hepatocyte nodules. We are also interested in the mechanisms of secretion of conjugated compounds to the bile and the reasons why glucuronidated compounds are excreted not in the bile but in the urine of nodule-bearing rats. Undoubtedly this gives the nodule-bearing rats the advantage of not being exposed a second time to compounds once excreted in the bile, deconjugated in the gut and reabsorbed into the portal blood for transportation to the liver[16].

DISCUSSION

What becomes increasingly intriguing, as more models of chemical carcinogenesis are being investigated, is the extensive degree of commonality in the profile of drug metabolizing enzymes in nodules produced by different protocols (*see* Ref. 39 for review). All nodules from rat liver, so far examined, in every parameter measured show the same alterations as has been given here for nodules produced using intermittent feeding of 2-acetylaminofluorene, and for nodules developed by selection after initiation by diethylnitrosamine as suggested by Solt and Farber[12]. Even nodules that have been promoted using a choline–methionine deficient diet or orotic acid have the same phenotype in this respect. It may be that this common biochemical phenotype is important not only for selection with certain drugs but also for the metabolism of endogenously formed toxic compounds, or the formation of growth stimulation factors, such as those derived from leukotrienes etc. necessary for the constant proliferation of nodular cells.

In Table 32.6 we have tabulated some differences between normal and nodular cells which correlate to drug resistance. In all parameters the nodules show alterations that protect them from exposure to toxic compounds or metabolites. Farber[39] suggests that these alterations may be a form of adaptation to a hazardous environment which enables the cells and the animal to survive an acute toxic exposure, and is combined with an increased tendency for cell proliferation. In support of this theory is the fact that most of the nodules formed do redifferentiate[11] to phenotypically normal appearing liver cells. As a disadvantage of this process of adaptation stands the risk of malignant transformation later in life. This negative consequence of an adaptive process appears in the post-reproductive period, which makes it a minor threat for the

Table 32.6 Possible mechanisms for resistance to the mitoinhibitory effect of 2-acetylaminofluorene (2-AAF)

Factor	*Change in nodules*
Portal blood supply	Decreased
Binding of 2-AAF to cytochrome P-450	Decreased
Metabolism of 2-AAF	Decreased
hydroxylation	
conjugation	Increased
Excretion of *N*-OH-2-AAF	Increased
Binding of reactive drug metabolites to macromolecules	Decreased
Enterohepatic circulation	Decreased

survival of the species. It is attractive to consider the complexity and the stereotypy of the alterations in preneoplastic liver lesions as a part of a biological programme for normal cell adaptation, switched on by the initiation procedure and maintained or selected for by the promotion, rather than the result of a series of specific mutations and permanent induction processes. Whether the initiation process contains a point mutation in a regulatory gene locus and is irreversible, or influences gene regulation in other ways and made irreversible by mutation-like events later on during the promotion, is not yet known.

Although the genetic programme for the regulation of drug-metabolizing enzymes in hepatocyte nodules is altered, the inducibility of the individual enzymes using different chemical inducers seems to be intact, with only one exception registered so far. Pickett *et al.*[29] have shown that the Ya/Yc subunits of glutathione-S-transferase cannot be induced in hepatocyte nodules using methylcholanthrene, while the Yb subunit does increase as in normal rat liver, after treatment with methylcholanthrene. This indicates that together with gene amplification in preneoplastic tissue gene defects in regulatory sites do exist.

In the case of hepatocyte nodules produced by 2-acetylaminofluorene exposure we believe that the ability of the cells to proliferate in the presence of this mitoinhibitor is due to the specific way these cells handle the drug, resulting in a low covalent interaction with cellular macromolecules. The specific properties in drug metabolism shown by the initiated cells in these models are, therefore, decisive for the development of hepatocyte nodules and the subsequent transformation to hepatocellular carcinomas. As far as 2-acetylaminofluorene is concerned the slow activation and the fast conjugation to glururonic acid seem to be the two most important factors.

ACKNOWLEDGEMENTS

This work is supported by grants from the Swedish Medical Research Council and the National Cancer Institute of Canada.

References

1. Farber, E. (1980). The sequential analysis of liver cancer induction. *Biochim. Biophys. Acta*, **605,** 149–66
2. Pitot, H. C. and Sirica, A. E. (1980). The stages of initiation and promotion in hepatocarcinogenesis. *Biochim. Biophys. Acta*, **605,** 191–215
3. Emmelot, P. and Scherer, E. (1980). The first relevant cell stage in rat liver carcinogenesis. A quantitative approach. *Biochim. Biophys. Acta*, **605,** 247–304
4. Popper, H., Sternberg, S. S., Oser, B. C. and Oser, M. (1960). The carcinogenic effect of aramite in rats. A study of hepatic nodules. *Cancer,* **13,** 1035–46
5. Epstein, S., Ito, N., Merkow, L. and Farber, E. (1967). Cellular analysis of liver carcinogenesis. The induction of large hyperplastic nodules in the liver with 2-fluorenylacetamide or ethionine and some aspects of their morphology and glycogen metabolism. *Cancer Res.*, **27,** 1702–11
6. Goldfarb, S. (1973). A morphological and histochemical study of carcinogenesis of the liver in rats fed 3-methyl-4-dimethylaminoazobenzene. *Cancer Res.*, **33,** 1119–28
7. Solt, D. B., Medline, A. and Farber, E. (1977). Rapid emergence of carcinogen-induced hyperplastic lesions in a new model for the sequential analysis of liver carcinogenesis. *Am. J. Pathol.*, **88,** 595–618
8. Pugh, T. D. and Goldfarb, S. (1978). Quantitative histochemical and autoradiographic studies of hepatocarcinogenesis in rats fed 2-acetylaminofluorine followed by phenobarbital. *Cancer Res.*, **38,** 4450–7
9. Farber, E. (1982). The biology of carcinogen-induced hepatocyte nodules and related liver lesions in the rats. *Toxicol. Pathol.*, **10,** 197–205
10. Farber, E., Parker, S. and Gruenstein, M. (1976). The resistance of putative pre-malignant liver cell populations, hyperplastic nodules, to the acute cytotoxic effects of some hepatocarcinogens. *Cancer Res.*, **36,** 3879–87
11. Tatematsu, M., Nagamine, Y. and Farber, E. (1983). Redifferentiation as a basis for remodeling of carcinogen-induced hepatocyte nodules to normal-appearing liver. *Cancer Res.*, **43,** 5049-58
12. Solt, D. and Farber, E. (1976). New principle for the analysis of chemical carcinogenesis. *Nature*, **263,** 702–3
13. Hayes, M. A. (1983). Failure of selective growth of liver nodules in rats given phenobarbitone during short-term feeding of 2-acetylaminofluorene. *Proc. Am. Assoc. Cancer Res.*, **24,** 85
14. Eriksson, L. C., Torndal, U.-B. and Andersson, G. N. (1983). Isolation and characterization of endoplasmic reticulum and Golgi apparatus from hepatocyte nodules in male Wistar rats, *Cancer Res.*, **43,** 3335–47
15. Solt, D., Hay, J. B. and Farber, E. (1977). Comparison of the blood supply to diethylnitrosamine-induced hyperplastic nodules and hepatomas and to the surrounding liver. *Cancer Res.*, **37,** 1686–91
16. Eriksson, L. C., Spiewak, J. A., Roomi, M. W. and Farber, E. (1983). Kinetic aspects of 2-acetylaminofluorene uptake, metabolism, excretion and enterohepatic circulation. In Rydström, J., Montelius, J. and Bengtsson, M. (eds.). *Extrahepatic Drug Metabolism and Chemical Carcinogenesis*, pp. 297–8. (Amsterdam: Elsevier)
17. Gravela, E., Feo, F., Canuto, R. A., Garcea, R. and Gabriel, L. (1975). Functional and structural alterations of liver ergastoplasmic membranes during DL-ethionine hepatocarcinogenesis. *Cancer Res.*, **35,** 3041–7
18. Cameron, R., Sweeney, G. D., Jones, K., Lee, G. and Farber, E. (1976). A relative deficiency of cytochrome P-450 and aryl hydrocarbon (benzo(a)pyrene) hydroxylase in hyperplastic nodules induced by 2-acetylaminofluorene in rat liver. *Cancer Res.*, **36,** 3888–93
19. Okita, K., Noda, K., Fukumoto, Y. and Takemoto, T. (1976). Cytochrome P-450 in hyperplastic liver nodules during hepatocarcinogenesis with 2-fluorenylacetamide in rats. *Gann*, **67,** 899–902
20. Feo, F., Canuto, R. A., Garcea, R., Brossa, O. and Caselli, G. C. (1978). Phenobarbital stimulation of cytochrome P-450 and aminopyrine *N*-demethylase in hyperplastic liver nodules during DL-ethionine carcinogenesis. *Cancer Lett.*, **5,** 25–30
21. Kaneko, A., Dempo, K., Kaku, T., Yokoyama, S., Satoh, M. and Onoe, T. (1980).

Effect of phenobarbital administration on hepatocytes constituting the hyperplastic nodules induced in rat liver by 3-methyl-4-dimethylaminoazobenzene. *Cancer Res.*, **40,** 1658–62

22. Sato, M., Yoshida, T., Suzuki, Y., Degawa, M. and Hashimoto, Y. (1981). Selective induction of microsomal 2-acetylaminofluorene *N*-hydroxylation by dietary 2-acetylaminofluorene in rats. *Carcinogenesis*, **2,** 571–4
23. Åström, A., De Pierre, J. W. and Eriksson, L. C. (1983). Characterization of drug-metabolizing systems in hyperplastic nodules from the livers of rats receiving 2-acetylaminofluorene in their diet. *Carcinogenesis*, **4,** 577–81
24. Roomi, M. W., Ho, R. K., Cameron, R. G., Sarma, D. S. R. and Farber, E. (1984). A novel biochemical pattern in hepatocyte nodules generated during liver carcinogenesis in five different models. *Proc. Am. Assoc. Cancer Res.*, **25,** 112
25. Bock, K. W., Lilienblum, W., Pfeil, H. and Eriksson, L. C. (1982). Increased uridine diphosphate-glucuronyltransferase activity in preneoplastic liver nodules and Morris hepatomas. *Cancer Res.*, **42,** 3747–52
26. Yin, Z., Sato, K., Tsuda, H. and Ito, N. (1982). Changes in activities of uridine diphosphate-glucuronyltransferases during chemical hepatocarcinogenesis. *Gann*, **73,** 239–48
27. Fischer, G., Ullrich, D., Katz, N. R., Bock, K. W. and Schauer, A. (1983). Immunohistochemical and biochemical detection of UDP-glucuronyltransferase activity in putative preneoplastic liver foci. *Virch. Arch. Cell Pathol.*, **42,** 193–200
28. Sato, K., Kitohara, A., Satoh, K., Ishihawa, T., Tatematsu, M. and Ito, N. (1984). The placental form of glutathione S-transferase as a marker protein for preneoplasia in rat chemical hepatocarcinogenesis. *Gann*, **75,** 199–202
29. Pickett, C. B., Williams, J. B., Lu, A. Y. H. and Cameron, R. G. (1984). Elevated levels of rat liver glutathione S-transferase and DT-diaphorase mRNAs in persistent hepatocyte nodules. *Proc. Am. Assoc. Cancer Res.*, **25,** 7
30. Schor, N. A., Ogawa, K., Lee, G. and Farber, E. (1978). The use of DT-diaphorase for the detection of foci of early neoplastic transformation in rat liver. *Cancer Lett.*, **5,** 167–71
31. Levin, W., Lu, A. Y. H., Thomas, P. E., Ryan, D., Kizer, D. and Griffin, M. J. (1978). Identification of epoxide hydrolase as the preneoplastic antigen in rat liver hyperplastic nodules. *Proc. Natl. Acad. Sci. USA*, **75,** 3240–3
32. Sharma, R. N., Gurtoo, H. L., Farber, E., Murray, R. K. and Cameron, R. G. (1981). Effects of hepatocarcinogens and hepatocarcinogenesis on the activity of rat liver microsomal epoxide hydrolase with observations on the electophoretic behavior of this enzyme. *Cancer Res.*, **41,** 3311–9
33. Oesch, F., Vogel-Bindel, U., Guenther, T. M., Cameron, R. and Farber, E. (1983). Characterization of microsomal epoxide hydrolase in hyperplastic liver nodules of rat. *Cancer Res.*, **43,** 313–9
34. Shirai, T. and King, C. M. (1982). Sulfotransferase and deacetylase in normal and tumor-bearing liver of CD-rats: Autoradiographical studies with *N*-hydroxy-2-acetylaminobiphenyl *in vitro* and *in vivo*. *Carcinogenesis*, **3,** 1385–91
35. Ringer, D. P., Kampschmidt, K., King, R. L. Jr., Jackson, S. and Kizer, D. E. (1983). Rapid decrease in *N*-hydroxy-2-acetylaminofluorene sulfotransferase activity of liver cytosols from rats fed carcinogen. *Biochem. Pharmacol.*, **32,** 315–9
36. Cameron, R., Kellen, J., Kolin, A., Malkin, A. and Farber, E. (1978). Gamma-glutamyltransferase in putative premalignant liver cell populations, during hepatocarcinogenesis. *Cancer Res.*, **38,** 823–9
37. Spiewak, J. A. (1984). The role of metabolism in rendering carcinogen-induced liver nodules resistant to the effects of 2-acetylaminofluorene. *Proc. Am. Assoc. Cancer Res.*, **25,** 113
38. Spiewak, J. A. and Eriksson, L. C. (1983). Pharmacokinetics of 2-acetylaminofluorene excretion in normal rats and rats with 2-acetylaminofluorene induced nodules. *Proc. Am. Assoc. Cancer Res.*, **24,** 76
39. Farber, E. (1984). The biochemistry of preneoplastic liver: A common metabolic pattern in hepatocyte nodules. *Can. J. Biochem.* (In press)
40. Ryzewski, C. N. and Malejka-Giganti, D. (1982). Systems for the separation of metabolites of the carcinogen, *N*-2-fluorenylacetamide, by high performance liquid chromatography. *J. Chromatogr.*, **237,** 447-56
41. Conway, J. G., Popp, J.A., Ji, S. and Thurman, R. G. (1983). Effect of size on portal circulation of hepatic nodules from carcinogen-treated rats. *Cancer Res.*, **43,** 3374–9

33
Increased UDP-glucuronosyl-transferase in preneoplastic liver foci

D. ULLRICH, G. FISCHER AND K. W. BOCK

ABSTRACT

Alterations in the pattern of drug-metabolizing enzymes were investigated in an initiation/promotion model of hepatocarcinogenesis. Development of adenosine triphosphatase-deficient foci was used to quantitate prestages. Activities of UDP-glucuronosyltransferase and arylhydrocarbon hydroxylase were determined in microdissections from focal and extrafocal liver tissue.

Initiation by a single administration of *N*-nitrosomorpholine (75 mg/kg, 24 h after partial hepatectomy) led to a 3–5-fold increase of UDP-glucuronosyltransferase activity in focal tissue, detected 180–330 days after initiation, whereas arylhydrocarbon hydroxylase was decreased by 50%. Similar alterations of the two enzymes were observed after feeding a diet containing 0.03% (w/v) 2-acetylaminofluorene. Chronic administration of the tumour-promoter phenobarbital (0.1 g/100 ml, in drinking water) further increased UDP-glucuronosyltransferase activity up to 9-fold, compared with untreated controls. However, this further increase of enzyme activity by phenobarbital was reversible.

The results indicate that (1) initiation leads to permanent alterations of drug-metabolizing enzymes, consistent with increased toxin-resistance of initiated hepatocytes and (2) chronic administration of the tumour-promoter phenobarbital markedly enhances gene expression in initiated hepatocytes.

INTRODUCTION

Numerous studies delineated at least two prestages of chemical carcinogenesis: initiation and promotion[1–4]. In hepatocarcinogenesis, initiated cell clones can be identified histochemically by enzyme alterations: for example, reduction of canalicular adenosine triphosphatase (ATPase)[5] or reappearance of the fetal enzyme γ-glutamyltranspeptidase[6]. In the presence of tumour promoters some focal lesions develop into hyperplastic nodules. These nodules appear to possess two options, remodelling or further development into hepatocellular carcinoma[3,7].

A large number of hepatic enzymes appear to be permanently altered after initiation, including enzymes involved in carbohydrate metabolism[8,9] and in drug metabolism[10–18]. Interestingly, cytochrome P-450 dependent reactions, often involved in the activation of carcinogens to ultimate carcinogens, are decreased in preneoplastic cells[10], whereas drug metabolizing enzymes mostly involved in the inactivation of drug metabolites, are markedly increased. The latter enzymes include microsomal epoxide hydrolase[11,12], microsomal UDP-glucuronosyltransferase (GT)[13–17], cytosolic glutathione S-transferase[17] and cytosolic DT-diaphorase[18]. This altered pattern of drug metabolizing enzymes appears to be a special phenotypic programme since it is found after treatment with many diverse initiating agents. The altered enzyme pattern is consistent with the general increase in resistance of initiated cells to the cytotoxicity of chemical carcinogens[7]. Based on this concept a model of tumour promotion was developed which includes chronic exposure to cytotoxins after initiation[3,19]. Toxin-injured normal liver cells lead to regenerative growth of resistant hepatocytes[20]. This 'resistant hepatocyte' model has been shown to be one of the most effective means of tumour promotion.

A second model of tumour promotion uses chronic enzyme induction by inducers of drug metabolizing enzymes such as phenobarbital, polychlorinated biphenyls or TCDD[4]. Tumour promotion may be associated with the inducing action of these compounds since they also lead to liver growth by both hypertrophy and hyperplasia in normal liver[21–23].

Recently we developed methods to determine GT both histochemically and biochemically in microdissections from focal and extrafocal tissues[15]. When applied to an initiation promotion model of hepatocarcinogenesis these methods offered the possibility to study, separately, the effects of initiators and promoters on this enzyme.

MONITORING OF PRESTAGES OF HEPATOCARCINOGENESIS

Histochemical detection of ATPase-negative foci has been shown to be a useful marker of putative preneoplastic rat liver lesions[5]. The increase of the intersectional area of these foci was used to monitor the development of cancer prestages (Figure 33.1). An initial phase of development (up to 280 days) was followed by an accelerated growth in which numerous hyperplastic nodules were found. At 450 days after initiation hepatocarcinomas could be detected (Figure 33.2).

Stereologic models have been developed to quantitate the number and size of foci[24]. These models are particularly useful when focal lesions are compared which differ widely in their mean diameters. As shown in Table 33.1, chronic administration of phenobarbital did not increase the number but significantly increased the size of foci. These findings are in agreement with previous observations[21].

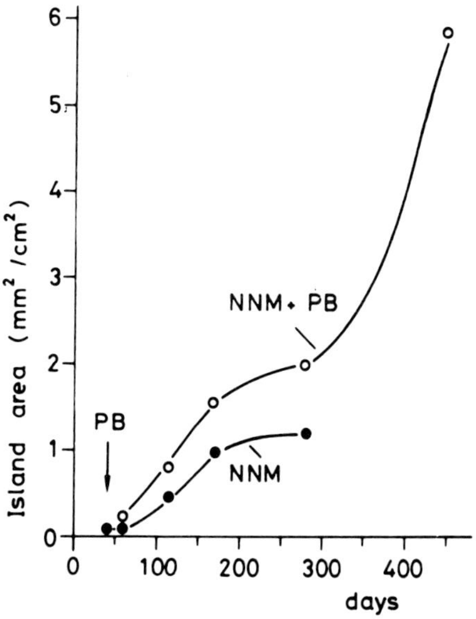

Figure 33.1 Development of ATPase-negative foci and hyperplastic nodules. Preneoplastic liver lesions were initiated in male Wistar rats by the administration of *N*-nitrosomorpholine (75 mg/kg, once intraperitoneally, 24 h after partial hepatectomy). After 3 weeks sodium phenobarbital (0.1 g/100 ml) was continuously administered in tap water. ATPase-negative lesions were visualized histochemically, and their area was determined by planimetry. Eight sections each from six animals per group were analysed

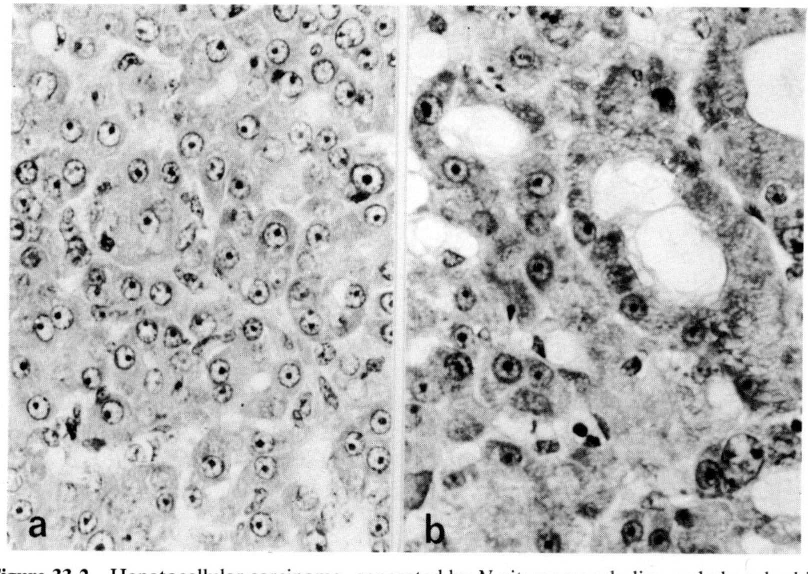

Figure 33.2 Hepatocellular carcinoma, generated by *N*-nitrosomorpholine and phenobarbital in an initiation/promotion model. The hepatocellular carcinoma was observed 450 days after initiation in the model described in Figure 33.1. Trabecular (**a**) and tubular (**b**) patterns of hepatocellular carcinomas were detectable

Table 33.1 Effect of phenobarbital on the development of ATPase-negative foci in rat liver, 180 days after initiation with *N*-nitrosomorpholine (NNM)[a]

Treatment	*No. of foci per cm³ of liver*	*Mean volume of foci* (mm³)	*Volume % of foci in liver*
NNM	194±40	0.07±0.03	1.1±0.5
NNM+phenobarbital	170±41	0.20±0.13*	2.6±0.9**

[a] ATPase-negative foci were produced and visualized as in Figure 33.1. Eight sections each (ca. 2 cm²) from six animals per group were analysed. Calculations are based on the model described by Campbell *et al.*[24]. The means ± SD are listed
* $p<0.05$; ** $p<0.005$

EFFECTS OF A SINGLE ADMINISTRATION OF *N*-NITROSOMORPHOLINE ON DRUG METABOLIZING ENZYMES

Adminisitration of a single dose of *N*-nitrosomorpholine, 24 h after partial hepatectomy, led to a persistent increase of GT activity toward 1-naphthol in foci (Figure 33.3). This increase was 5-fold at 330 days after initiation. In contrast arylhydrocarbon hydroxylase activity was decreased by 50% in focal tissue. Similar alterations in the pattern of drug metabolizing enzymes were observed after feeding 2-acetylaminofluorene[10,13,17]. GT was also increased in liver foci produced by chronic administration of metapyrilene[16] or diethylnitrosamine (unpublished results). These results indicate that GT belongs to the group of enzymes which are permanently increased after initiation. This increase of enzyme activity has been operationally termed 'permanent induction' in order to distinguish it from regular induction which is reversible.

Epoxide hydrolase is another enzyme which is permanently increased after initation of hepatocarcinogenesis[11,12]. In studies with this enzyme a sustained increase of its messenger ribonucleic acid was observed in hepatocytes after the administration of 2-acetylaminofluorene[25], indicating that the increased enzyme activity was due to increased transcription.

GT consists of a family of isoenzymes. It was shown previously, based on functional criteria, that it is the isoenzyme termed GT_1 or GT_{MC} which is preferentially increased in preneoplastic foci[13] (*see* Chapter 6).

The altered pattern of drug metabolizing enzymes leads to decreased activation and more efficient conjugation and excretion of toxins, and can be related to an increased resistance to the cytotoxic actions of carcinogens[3,7,19]. Hence under the conditions of chronic exposure, resistant hepatocytes gain a growth advantage over normal hepatocytes.

Increased GT activity in focal tissue should lead to a shift from sulphation to glucuronidation, two reactions which often compete in the conjugation of phenols. This shift has actually been demonstrated in organ cultures of human tumorous tissue from lung and colon[26,27] and in bronchial carcinoma cell lines[28]. These findings suggest that the altered pattern of drug metabolizing enzymes may also be important in human carcinogenesis.

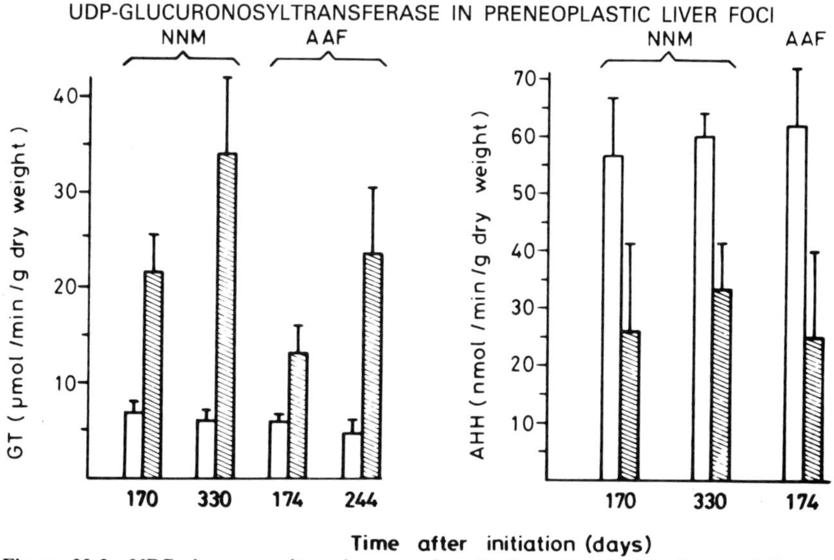

Figure 33.3 UDP-glucuronosyltransferase and arylhydrocarbon hydroxylase activities in focal and extrafocal liver tissue. Microdissection was carried out using an exact optical projection of a section stained for ATPase onto an unstained lyophilized serial section[15]. Enzyme activities were determined in lyophilized sections from focal tissue (hatched bars) and extrafocal tissue (open bars). Rats were treated by either a single administration of *N*-nitrosomorpholine (NNM), as described in Figure 33.1, or by continuous feeding of 2-acetylaminofluorene (AAF)[15]. The means ± SD are shown. Determination of GT activity in studies with NNM and AAF, $n=12$ and 8, respectively. Determination of arylhydrocarbon hydroxylase (AHH) activity, $n=4$

EFFECTS OF THE TUMOUR PROMOTER PHENOBARBITAL ON UDP-GLUCURONOSYLTRANSFERASE IN PRENEOPLASTIC LIVER FOCI

GT activity was compared in focal tissue from animals which either remained untreated after initiation or received phenobarbital chronically in drinking water. As shown in Table 33.2, phenobarbital treatment led to a further increase of GT activity in focal tissue (up to 9-fold, compared with extrafocal tissue from animals which remained untreated after initiation). However, this increase above 'permanent induction' was reversible since GT activity was reduced when phenobarbital was withdrawn 14 days before the analysis. An enzyme level was reached which was similar to that found in animals which received the initiator only. Some animals received 3-methylcholanthrene 4 days before the analysis in addition to phenobarbital, since 3-methylcholanthrene is the preferential inducer of GT activity towards 1-naphthol. This preferential induction is clearly seen in extrafocal tissue. However, in focal tissue enzyme activity could not be further increased by 3-methylcholanthrene. This finding suggests that gene expression in focal tissue could not be further increased under these conditions. The percentage increase of GT activity induced by phenobarbital was similar in focal and extrafocal tissue. However, the inducing action of phenobarbital may be greater in focal tissue, as suggested by the larger difference in enzyme activity.

Table 33.2 Effects of phenobarbital and 3-methylcholanthrene on UDP-glucuronosyltransferase activities in focal and extrafocal tissue (330 days after initiation)

Treatment after initiation with N-nitrosomorpholine	*UDP-glucuronosyltransferase activity*[a] (μmol min^{-1} g dry weight^{-1}) *Extrafocal tissue*	*Focal tissue*
None	6.3±1.4	33.9± 8.1
Phenobarbital	12.1±1.4	55.6±11.3
Phenobarbital withdrawn 14 days before sacrifice	6.9±0.5	28.7± 3.1
Phenobarbital+3-methylcholanthrene (4 days before sacrifice)	23.2± 3.3	60.6±12.7

[a] Focal lesions were produced as in Figure 33.1. 3-Methylcholanthrene was administered as a single dose (40 mg/kg, dissolved in olive oil). GT activity toward 1-naphthol was determined as described in Figure 33.3. The means ± SD of 12 determinations are listed

Increased GT activity in nodular tissue or in normal liver after the administration of inducers was correlated with an increased level of enzyme protein[13,29]. Moreover, studies with hepatoma cells suggest that increased GT activity after the administration of inducers is due to an increased gene expression of the enzyme[30]. Based on these observations our findings suggest that phenobarbital markedly enhances gene expression in focal tissue. Chronic administration of inducing agents at high doses lead to liver growth, due to both hypertrophy and hyperplasia[21–23]. The biochemical basis of this adaptive hyperplasia remains to be elucidated. However, it is conceivable that the strong negative growth control in a resting tissue such as liver is relieved in preneoplastic hepatocytes. Hence the adaptive hyperplasia may be exaggerated in focal tissue. This may be the basis for the tumour promoting effects of inducing agents.

ACKNOWLEDGEMENTS

We are grateful to Mrs U. Jongepier, Mrs E. Spangenberg, and Mrs G. Voltmer for expert technical assistance. We also acknowledge financial support by the Deutsche Forschungsgemeinschaft (D.U. and K.W.B.) and the Bundesministerium für Forschung und Technologie (G.F.).

References

1. Berenblum, I. and Shubik, P. (1947). The role of croton oil applications, associated with a single painting of a carcinogen, in tumour induction of the mouse's skin. *Br. J. Cancer*, **1**, 379–82
2. Emmelot, P. and Scherer, E. (1980). The first relevant cell stage in rat liver carcinogenesis. *Biochim. Biophys. Acta*, **605**, 247–304
3. Farber, E. and Cameron, R. (1980). The sequential analysis of cancer development. *Adv, Cancer Res.*, **31**, 125–226
4. Pitot, H. C. and Sirica, A. E. (1980). The stages of initiation and promotion in hepatocarcinogenesis. *Biochim. Biophys. Acta*, **605**, 191–215
5. Schauer, A. and Kunze, E. (1968). Enzymhistochemische und autoradiographische Untersuchungen während der Cancerisierung der Rattenleber mit Diäthylnitrosamin. *Z. Krebsforsch.*, **70**, 252–66

6. Cameron, R., Kellen, J., Kolin, A., Malkin, A. and Farber, E. (1978). γ-Glutamyltransferase in putative premalignant liver cell populations during hepatocarcinogenesis. *Cancer Res.*, **38,** 823–9
7. Farber, E. (1984). Chemical carcinogenesis: a current biological perspective. *Carcinogenesis*, **5,** 1–5
8. Hacker, H. J., Moore, M. A., Mayer, D. and Bannasch, P. (1982). Correlative histochemistry of some enzymes of carbohydrate metabolism in preneoplastic and neoplastic lesions in the rat liver. *Carcinogenesis*, **3,** 1265–72
9. Weinhouse, S. (1983). Isoenzyme alterations, gene regulation and the neoplastic transformation. *Adv. Enz. Regul.*, **21,** 369–86
10. Cameron, R., Sweeney, G. D., Jones, K., Lee, G. and Farber, E. (1976). A relative deficiency of cytochrome P-450 and aryl hydrocarbon (benzo(a)pyrene) hydroxylase in hyperplastic nodules induced by 2-acetylaminofluorene in rat liver. *Cancer Res.*, **36,** 3888–93
11. Levin, W., Lu, A. Y. H., Thomas, P. E., Ryan, D., Kizer, D. E. and Griffin, M. J. (1978). Identification of epoxide hydrase as the preneoplastic antigen in rat liver hyperplastic nodules. *Proc. Natl. Acad. Sci. USA*, **75,** 3240–3
12. Kuhlman, W. D., Krischan, R., Kunz, W., Guenthner, T. M. and Oesch, F. (1981). Focal elevation of liver microsomal epoxide hydrolase in early preneoplastic stages and its behaviour in the further course of hepatocarcinogenesis. *Biochem. Biophys. Res. Commun.*, **98,** 417–23
13. Bock, K. W., Lilienblum, W., Pfeil, H. and Eriksson, L. C. (1982). Increased uridine diphosphate-glucuronyltransferase activity in preneoplastic liver nodules and Morris hepatomas. *Cancer Res.*, **42,** 3747–52
14. Yin, Z., Sato, K., Tsuda, H. and Ito, N. (1982). Changes in activities of uridine diphosphate-glucuronyltransferases during chemical hepatocarcinogenesis. *Gann*, **73,** 239–48
15. Fischer, G., Ullrich, D., Katz, N., Bock, K. W. and Schauer, A. (1983). Immunohistochemical and biochemical detection of uridine-diphosphate-glucuronyltransferase (UDP-GT) activity in putative preneoplastic liver foci. *Virch. Arch. Cell Pathol.*, **42,** 193–200
16. Fischer, G., Schauer, A., Bock, K. W., Ullrich, D. and Katz, N. (1983). Immunohistochemical demonstration of increased UDP-glucuronyltransferase in putative preneoplastic liver foci. *Naturwissenschaften*, **70,** 153–4
17. Aström, A., DePierre, J. W. and Eriksson, L. (1983). Characterization of drug-metabolizing systems in hyperplastic nodules from the livers of rats receiving 2-acetylaminofluorene in their diet. *Carcinogenesis*, **5,** 577–81
18. Schor, N. A., Ogawa, K., Lee, G. and Farber, E. (1978). The use of the D-T diaphorase for the detection of foci of early neoplastic transformation in rat liver. *Cancer Lett.*, **5,** 167–71
19. Solt, D. and Farber, E. (1976). New principle for the analysis of chemical carcinogenesis. *Nature*, **263,** 701–3
20. Ying, T. S., Sarma, D. S. R. and Farber, E. (1981). Role of acute hepatic necrosis in the induction of early steps in liver carcinogenesis by diethylnitrosamine. *Cancer Res.*, **41,** 2096–102
21. Barka, T. and Popper, H. (1967). Liver enlargement and drug toxicity. *Medicine*, **46,** 103–8
22. Bock, K. W. and Remmer, H. (1978). Induction of hepatic hemoproteins. In De Matteis, F. and Aldridge, W. N. (eds.) *Handbook of Experimental Pharmacology*. Vol. 44, pp. 49–80. (Berlin-Heidelberg-New York: Springer-Verlag)
23. Schulte-Hermann, R., Ohde, G., Schuppler, J. and Timmermann-Trosiener, I. (1981). Enhanced proliferation of putative preneoplastic cells in rat liver following treatment with the tumour promoters phenobarbital, hexachlorocyclohexane, steroid compounds, and nafenopin. *Cancer Res.*, **41,** 2556–62
24. Campbell, H. A., Pitot, H. C., Potter, V. R., and Laishes, B. A. (1982). Application of quantitative stereology to the evaluation of enzyme-altered foci in rat liver. *Cancer Res.*, **42,** 465–72
25. Gonzalez, F. J., Samore, M., McQuiddy, P. and Kasper, C. B. (1982). Effects of 2-acetylaminofluorene and *N*-hydroxy-2-acetylaminofluorene on the cellular levels of epoxide hydratase, cytochrome P-450b, and NADPH-cytochrome c (P-450) oxidoreductase messenger ribonucleic acids. *J. Biol. Chem.*, **257,** 11032–6

26. Gibby, E. M., Mehta, R., Ellison, M. and Cohen, G. M. (1981). Conjugation pathways in human bronchial carcinoma cell lines. *Biochem. Pharmacol.*, **30,** 3333–6
27. Cohen, G. M, Grafstrom, R. C., Gibby, E. M., Smith, L., Autrup, H. and Harris, C. C. (1983). Metabolism of benzo(a)pyrene and 1-naphthol in cultured human tumorous and nontumorous colon. *Cancer Res.*, **43,** 1312–5
28. Cohen, G. M., Gibby, E. M. and Mehta, R. (1981). Routes of conjugation in normal and cancerous tissue from human lung. *Nature*, **291,** 662–4
29. Pfeil, H. and Bock, K. W. (1983). Electroimmunochemical quantification of UDP-glucuronosyltransferase in rat liver microsomes. *Eur. J. Biochem.*, **131,** 619–23
30. Malik, M., Koteen, G. M. and Owens, I. S. (1979). Induction of UDP-glucuronosyltransferase activity in the Reuber H-4-II-E hepatoma cell culture. *Molec. Pharmacol.*, **16,** 950–60

34
Alterations in glucuronic acid and sulphate ester conjugation in normal and tumour tissues

E. M. GIBBY, M. D'ARCY DOHERTY AND G. M. COHEN

ABSTRACT

The ability of a variety of different normal and tumour tissues from patients to conjugate 1-naphthol has been assessed. Normal human bronchus, lung and colon, maintained in short-term organ culture, metabolized 1-naphthol (20 μmol/l) predominantly to its sulphate ester conjugate, 1-naphthyl sulphate. In constrast, corresponding tumour tissues from the same patients metabolized 1-naphthol primarily to its glucuronic acid conjugate, 1-naphthyl-β-D-glucuronide. In addition, a number of other model tumour systems, including xenografts, human tumour cell lines and mouse leukaemic L1210 cells also formed 1-naphthyl-β-D-glucuronide predominantly. The predominance of glucuronic acid conjugation when compared to sulphate ester conjugation in tumour tissue may be exploitable in the design of selectively toxic anticancer agents.

INTRODUCTION

The metabolism of xenobiotics is generally considered to occur primarily, although not exclusively, in the liver in two phases, i.e. Phase I and Phase II reactions[1]. Most studies on the xenobiotic metabolizing enzymes in normal and tumour tissues have concentrated on Phase I oxidative reactions, most commonly in rodent hepatomas of different growth rates[2–4]. In general, these studies demonstrate the presence of cytochrome P-450 mixed function oxidase activities in such tumours, although the activities are generally much lower than from corresponding controls and do not appear to correlate with the growth rate of the hepatoma[4]. A recent study has shown that aryl hydrocarbon hydroxylase is also significantly lower in homogenates from tumours of patients with lung cancer than from corresponding 'normal' lung tissue from the same patients[5].

Only a small number of investigations have studied Phase II conjugation reactions in tumour tissues. Various rodent hepatomas exhibit increased UDP-glucuronosyltransferase activity when compared with the corresponding normal tissue using 1-naphthol, *p*-nitrophenol and *o*- and *p*-aminophenol as substrates[4,6–9]. In the Reuber H-35 hepatoma, the increase in glucuronic acid conjugation was accompanied by a greatly decreased phenol sulphotransferase activity to *p*-nitrophenol[8]. Human mammary neoplasms have a variable pattern of steroid-sulphating activity which differ from either normal breast tissue or normal liver[10].

Current studies in our laboratory have concentrated on the conjugation of 1-naphthol in a number of different normal and tumour tissues obtained from patients at surgery. Most of the normal tissues studied, including lung, bronchus and colon, metabolized 1-naphthol predominantly to its sulphate ester conjugate, 1-naphthyl sulphate, whereas the corresponding tumour tissue from the same patient formed, predominantly, the glucuronic acid conjugate, 1-naphthyl-β-D-glucuronide.

METABOLISM STUDIES

Short-term organ culture of human lung, bronchus and tumour tissue

Peripheral lung tissue and tumours, obtained at surgery from patients with lung cancer, were transported to the laboratory at 4°C in either phosphate buffered saline (lacking calcium and magnesium salts) or in Leibovitz L-15 medium (Gibco Biocult, Paisley, Scotland), and cultured within 3 hours of surgical removal. When short-term organ cultures of peripheral human lung were incubated with [1-^{14}C]-1-naphthol, the major metabolite formed was the sulphate conjugate, 1-naphthyl sulphate, with little or no glucuronic acid conjugate being formed (Figure 34.1)[11]. However, in contrast to the results with peripheral human lung tissue where sulphate ester conjugates were the major metabolites, with tumour tissue the metabolism of 1-naphthol varied with the histological classification of the tumour[12]. Particularly striking was the finding that tumour tissue, from all the patients with squamous cell carcinomas, metabolized 1-naphthol predominantly to its glucuronic acid conjugate, with very little or no sulphate conjugate being formed (Figure 34.1)[12]. Limited results, from other types of lung tumours prevent detailed analysis but these other tumours appeared to show a greater variability in the routes of conjugation[12]. These results are in good agreement with our studies using human lung tumour cell lines where cultures derived from squamous cell carcinomas also showed extensive formation of 1-naphthyl glucuronide with little or no sulphate conjugation[13]. Thus there appeared to be a major biochemical difference in the routes of conjugation of 1-naphthol between normal peripheral lung and squamous tumour tissue which may be exploitable in chemotherapy.

Squamous carcinoma of the lung is thought to arise from the bronchial epithelium. Thus, it was important to determine if the conjugation pathways

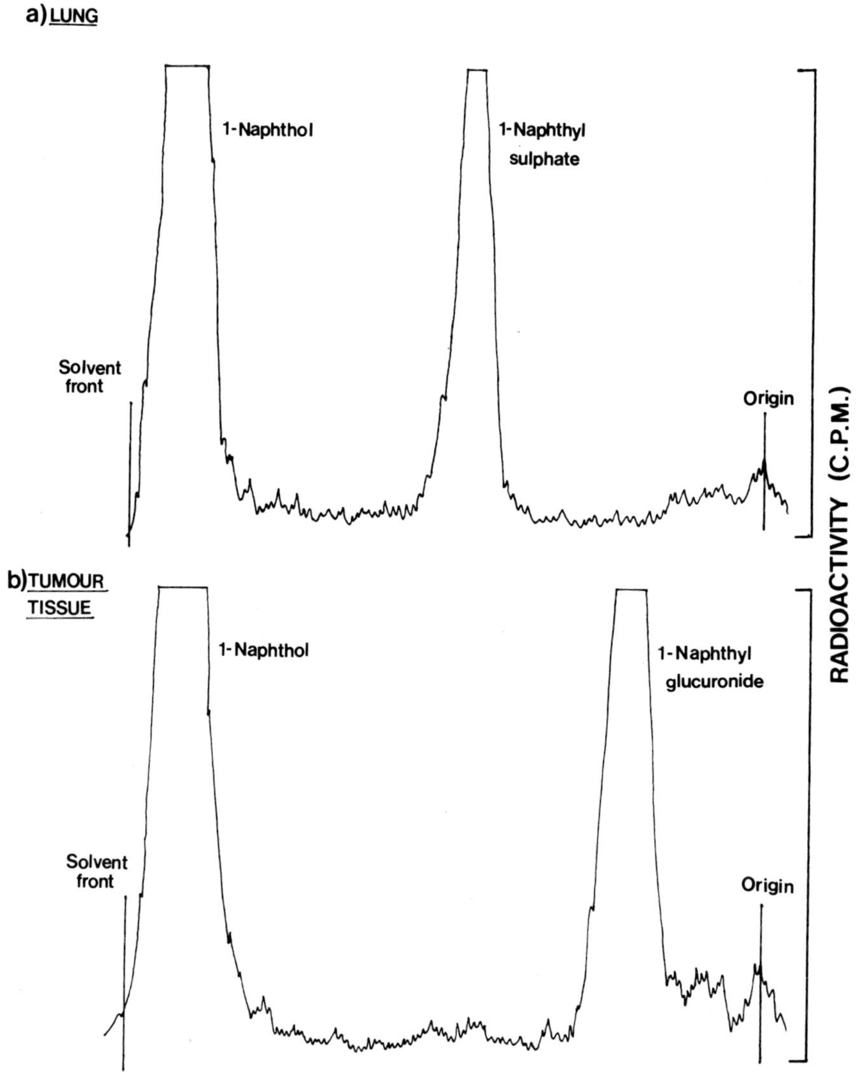

Figure 34.1 Thin layer chromatographic separation of 1-naphthol and its conjugates after short-term organ culture of [1-^{14}C]-1-naphthol with (**a**) human peripheral lung and (**b**) tumour tissue from a patient with a poorly differentiated squamous cell carcinoma. The metabolites were separated by thin layer chromatography as described previously[11] and detected by radiochromatogram scanning. The identity of metabolites was established in part by co-chromatography with authentic standards

present in the tumour are the same or different from the bronchial epithelium from which the tumours have originated. Human bronchus, in short-term explant culture, metabolized 1-naphthol to both its sulphate ester and glucuronic acid conjugates[14]. At low concentrations of 1-naphthol (20 μmol/l), more

1-naphthyl sulphate than 1-naphthyl-β-D-glucuronide was formed. Thus the intact normal bronchus conjugates 1-naphthol differently from tumour tissue. Considerable interindividual variation was observed both in the total extent of conjugate formation and in the relative amounts of the different conjugates formed[14].

Short-term organ cultures of human colon and colorectal tumour tissue

Normal human colon and tumour tissues were obtained at the time of surgery and transported to the laboratory in Leibovitz L-15 medium containing the antibiotics, gentamicin sulphate (50 μg/ml, Sigma), fungizone (50 μg/ml, Gibco Biocult), penicillin (100 units/ml) and streptomycin (100 μg/ml, Gibco Biocult). Short-term organ cultures of normal colon and tumour tissues were maintained essentially as previously described[15]. Tissue explants on Gelfoam sponge, in petri dishes, were placed in a Bellco incubator (Bellco Glass Inc., New Jersey, USA), gassed with filtered 95% O_2 and 5% CO_2 and rocked at 10 cyles/minute for 24 hours so that the explants were in the medium for 50% of each cycle.

Short-term organ cultures of normal human colon metabolized 1-naphthol to both its sulphate ester and glucuronic acid conjugates[16,17]. At low concentrations of 1-naphthol (20 μmol/l), normal colon formed significantly more 1-naphthyl sulphate than 1-naphthyl-β-D-glucuronide (Figure 34.2a)[17]. Considerable interindividual variation in the amounts of both conjugates formed was observed, ranging from 3.8 to 32.8 and 0.8 to 14.9 nmoles formed mg protein^{-1} 24 hour^{-1} for 1-naphthyl sulphate and 1-naphthyl-β-D-glucuronide, respectively[17]. At higher concentrations of 1-naphthol (100 μmol/l), the normal colon still formed significantly more sulphate ester than glucuronic acid conjugates, although at this concentration, glucuronic acid conjugates represented a higher percentage of the total metabolites formed.

Short-term organ cultures of colonic tumour tissue from the same patients also metabolized 1-naphthol (20 μmol/l) to both sulphate ester and glucuronic acid conjugates (Figure 34.2b). The most striking observation was the decrease in sulphate ester conjugate formed by the tumour tissue when compared with the normal[17] (compare Figures 34.2a and 2b). The amount of 1-naphthyl-β-D-glucuronide formed by the tumour tissue was significantly greater than with normal colonic tissue. However, the overall metabolism of 1-naphthol to conjugates was lower in the tumour tissue when compared with the normal because the decrease in 1-naphthyl sulphate formation was greater than the increase in 1-naphthyl-β-D-glucuronide. A marked interindividual variation in the ability of both normal and tumour tissues to conjugate chemicals was observed. This variability may be of importance in determining individual susceptibility to chemically induced damage.

The shift, from sulphate ester to glucuronic acid conjugation observed with the colonic tumour tissue when compared with the normal colon, was also in agreement with our results using human colonic tumour cell lines and human colonic adenocarcinoma xenografts which both formed predominantly 1-naphthyl-β-D-glucuronide[17].

The changes in sulphate ester and glucuronic acid conjugation (Figures 34.1

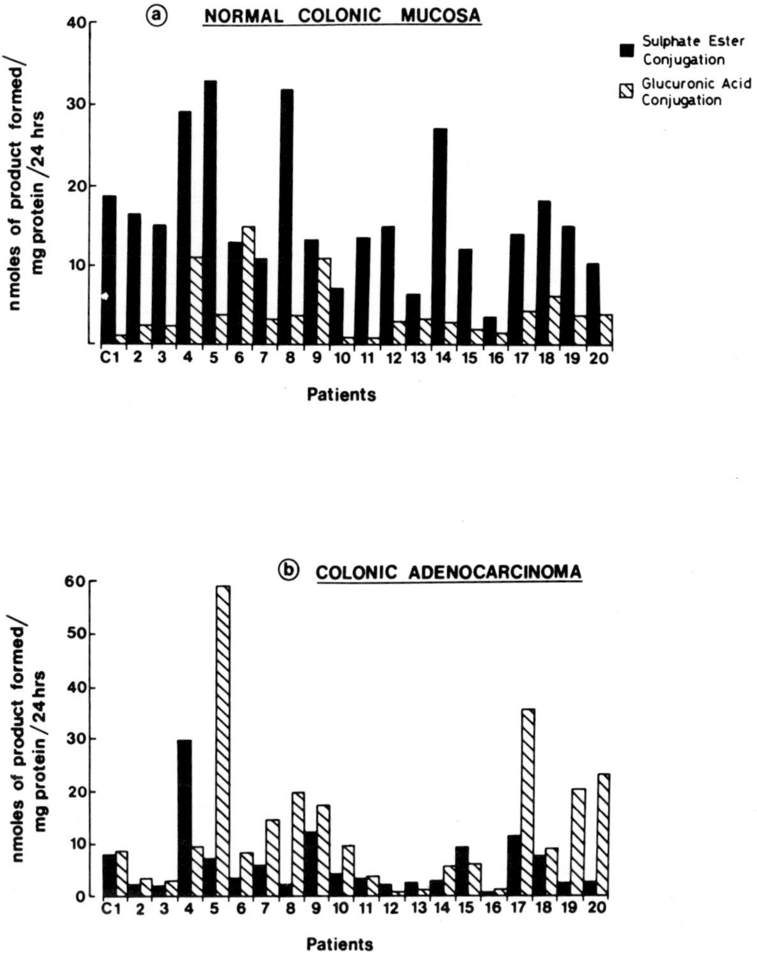

Figure 34.2 Conjugation of 1-naphthol by short-term organ culture of (**a**) normal colonic mucosa and (**b**) colonic adenocarcinomas from the same patients. Short-term organ cultures of normal-appearing human colonic tissue and tumour tissue, obtained at surgery, were cultured for 24 hours at 37°C in 1.0 ml of a supplemented CMRL-1066 medium. The culture medium was then replaced by one containing [1-^{14}C]-1-naphthol (20 μmol/l), and incubated for a further 24 hours when the medium was removed and analysed for conjugates by thin layer chromatography. The amount of radioactivity in the medium at the end of the culture was, on average, approximately 70% of the total radioactivity. The results in Figure 34.2a and 2b are expressed as mean values of 2–4 determinations (dishes)

and 2) observed between normal and tumour tissue in both the lung and the colon may be affected by alterations in the level or activities of the hydrolytic enzymes, β-glucuronidase and arylsulphatase. Thus the lower sulphate ester conjugate production in tumour tissue could be caused by an increased activity of arylsulphatase. Such increases have been reported in several solid human carcinomas, including colorectal carcinoma[18,19]. Recently, however Morgan *et al.*[20] demonstrated that only 24% of tumours from patients with adenocarcinoma of the colorectal regions had elevated levels of arylsulphatase B. Thus, alterations in the hydrolytic enzymes cannot apparently explain the differences in conjugation observed at least between normal colon and tumour tissues. Such differences may be explained by alterations in enzyme protein(s) or in the generation of the appropriate cofactors. Both UDP-glucuronosyltransferase[21] and sulphotransferase[22] exist in multiple forms, and as yet it is not known if similar changes in conjugation occur with other substrates. Although the significance of such alterations in conjugation is not clear, this may be related to changes in mucus secretion. A large proportion of colonic mucins from normal human colon consists of sulphomucins, whereas in colonic tumours a marked decrease or absence of sulphomucins is accompanied by an increase in sialomucins[23]. However, it has also been found that normal colonic mucosa adjacent to and remote from colon carcinomas show a shift towards sialomucins[24,25].

Short-term organ culture of human melanoma xenografts

We have also studied the metabolism of 1-naphthol (20–1000 μmol/l) in a series of human melanoma xenografts, which had been maintained in nude mice. Short-term organ cultures of human melanoma xenografts metabolized 1-naphthol to both its sulphate ester and glucuronic acid conjugates. Four-fifths of the melanomas formed significantly more glucuronic acid than sulphate ester conjugates, but the other melanoma formed more sulphate ester conjugate.

Metabolism of 1-naphthol by mouse leukaemic L1210 cells

Recently we have found that 1-naphthol is selectively toxic to short-term organ cultures of human colonic tumour tissue when compared with normal colon from the same patients[26]. This suggested that 1-naphthol may be of potential value as an antitumour agent. As part of an investigation of its antitumour activity, we have studied the metabolism of 1-naphthol both in mice infected with L1210 cells and also in L1210 cells in culture. [1-^{14}C]-1-Naphthol (70 mg/kg, 10 μCi/mouse in 50% propylene glycol in saline) was injected i.p. into mice, infected 5 days earlier with 10^5 L1210 cells (i.p.). When serial samples of ascites fluid were withdrawn 20 minutes to 6 hours following injection with [1-^{14}C]-1-naphthol, it was found that there was a very rapid clearance of radioactivity from the ascitic fluid within the first 20 minutes. Assuming that each mouse had 1 ml of ascitic fluid, only 6–7% of the radioactivity remained in the ascitic fluid 20 minutes after injection. The majority of the radioactivity (78–96%) in the ascitic fluid at this and later time points was associated with Phase II metabolites of 1-naphthol. At each time point studied there was an excess of 1-naphthyl sulphate over 1-naphthyl-β-D-glucuronide present in the ascitic fluid, the ratio of these conjugates increasing from 1.2 at 20 minutes to 11.5 after 6 hours. In order to assess whether this pattern of Phase II metabolites was due to the metabolism of 1-naphthol by the tumour cells, *in vitro* experiments were carried out. Only very low levels of Phase II metabolism were observed when [1-^{14}C]-1-naphthol (20 μmol/l) was incubated (90 minutes) with

L1210 cells in ascitic fluid taken directly from an infected mouse (Table 34.1).

Table 34.1 Metabolism of [1-^{14}C]-1-naphthol (20 μmol/l) by L1210 cells *in vitro*

Source of L1210 cells	*Incubation medium*	*Length of incubation* (hours)	*nmoles Conjugate formed/10⁶ cells* *1-naphthyl-β-D-glucuronide*	*1-naphthyl sulphate*
Ascitic fluid taken directly from a mouse	Ascitic fluid	1.5	<0.13 (<3)*	<0.02 (<1)*
	0.9% saline	1.5	<0.12 (<3)	<0.04 (<1)
Isolated from ascitic fluid and passaged 3 times *in vitro*	RPMI	24.0	27.9 (29)	ND (0)
An established L1210 cell line (Flow Labs Ltd)	RPMI	24.0	30.0 (29)	ND (0)

ND: Not detectable
* Percentage of radioactivity present in the culture medium comigrating with authentic 1-naphthyl-β-D-glucuronide and 1-naphthyl sulphate on TLC plates. L1210 cells were obtained either directly from the ascitic fluid of a mouse infected 7 days earlier with 10^5 L1210 cells or from L1210 cell lines either set up in our laboratory or purchased from Flow Labs Ltd. The cells derived from fresh ascitic fluid were either incubated with [1-^{14}C]-1-naphthol (20 μmol/l, 56 μCi/μmole) directly or washed in 0.2% saline, to lyse red blood cells prior to incubation with an equimolar concentration of [1-^{14}C]-1-naphthol in 0.9% saline (2.1–3.7 × 10^7 cells/ml). The L1210 cell lines were cultured in RPMI medium in the presence of [1-^{14}C]-1-naphthol (20 μmol/l, 56 μCi/μmole) at a cell concentration of 1.9–2.1 × 10^5 cells/ml. The incubations were for the times stated at 37°C under 5% CO_2. The medium was then analysed by TLC

Lysis of red blood cells in the ascitic fluic by pretreatment of the cells with 0.2% saline had little effect. The low level of metabolism, less than 4% conversion to Phase II metabolites, observed in these experiments suggests that the rapid metabolism observed in ascitic fluid *in vivo* is probably host mediated. In support of this theory, the only metabolite of [1-^{14}C]-1-naphthol (20 μmol/l) detected in continuous cultures of L1210 cells was 1-naphthyl-β-D-glucuronide (Table 34.1). This is in marked contrast to the excess of 1-naphthyl sulphate over 1-naphthyl-β-D-glucuronide observed in peritoneal fluid *in vivo*.

COMMENTS

Our studies, together with those from a number of other laboratories, suggest marked alterations in the ability of tumour tissue to conjugate xenobiotics. We have attempted to summarize some of these studies, particularly those involving human tissues in Table 34.2.

Generally, it would appear that in tumour tissues, there is an increase in glucuronic acid conjugation and a decreased sulphate ester conjugation. However, exceptions to this have been noted, and the histological classification of the tumour would also appear to be of importance. The reasons for these

Table 34.2 Alteration of conjugation pathways in tumours

Species	*Tumour tissue*	*Enzyme activity compared to normal*	*Substrate*	*Reference*
Human	breast	low steroid sulphation	17-β-oestradiol	10, 27
		high steroid sulphation*	17-β-oestradiol	27
Human	squamous carcinoma of the lung	marked increase in UDP-GT**	1-naphthol	12, 13
		Marked decrease in phenol sulphotransferase	1-naphthol	12, 13
	other lung carcinomas	generally decreased phenol sulphotransferase	1-naphthol	12, 13
Human	lung adeno-carcinomas	increased cerebroside sulphotransferase	Galactocere-broside	28
Human	squamous carcinoma of the lung	unchanged cerebroside sulphotransferase	Galactocere-broside	28
Human	colonic adeno-carcinomas	increased UDP-GT	1-naphthol	16, 17
		Decreased phenol sulphotransferase	1-naphthol	16, 17
Rodent	hepatoma	increased UDP-GT	1-naphthol *p*-nitrophenol *o*- & *p*-nitrophenol	4,6–9
Rodent	Reuber H-35 hepatoma	increased UDP-GT Decreased phenol sulphotransferase	*p*-nitrophenol	8
Rat	preneoplastic liver nodules	increased UDP-GT	1-naphthol, 4-methylumbellife-rone, 3-hydroxy -benzo(a)pyrene and *o*-aminophenol	29, 30

* Apparent correlation with oestrogen receptor status
** UDP-GT = UDP-glucuronosyltransferase

changes in conjugation are not clear but may be related to changes in (1) the hydrolytic enzymes; (2) the ability to generate cofactors for conjugation; (3) conjugating enzymes; (4) energy metabolism in tumour cells and (5) cell-surface glycosaminoglycans.

Although conjugation of drugs is generally considered to be a detoxification process, there are examples of conjugation, including glucuronidation, which lead to more reactive metabolites. Based on the biochemical differences observed here, it may be possible to design drugs, activated by glucuronic acid conjugation but not by sulphate conjugation, which would be selectively toxic to the tumour cells. Alternatively, it may be possible, by supplying substrates which will be extensively glucuronidated, to selectively deplete tumour cells of UDPGA, thus leading to cell death.

The reasons for the apparent alteration in conjugation observed in these studies and their implications for cancer chemotherapy require further investigation.

ACKNOWLEDGEMENTS

We would like to thank the Cancer Research Campaign of Great Britain for a grant to support this work. We thank Mrs M. Fagg for typing the manuscript.

References

1. Williams, R. T. (1959). *Detoxication Mechanisms*, 2nd Edn. (London: Chapman and Hall)
2. Adamson, R. H. and Fouts, J. R. (1961). The metabolism of drugs by hepatic tumors. *Cancer Res.*, **21,** 667–72
3. Miyake, Y., Gaylor, J. L. and Morris, H. P. (1974). Abnormal microsomal cytochromes and electron transport in Morris hepatomas. *J. Biol. Chem.*, **249,** 1980–7
4. Zimmerman, J. J., Gorski, J. P. and Kasper, C. B. (1976). Quantitative relationship of UDP-glucuronosyltransferase to the NADPH and NADH electron-transport systems in Morris hepatomas with varying growth rates. *Drug Metab. Disp.*, **5,** 572–8
5. Sabadie, N., Richter-Reichhelm, H. B., Saracci, R., Mohr, U. and Bartsch, H. (1981). Studies on inter-individual differences in oxidative benzo(a)pyrene metabolism by normal and tumorous surgical lung specimens from 105 lung cancer patients. *Int. J. Cancer.*, **27,** 417–26
6. Lueders, K. K., Dyer, H. M., Thompson, B. and Kuff, E. L. (1973). Glucuronyltransferase activity in transplantable rat hepatomas. *Cancer Res.*, **30,** 274–9
7. Winsnes, A. and Rugstad, H. E. (1973). Different properties of microsomal UDP-glucuronyltransferase in Buffalo rat liver and a clonal strain of rat hepatoma cells derived from the same rat strain. *Acta Pharmacol. Toxicol.*, **33,** 161–6
8. Gessner, T. (1974). Studies of glucuronidation and sulfation in tumor-bearing rats. *Biochem. Pharmacol.*, **23,** 1809–16
9. Bock, K. W., Lorch, F. and Van Ackeren, G. (1975). Substrate specificity of UDP-glucuronyltransferase in rat liver and in Morris hepatomas: studies on a connection with the mono-oxygenase epoxide hydrase system. *Naun. Schiemd. Arch. Pharmacol.*, **287,** (Suppl.) R77
10. Dao, T. L. and Libby, P. R. (1968). Conjugation of steroid hormones by normal and neoplastic tissues. *J. Clin. Endocrinol. Met.*, **28,** 1431–9
11. Mehta, R. and Cohen, G. M. (1979). Major differences in the extent of conjugation with glucuronic acid and sulphate in human peripheral lung. *Biochem. Pharmacol.*, **28,** 2479–82
12. Cohen, G. M., Gibby, E. M. and Mehta, R. (1981). Routes of conjugation in normal and cancerous tissue from human lung. *Nature*, **291,** 662–4
13. Gibby, E. M., Mehta, R., Ellison, M. and Cohen, G. M. (1981). Conjugation pathways in human bronchial carcinoma cell lines. *Biochem. Pharmacol.*, **30,** 3333–6
14. Gibby, E. M. and Cohen, G. M. (1984). Conjugation of 1-naphthol by human bronchus and bronchoscopy samples. *Biochem. Pharmacol.*, **33,** 739–43
15. Autrup, H. (1980). Explant culture of human colon. In Harris, C. C., Trump, B. F. and Stoner, G. D. (eds.). *Methods in Cell Biology*. Vol. 21, pp. 385–401. (New York: Academic Press)
16. Cohen, G. M., Grafstrom, R. C., Gibby, E. M., Smith, L., Autrup, H. and Harris, C. C. (1983). Metabolism of benzo(a)pyrene and 1-naphthol in cultured human tumorous and non-tumourous colon. *Cancer Res.*, **43,** 1312–15

17. Gibby, E. M. and Cohen, G. M. (1984). Conjugation of 1-naphthol by human colon and tumour tissue using different experimental systems, *Br. J. Cancer.*, **49,** 645–51
18. Fishman, W. H. and Anlyan, A. J. (1947). β-Glucuronidase activity in human tissues: some correlations with processes of malignant growth and with the physiology of reproduction. *Cancer Res.*, **7,** 808–17
19. Dzialoszynski, L. M., Frohlich, A. and Kroll, J. (1966). Cancer and arylsulphatase activity. *Nature*, **212,** 733
20. Morgan, L. R., Samuels, M. S., Thomal, W., Krementx, E. T. and Meeker, W. (1975). Arylsulfatase B in colorectal cancer. *Cancer Suppl.*, **36,** 2337–45
21. Dutton, G. and Burchell, B. (1977). Newer aspects of glucuronidation. In Bridges, J. W. and Chasseaud, L. F. (eds.). *Progress in Drug Metabolism*, Vol. 2, pp. 1–70. (Chichester: Wiley & Sons)
22. Mulder, G. J., Caldwell, J., Van Kempen, G. M. J. and Vonk, R. J. (eds.). (1982). *Sulfate Metabolism and Sulfate Conjugation.* (London: Taylor & Francis)
23. Filipe, I. (1979). Mucins in the human gastrointestinal epithelium: A review. *Invest. Cell Pathol.*, **2,** 195–216
24. Filipe, M. I. and Branfoot, A. C. (1974). Abnormal patterns of mucus secretion in apparently normal mucosa of large intestine with carcinoma. *Cancer*, **34,** 282–90
25. Shamsuddin, A. K. M., Weiss, L., Phelps, P. C. and Trump, B. F. (1981). Colon epithelium IV. Human colon carcinogenesis. Changes in human colon mucosa adjacent to and remote from carcinomas of the colon, *J. Natl. Cancer Inst.*, **66,** 413-19
26. Cohen, G. M., Wilson, G. D., Gibby, E. M., Smith, M. T., Doherty, M. d'A. and Connors, T. A. (1983). 1-Naphthol: A potential selective antitumour agent. *Biochem. Pharm.*, **15,** 2363-5
27. Adams, J. B., Pewnim, T., Chandra, D. P., Archibald, L. and Foo, M. S. (1979). A correlation betwen estrogen sulfotransferase levels and estrogen receptor status in human primary breast carcinoma. *Cancer Res.*, **39,** 5124–6
28. Gasa, S., Makita, A., Hirama, M. and Kawabata, M. (1979). Cerobroside sulfotransferase activity in human lung tissues. An elevated level in lung adenocarcinoma. *J. Biochem.*, **86,** 265–7
29. Yin, Z., Sato, K., Tsuda, H. and Ito, N. (1982). Changes in activities of uridine diphosphate-glucuronyltransferases during chemical hepatocarcinogenesis. *Gann*, **73,** 239–48
30. Bock, K. W., Lilienblum, W., Pfeil, H. and Eriksson, L. C. (1982). Increased uridine diphosphate-glucuronyltransferase activity in preneoplastic liver nodules and Morris hepatomas. *Cancer Res.*, **42,** 3747–52

Section 9
Pathophysiological Aspects

Chairman: R. Preisig

35
Clinical toxicological aspects of glucuronide conjugation

L. F. PRESCOTT

INTRODUCTION

Conjugates usually have little or no biological activity, and conjugation makes an important contribution to the termination of action and rapid elimination from the body of many drugs. As such, it often plays an important role in recovery from drug overdose and poisoning. In this context, glucuronide conjugation is of particular significance, since it represents a removal process of a potentially very large capacity for the direct Phase 2 metabolism of many lipid soluble compounds which possess free hydroxyl, phenolic, carboxylic acid and amino groups[1].

THE SIGNIFICANCE AND LIMITATIONS OF GLUCURONIDE CONJUGATION

Unfortunately, there is a paucity of clinical toxicological data which relate specifically to glucuronide conjugation. The detailed investigation of drug metabolism and kinetics in poisoned patients is often difficult because of the circumstances of emergency and factors such as mulitiple overdosage, uncertainty concerning the dose absorbed and abnormal drug absorption, distribution, metabolism and excretion. Drug disposition is altered unpredictably by complications such as hypoxia, acidosis, hypothermia, slow gastric emptying, reduced plasma protein binding and low cardiac output with circulatory failure, reduced tissue perfusion and reduced hepatic and renal blood flow. To complicate matters, these factors are often continuously changing during the course of the intoxication.

Nevertheless, many poisons and drugs which are taken in overdosage would be expected to undergo glucuronide conjugation and this process is undoubtedly of importance for their elimination. Glucuronide conjugates are very polar and they thus have a small, largely extracellular distribution with relatively high concentrations in the plasma. At the same time, they are often actively secreted into bile and urine and may, therefore, have a very high clearance. Since the halflife of a drug or metabolite is directly related to the volume of distribution and inversely related to its clearance, glucuronide conjugates can be eliminated very rapidly. The capacity for glucuronide conjugation of some compounds is very large, so that this process can be a very efficient mechanism for the mass removal of drugs and poisons from the body.

On the other hand, several factors may limit the rate and extent of removal of drugs from the body by glucuronide conjugation. Enterohepatic circulation of conjugates, and subsequent hydrolysis in the gastrointestinal tract may result in reabsorption of the parent compound with consequent prolongation of intoxication. It is not known to what extent this applies in man following drug overdosage, but repeated oral administration of adsorbents such as activated charcoal may greatly enhance the elimination of some potential substrates for glucuronide conjugation[2].

With some substrates, glucuronyltransferase readily becomes saturated, thus limiting the contribution of conjugation to detoxification and rapid elimination. Perhaps the best known example is the saturation of the phenolic glucuronidation of salicylate even within the therapeutic dose range[3]. However, this is only a minor pathway of salicylate removal, and is of no practical significance in the recovery from salicylate intoxication. The dose-dependent elimination of diflunisal may also represent saturation of glucuronyltransferase[4]. Sulphate conjugation is often limited by depletion of inorganic sulphate, but it is not known whether glucuronide conjugation in man is ever similarly restricted by the availability of uridine diphosphoglucuronic acid (UDPG). However, the acute LD_{50} of paracetamol in mice is increased by the intravenous administration of UDPG[5], and its availability could conceivably be a limiting factor in some circumstances.

PARACETAMOL POISONING

Paracetamol (acetaminophen) is normally a very safe drug, but if taken in overdosage it may produce acute hepatic necrosis through the conversion of a small fraction of the dose to a reactive arylating intermediate which binds covalently to liver cells causing necrosis. The toxic metabolite is normally rapidly inactivated by conjugation with glutathione, and liver damage does not occur unless glutathione is depleted[6]. Glucuronide conjugation is the major route of paracetamol metabolism in man and it accounts for 60–65% of both therapeutic and toxic doses. About 30% of a therapeutic dose is conjugated with sulphate, but following overdosage this pathway is completely saturated and it contributes little to removal of the drug[7]. The glucuronide conjugation of paracetamol, therefore, plays a crucial protective role by promoting its rapid elimination and shunting the drug away from the route of hepatotoxic metabolic activation. Glucuronyltransferase is inducible, and the rate of elimination of paracetamol is significantly increased in patients who have been taking inducers of hepatic microsomal enzymes, such as anticonvulsants and rifampicin[8]. However, the increase is small and of doubtful clinical significance.

It has been suggested that paracetamol causes liver damage following overdosage because glucuronide conjugation becomes saturated, so that proportionately more drug undergoes metabolic activation[9]. However, there is no good evidence to support this hypothesis. The plasma paracetamol halflife after a therapeutic dose is 2–2.5 h, and in the absence of severe liver damage following overdosage there is only a minor prolongation to 3–3.5 h. This small change can be accounted for entirely by the saturation of sulphate conjugation, and there is no evidence of transition from zero to first order kinetics as plasma concentrations fall (Figure 35.1). The plasma paracetamol halflife is only increased beyond 4 h when conjugation is impaired because of hepatic necrosis[7]. As shown in Figures 35.1 and 2, glucuronide conjugation is maintained without saturation even in severely poisoned patients with high plasma paracetamol concentrations, in whom liver damage has been prevented by the early administration of the glutathione precursor *N*-acetylcysteine.

Quite exceptionally, a patient may be encountered with extremely high plasma paracetamol concentrations of the order of 1000 μg/ml, and in such

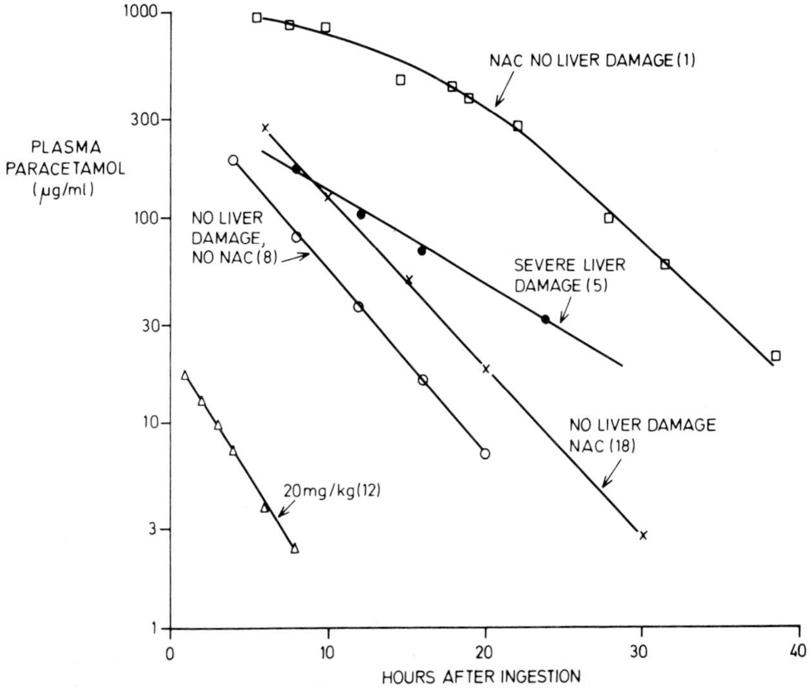

Figure 35.1 Plasma paracetamol concentrations after a therapeutic dose (20 mg/kg) in healthy subjects (△—△), overdosage without *N*-acetylcysteine (NAC) treatment and no liver damage (○—○), overdosage with NAC treatment and no liver damage (×—×), overdosage with severe liver damage (●—●) and massive overdosage with NAC treatment and no liver damage (□—□). Numbers in parentheses indicate the number of patients or subjects in each group

circumstances glucuronide conjugation may become saturated[1]. The data from one such patient who absorbed about 900 mg/kg, and would inevitably have died in liver failure but for early treatment with *N*-acetylcysteine, is included in Figures 35.1 and 2. Liver function tests remained normal, but the initial zero order and subsequent first order pattern of decline in plasma paracetamol concentrations (Figure 35.1), and the almost constant 'plateau' concentrations of the glucuronide conjugate during the first 24 hours (Figure 35.2) are consistent with saturation.

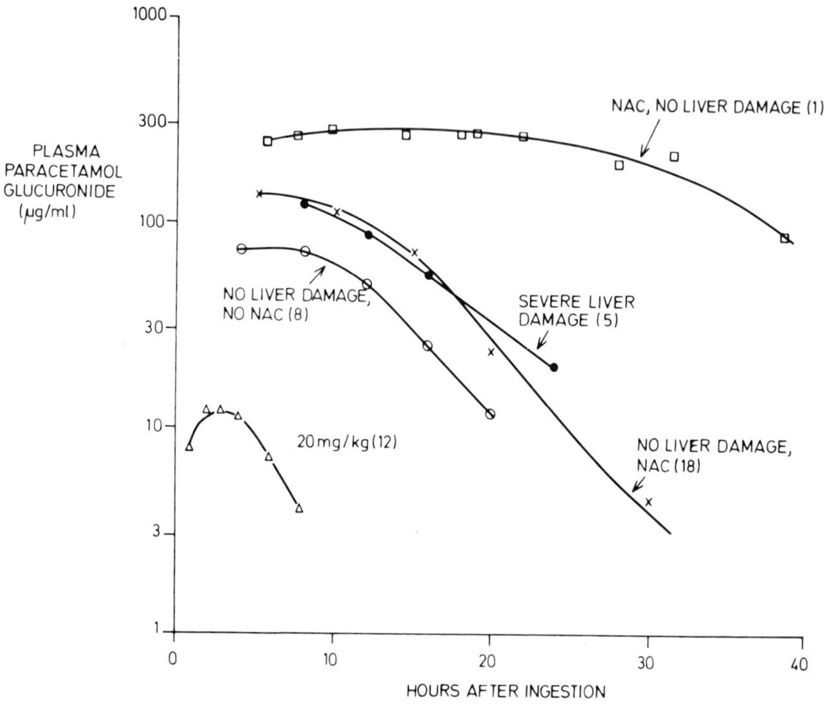

Figure 35.2 Plasma paracetamol glucuronide concentrations (expressed as paracetamol equivalents) in the same patients and subjects as shown in Figure 35.1

We recently had the opportunity to study the capacity for glucuronide conjugation in a neonate who was delivered at 36 weeks by Caesarian section shortly after his 25-year-old mother took an overdose of paracetamol[10]. The plasma paracetamol concentration in cord blood on delivery, about 2.5 h after overdosage, was 144 μg/ml, and the pattern of decline was consistent with saturation at concentrations above 80–100 μg/ml. In addition, the rates of glucuronide formation and excretion were abnormally slow in the infant, as shown by marked prolongation of the plasma paracetamol halflife (10 h compared with 2.5 h in the mother), and a delay of about 20 hours before maximum plasma concentrations of the glucuronide conjugate were achieved (Figure 35.3). As judged by the ratios of urinary metabolite concentrations, paracetamol metabolism in the infant was quantitatively similar to that in the mother,

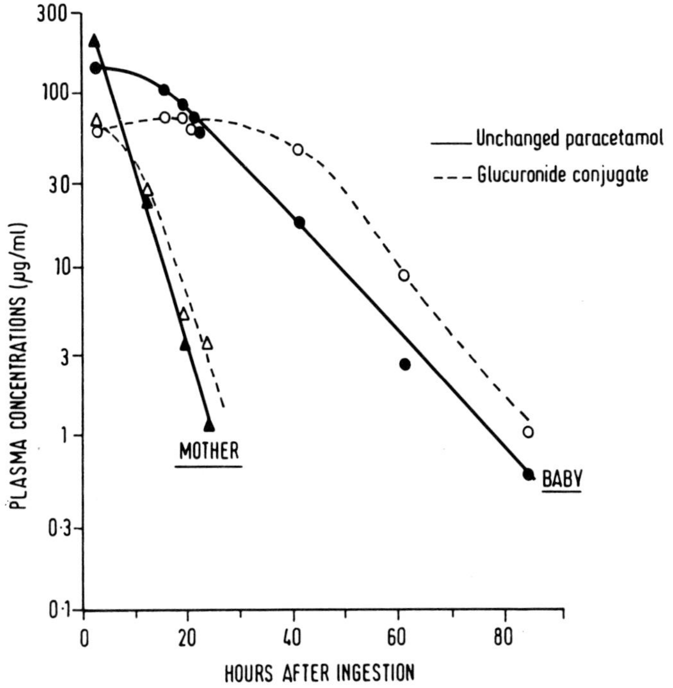

Figure 35.3 Plasma concentrations of paracetamol and paracetamol glucuronide following overdosage in a 25-year-old mother and in her infant delivered by Caesarian section 2.5 h later

although proportionately less mercapturic acid and cysteine conjugates were produced.

PHENOXY ACID HERBICIDES

2,4-Dichlorophenoxyacetic acid (2,4-D) and 2-methyl-4-chlorophenoxypropionic acid (mecoprop) belong to the class of hormone weedkillers, and can cause serious and lethal toxicity when taken in large amounts. 2,4-D is excreted in the urine largely unchanged, while mecoprop undergoes slow glucuronide conjugation. We recently studied the disposition and kinetics of these herbicides following severe poisoning in a 39-year-old man[11]. The patient was extremely ill with initial plasma concentrations of 2,4-D and mecoprop of 400 and 751 μg/ml, respectively. Over the next 2 days there was no change in his condition, and the plasma concentration of 2,4-D remained essentially unchanged while mecoprop concentrations fell slowly with a halflife of 40 h. At this point, the urine was made alkaline by infusion of sodium bicarbonate, in an attempt to increase the renal clearance of the weedkiller as an alternative route of elimination. There was only about a 50% reduction in the halflife of mecoprop, but plasma 2,4-D concentrations fell precipitously and the patient made a rapid recovery. The renal clearances of 2,4-D and mecoprop increased by factors of 5 and 2, respectively for each increase in urine pH of one unit, and about 10% of the 2,4-D and 65% of the mecoprop were excreted as conjugates. These observations illustrate the problems of prolonged intoxication with phenoxy acid herbicides in the absence of rapid glucuronide conjugation, and the value of opening up alternative routes of elimination to enhance removal from the body.

CONCLUSIONS

Glucuronide conjugation is probably important for recovery following overdosage with many therapeutic and toxic agents. Although saturation may occur readily with some substrates, with others the capacity for glucuronide conjugation is very large, and this reaction represents an important mechanism for detoxification and the mass removal of drugs and poisons from the body. In the case of paracetamol poisoning, glucuronide conjugation also plays a vital role in shunting the drug away from the pathway of hepatotoxic metabolic activation. Information concerning the relevance of glucuronide conjugation following drug overdosage in man is limited, and further studies are required.

References

1. Prescott, L. F. (1984). Drug conjugation in clinical toxicology. *Biochem. Soc. Trans.*, **12,** 96–9
2. Neuvonen, P. J. (1982). Clinical pharmacokinetics of oral activated charcoal in acute intoxications. *Clin. Pharmacokin.*, **7,** 465–89
3. Levy, G., Tsuchiya, T. and Amsel, L. P. (1972). Limited capacity for salicyl phenolic glucuronide formation and its effect on the kinetics of salicylate elimination in man. *Clin. Pharmacol. Therap.*. **13,** 258–68
4. Tocco, D. J., Breault, G. O., Zacchei, A. G., Steelman, S. L. and Perrier, C. V. (1975). Physiological disposition and metabolism of 5-(2′,4′- difluorophenyl)salicylic acid, a new salicylate. *Drug Metab. Disp.*, **3,** 453–66
5. Galatulas, I. and Montanari, P. (1976). Effect of pretreatment with UDPG on acute toxicity of paracetamol in mice. *IRCS Med. Sci. Biochem. Drug Metab. Toxicol. Pharmacol.*, **4,** 92
6. Mitchell, J. R., Thorgeirsson, S. S., Potter, W. Z., Jollow, D. J. and Keiser, H. (1974). Acetaminophen-induced hepatic injury: protective role of glutathione in man and rationale for therapy. *Clin. Pharmacol. Therap.*, **16,** 676–84
7. Prescott, L. F. (1980). Kinetics and metabolism of paracetamol and phenacetin. *Br. J. Clin. Pharmacol.*, **10,** 291–8S
8. Prescott, L. F., Critchley, J. A. J. H., Balali-Mood, M. and Pentland, B. (1981). Effects of microsomal enzyme induction on paracetamol metabolism in man. *Br. J. Clin. Pharmacol.*, **12,** 149–53
9. Slattery, J. T. and Levy, G. (1979). Acetaminophen kinetics in acutely poisoned patients. *Clin. Pharmacol. Therap.*, **25,** 184–95
10. Roberts, I., Robinson, M. J., Mughel, M. Z., Ratcliffe, J. G. and Prescott, L. F. (1984). Paracetamol metabolites in the neonate following maternal overdosage. *Br. J. Clin. Pharmacol.*, **18,** 201–6
11. Prescott, L. F., Park, J. and Darrien, I. (1979). Treatment of severe 2,4-D and mecoprop intoxication with alkaline diuresis. *Br. J. Clin. Pharmacol.*, **7,** 111–6

36
Differential hepatic glucuronidation of (−)- and (+)- morphine in the rat and the human fetus

B. GAWRONSKA-SZKLARZ, J.-O. SVENSSON, J. WIDÉN AND A. RANE

INTRODUCTION

Many drugs are available as racemic preparations, the enantiomers of which have different potencies and metabolism[1-4]. Several members of the opiates exist as enantiomers, with only one form active as an analgesic because of steric hindrance at the receptor site. Such stereoselective activity has been demonstrated for levorphanol[5-7] and levomethorphan[5] by conformation analysis.

The natural morphine is levo-rotating and designated (−)-morphine. (+)-Morphine is the unnatural enantiomer, and is virtually devoid of analgesic effect[8]. With the improved synthesis of (+)-morphine[9] and high performance liquid chromatography for analysis of morphine glucuronides[10] it was possible to study the UDP-glucuronyltransferase catalysed metabolism of (+)-morphine, and relate it to the corresponding metabolism of the active (−)-morphine.

The UDP-glucuronyltransferase activity with (−)- or (+)-morphine as substrate was investigated in liver preparations from Sprague-Dawley rats and Rhesus monkey. The metabolism pattern was compared with that in human fetal liver microsomes, which have a unique capacity to catalyse the conjugation of natural (−)-morphine but not several other drug molecules investigated so far[11]. Therefore, it was of interest to study the metabolism of (+)-morphine since stereo- and regio-selective metabolism by hepatic enzymes may help to explain the development of the different UDP-glucuronyltransferases[12] during ontogenesis[13].

MATERIALS AND METHODS

Male Sprague-Dawley rats (180–200 g) were used for isolation of liver microsomes as described previously[11]. Phenobarbital was given intraperitoneally (i.p.) in a dose of 40 mg/kg twice daily for 3 days. Morphine–HC1 was administered daily, i.p., for 14 days, with an initial dose of 20 mg kg^{-1} day^{-1} which was increased every second day until the rats received 125 mg kg^{-1} day^{-1} (20, 30, 45, 60, 80, 100, 125 mg/kg). The control rats received i.p. injections of isotonic saline.

The rats were sacrificed by a blow on the head. The liver was immediately removed and cooled, minced and rinsed in 0.3 mol/l sucrose. Homogenization was carried out in a Potter–Elvehjem glass-Teflon homogenizer in 3 parts (w/v) of 0.3 mol/l sucrose. The homogenate was centrifuged at 9000 *g* for 10 min at 4°C. The supernatant was further centrifuged for 60 min at 105 000 *g* and 4°C. The resulting microsomal pellets were resuspended in 0.3 mol/l sucrose. The morphine glucuronidation assay was essentially similar to that described by Bock *et al.*[14] as modified by Pacifici *et al.*[11].

Incubation mixtures (100 μl final volume) contained 50 μl of a mixture consisting of equal parts of 1 mol/l Tris–HCl (pH 7.4), 50 mmol/l $MgCl_2$, and 18 mmol/l (or lower) morphine (to give a final concentration of 3 mmol/l morphine, or lower), 40 μl of a microsomal suspension (to give a protein concentration of 1.2–1.6 mg/ml incubation mixture) and 10 μl of uridine diphospho- glucuronic acid (UDPGA, to give a final concentration of 15 mmol/l).

The substrate (+)- or (−)-morphine (available as base and HCl salt, respectively) was dissolved in water with 20 μl 2.5% H_3PO_4 in order to acidify the solution and increase the solubility of the (+)-morphine base (20 μl was added to about 0.6 ml 18 mmol/l (+)-morphine).

The reaction was performed under conditions that were linear with respect to protein concentration and time. Incubations were carried out at 37°C for 20 min. The reaction was stopped by freezing the samples on dry ice.

The UDP-glucuronyltransferase activity was calculated as the rate of formation of morphine-3-glucuronide (M3G) and morphine-6-glucuronide (M6G). The metabolite concentrations were determined by reversed phase ion-pair high performance liquid chromatography according to Svensson *et al.*[10].

RESULTS

(−)-Morphine glucuronidation was catalysed by rat liver microsomes only at the aromatic 3-OH-group (Table 36.1 and Figure 36.2). Occasionally a small peak at the position of M6G was observed in the chromatogram, but this was below the detection limit. The glucuronidation pattern was different with (+)-morphine as substrate. Both OH- groups were conjugated with glucuronic acid with preference for the formation of (+)-M6G. The rate of formation of this metabolite was considerably higher than the rate of formation of (+)-M3G. Only 23–39% (average 28%) of the total glucuronide formation was accounted for by the formation of the (+)-M3G.

The glucuronidation was also studied in liver microsomal preparations from four human fetuses. The reaction was linear with time and protein concentration for the formation of (−)-M3G, (+)-M6G and (+)-M3G as is demonstrated in Figure 36.1

Table 36.1 Regioselective and stereoselective glucuronidation of (−)- and (+)-morphine to the morphine-3- (M3G) and 6-glucuronides (M6G) in liver microsomes from human fetuses, from rats and Rhesus monkey

Enzyme origin	*UDP-glucuronyltransferase activity* (nmol mg protein^{-1} min^{-1}) *(−)-Morphine*		*(+)-Morphine*	
	M3G	*M6G*	*M3G*	*M6G*
Human fetuses ($n = 4$)	0.016	NM	0.007	0.118
	0.053	0.011	0.027	0.460
	0.050	0.009	0.025	0.256
	0.010	NM	0.008	0.049
Rats ($n = 4$–5)	1.98	NM	0.38	0.93
Rhesus monkey ($n = 1$)	1.13	0.02	0.26	0.13

NM = not measurable

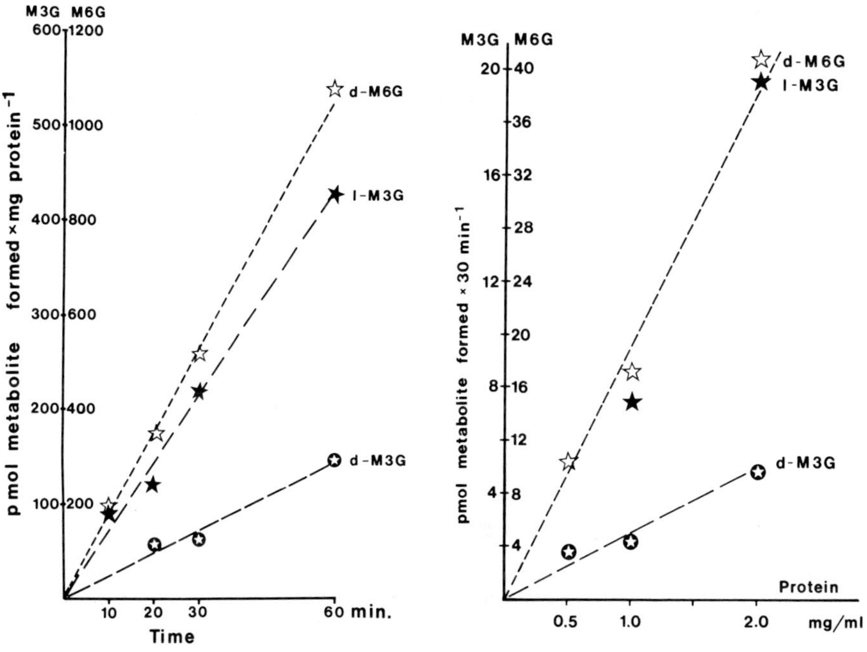

Figure 36.1 Glucuronidation of (−)- and (+)-morphine in liver microsomes from a human fetus. Linearity with time and protein concentration. The formation of the 3-OH- and 6-OH-glucuronides of the two enantiomers [(−)-M3G, (−)-M6G, (+)-M3G, (+)-M6G] was measured. The enantiomers are denoted as l-(−) and d-(+)-morphine in the figure

In human fetal liver microsomes (−)-morphine was virtually only conjugated at the 3-OH-group, although in two of the preparations trace amounts of (−)-M6G were formed (Table 36.1 and Figure 36.2). The reverse was observed for (+)-morphine which was almost solely metabolized to (+)-M6G. Formation of (+)-M3G accounted for less than 13% (average 8%) of the total glucuronide formation from (+)-morphine.

The UDP-glucuronyltransferase activity with (−)- and (+)-morphine as substrates was also studied in liver microsomes from one Rhesus monkey. Similar to the human fetal liver, there was minimal formation of (−)-M6G. However, in contrast to the previous results, there was more (+)-M3G than (+)-M6G formed from (+)-morphine (Figure 36.2).

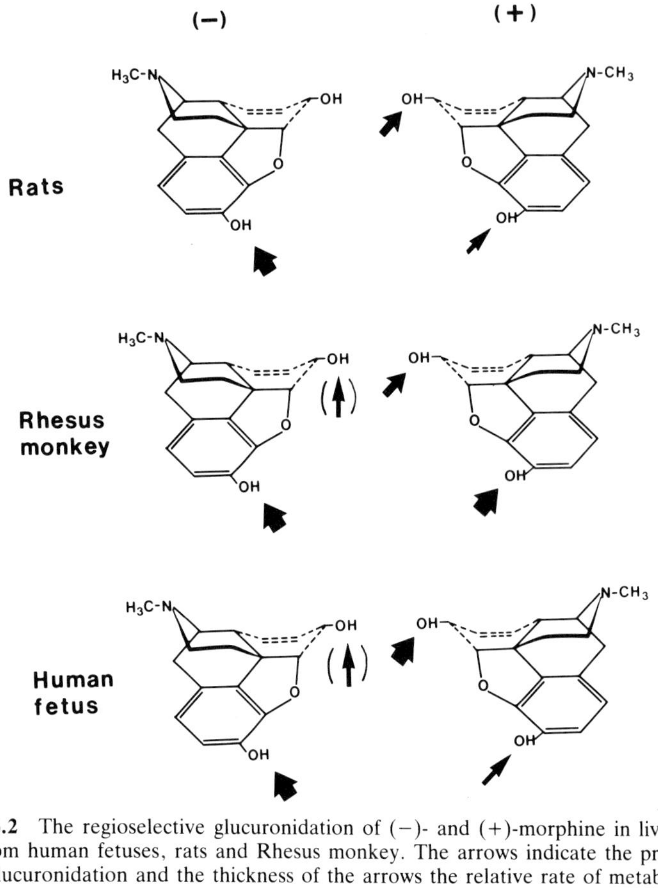

Figure 36.2 The regioselective glucuronidation of (−)- and (+)-morphine in liver microsomes from human fetuses, rats and Rhesus monkey. The arrows indicate the preferential sites of glucuronidation and the thickness of the arrows the relative rate of metabolism

DISCUSSION

The unnatural (+)-enantiomer of morphine is devoid of the analgesic properties of its natural (−)-form after injection into the periaqueductal grey matter in rats[8]. The complete (or almost complete) absence of analgesic effect of the (+)-forms of several other members of the methylmorphinan group of drugs[15], such as detrorphan[5,6] and dextromethorphan[6], seems to be a unique feature for these members of the opiate group. Many other drugs such as hexobarbital[2], propranolol[3], warfarin[1] and verapamil[4] exist as enantiomers which are both active although with different potencies. While these drugs are oxidized by the cytochrome P-450 enzyme system, which has some degree of stereoselectivity, it seemed of interest to study the liver microsomal UDP-glucuronyltransferase in this respect with the two morphine enantiomers.

In the human fetal liver there was a conspicuous dissociation between glucuronidation at the 3-OH- and 6-OH-groups of the two morphine enantiomers. Whilst the natural (−)-form is virtually only conjugated in the 3-OH position (more than 83% of the total conjugation), the unnatural (+)-form was almost only conjugated in position 6 (more than 87% of total conjugation).

With (−)-morphine only (−)-M3G formation was catalysed in adult rat liver microsomes, and M6G was not present in measurable amounts in the incubates. With (+)-morphine as substrate, about 70% of the glucuronide formed was present as (+)-M6G.

In the single sample of Rhesus monkey liver microsomes the conjugation of (+)-morphine was more evenly distributed between the two OH-groups.

Irrespective of species, there was an overwhelming preference for glucuronidation of the 3-OH group of the natural (−)-morphine. In contrast, (+)-morphine was preferentially glucuronidated to (+)-M6G, particularly in the human fetal liver. Current studies with human adult liver will reveal whether the high degree of regioselectivity in glucuronidation of (+)-morphine is unique for man. Both the rat and the Rhesus monkey seem to lack this degree of regioselectivity. Previous work in our laboratory[16,17] has demonstrated a consistency between the plasma levels of (−)-M3G and (−)-M6G after oral dosing, and their relative rates of formation *in vitro* in liver microsomes and the results are in agreement with the present human and Rhesus monkey data, i.e. the Rhesus monkey forms relatively less (−)-M6G than man.

The compiled previous and present data indicate a species difference between the human fetus and the investigated animals in the metabolism of morphine, particularly the (+)-form. Current studies in our laboratory aim to investigate whether this difference bears any relevance to the ontogenetic differentiation[11,13] of the UDP-glucuronyltransferases in man and the rat.

ACKNOWLEDGEMENTS

This work was supported by grants from the Swedish Medical Research Council (14x-04496), the Expressen Prenatal Research Foundation and the Swedish Cancer Society. d(+)-morphine was kindly donated from the National Institute on Drug Abuse, Rockville, Md, USA.

References

1. Pohl, L. R., Porter, W. R. and Trager, W. (1977). Stereochemical biotransformation of warfarin as a probe of the homogeneity and mechanisms of microsomal hydroxylates. *Biochem. Pharmacol.*, **26**, 109–14

2. Miyano, K., Fujii, K. and Toki, S. (1980). Stereoselective hydroxylation of hexobarbital enantiomers by rat liver microsomes. *Drug Metab. Dispos.*, **7,** 351–5
3. von Bahr, C., Hermansson, J. and Lind, M. (1982). Oxidation of (R)- and (S)-propranolol in human and dog liver microsomes. Species differences in stereoselectivity. *J. Pharmacol. Exp. Ther.*, **222,** 458–62
4. Eichelbaum, M., Mikus, G. and Vogelgesang, B. (1984). Pharmacokinetics of (+)-, and (−)- and (±)-verapamil after intravenous administration. *Br. J. Clin. Pharmacol.*, **17,** 453–8
5. Randall, L. O. and Lehmann, G. (1950). Analgesic action of 3-hydroxy-*N*-methylmorphinan hydrobromide (Dromoran). *J. Pharmacol. Exp. Ther.*, **99,** 163–70
6. Benson, W. M., Stefko, P. L. and Randall, L. O. (1953). Comparative pharmacology of levorphan, racemorphan and dextrorphan and related methyl ethers. *J. Pharmacol. Exp. Ther.*, **109,** 189–200
7. Beckett, A. H. and Casy, A. F. (1954). Synthetic analgesics: stereochemical considerations. *J. Pharm. Pharmacol.*, **6,** 986–1001
8. Jacquet, Y. F., Klee, W. A., Rice, K. C., Iijima, I. and Minamikawa, J. (1977). Stereospecific and nonstereospecific effects of (+) and (−)-morphine: Evidence for a new class of receptors? *Science*, **198,** 842–4
9. Iijima, I., Minamikawa, J., Jacobson, A. E., Brossi, A. and Rice, K. C. (1978). Studies in the (+)-morphinan series. 4. A markedly improved synthesis of (+)-morphine. *J. Org. Chem.*, **43,** 1462–3
10. Svensson, J.-O., Rane, A., Säwe, J. and Sjöqvist, F. (1982). Determination of morphine, morphine-3-glucuronide and (tentatively) morphine-6-glucuronide in plasma and urine using ion-pair high-performance liquid chromatography. *J. Chromatogr.*, **230,** 427–32
11. Pacifici, G. M., Säwe, J., Kager, L. and Rane, A. (1982). Morphine glucuronidation in the human fetal and adult liver. *Eur. J. Clin. Pharmacol.*, **22,** 553–8
12. Bock, K. W., Burchell, B., Dutton, G. J., Hänninen, O., Mulder, G. J., Owens, I. S., Siest, G. and Tephly, T. R. (1983). UDP-glucuronosyltransferase activities. Guidelines for consistent interim terminology and assay conditions. *Biochem. Pharmacol.*, **32,** 953–5
13. Wishart, G. J. and Dutton, G. J. (1978). Induction by natural and xenobiotic compounds of UDP-glucuronyltransferase activities during the perinatal period. In Neubert, D., Merker, H.-J., Nau, H. and Langman, J. (eds.) *Role of Pharmacokinetics in Prenatal and Perinatal Toxicology*, pp. 215–24. (Stuttgart: Georg Thieme)
14. Bock, K. W., Brunner, G., Hoensch, M., Huber, E. and Josting, D. (1978). Determination of microsomal UDP-glucuronyltransferase in needle-biopsy specimens of human liver. *Eur. J. Clin. Pharmacol.*, **14,** 367–73
15. Radouco-Thomas, C. (1956). Contribution to the study of synthetic analgesic narcotics. *Bull. Narcot.*, **8,** 18–25
16. Rane, A., Säwe, J., Lindberg, B., Svensson, J.-O., Garle, M., Jorulf, H. and Erwald, R. (1984). Morphine glucuronidation in the Rhesus monkey: A comparative *in vivo* and *in vitro* study. *J. Pharmacol. Exp. Ther.*, **229,** 571–6
17. Säwe, J., Kager, L., Svensson, J.-O. and Rane, A. (1984). Oral morphine in cancer patients: *In vivo* kinetics and *in vitro* hepatic glucuronidation in the individual patient. Manuscript

37
Nuclear and microsomal UDP-glucuronyltransferase in human liver

G. M. PACIFICI, C. COLIZZI, L. GIULIANI AND A. RANE

INTRODUCTION

In 1970, Franke and co-workers described a procedure to isolate nuclei from mammalian liver[1]. One year later, Kasper described the activity of the aryl hydrocarbon hydroxylase and the content of cytochrome P-450 in rat liver nuclei[2]. In 1974, the first demonstration of nuclear UDP-glucuronyltransferase (GT) was provided by Amar-Costesec *et al.*[3]. These authors measured the rate of glucuronidation of 4-methyl umbelliferone and bilirubin in the nuclear fraction from rat liver. Recently, a number of studies have been published, and it appears that the nuclear membranes of rat liver catalyse reactions which were considered to be catalysed by the microsomes only[4]. Very little is known about drug metabolism in the nuclei from the human[5] and primate tissues[6,7].

The cell nucleus is the site where the genetic material resides, and thus, it is also the putative target of carcinogens and mutagens. Conjugative pathways play a major role in the detoxification of xenobiotics. Drugs and chemicals (food additives, environmental pollutions, insecticides and other products) that are foreign to the body undergo enzymatic conjugation, which usually results in loss of pharmacologic and toxicologic activities. Among the conjugative reactions, glucuronide formation is one of the most common routes of drug metabolism.

After entry into the cell, part of the compound or part of its reactive metabolites may escape from the cytoplasmic detoxificating system, and penetrate the nucleus. Thus, the GT located in the nuclear envelope seems to occupy a strategic position for proximity with the genetic material. Since no information was available on GT in the nuclear fraction of human liver, we studied the glucuronidation of 1-naphthol in human hepatic nuclear membranes.

MATERIALS AND METHODS

Radioactive substrates

1-[1-^{14}C]Naphthol (56 mCi/mmol) and [7-^{3}H]styrene-7,8-oxide (137 mCi/mmol) were purchased from The Radiochemical Centre (Amersham, England).

Unlabelled substrates and chemicals

Uridine 5′-diphosphoglucuronic acid (UDPGA), 1-naphthol, 4-4′-hydroxybiphenyl, umbelliferone (7-hydroxycoumarin), *p*-nitrophenol and salicylic acid were obtained from Sigma (St. Louis, MO, USA). Styrene oxide, styrene glycol and 2-hydroxy-biphenyl were purchased from Aldrich (Bersee, Belgium). Oxazepam was kindly supplied by Roche (Milan, Italy). Morphine was a gift from the Department of Forensic Medicine of this University. TLC plates (19 channel LK5DF) were from Whatman Inc. (Milan, Italy).

Patients

Fourteen patients of both sexes and aged between 34 and 69 years ($\bar{x} \pm$ SEM $= 50.2 \pm 3.0$), submitted to abdominal surgery for curative purposes, were included in the study. Wedge biopsies of human liver were obtained for diagnostic purposes. Part of the tissue surplus to histological investigation was used for the isolation of the nuclear and microsomal fractions. All liver specimens used had normal cell architecture. Liver specimens were immediately frozen at −80°C and stored at this temperature for 3–20 days.

Preparation of the subcellular fractions

The nuclear and microsomal fractions were isolated from the same biopsy specimen using differential centrifugation. The procedure for the isolation of nuclei and microsomes has previously been described in detail[5]. Each nuclear preparation was examined by phase-contrast microscopy (Leitz, Wetzlor, Germany, mod. Orthoplan; magnification × 400). The nuclear preparations appeared free from cytoplasmic contaminants.

Assays

The activity of GT was assayed with 1-naphthol as substrate as described elsewhere[8], with minor modifications. An aliquot of the nuclear or microsomal fraction was used instead of the total liver homogenate. Final volume of the incubation mixture was 0.1 ml. In the standard incubation, the concentration of UDPGA was 5 mmol/l and that of 1-naphthol 0.5 mmol/l. Incubations were carried out at 37°C for 10 min; pH 7.4. Reactions were started by adding 1-naphthol (200 000 c.p.m.) in 5 μl of dimethylsulphoxide. For the velocity versus substrate concentration curves, the concentration of 1-naphthol was kept constant at 0.5 mmol/l, whereas that of UDPGA varied from 0.32 to 10 mmol/l. Alternatively, the UDPGA concentration was kept constant at 5 mmol/l, and that of 1-naphthol ranged between 0.032 and 1 mmol/l. The inhibition study was made by adding each inhibitor in 5 μl of dimethylsulphoxide. The pH was adjusted to 8.7 in order to have the highest activity. Each sample was assayed in duplicate. Each assay was provided with two blanks which were treated as the samples, but UDPGA was replaced by water. The activity of styrene oxide hydrolase was measured in the nuclear and microsomal fractions as described elsewhere[5]. Protein concentration was measured using the method by Lowry *et al.*[9].

RESULTS

The nuclear and microsomal activities of GT are shown in Table 37.1. The effects of UDPGA and 1-naphthol concentrations on GT activity were studied in the nuclear and microsomal fractions obtained from three livers. The results are depicted in Figures 37.1 and 2. These figures also show the transformation of the enzymatic activities into Eadie–Hofstee plots. The kinetic parameters of GT are shown for each subcellular fraction and substrate. The data are summarized in Tables 37.2, 3, 4 and 5.

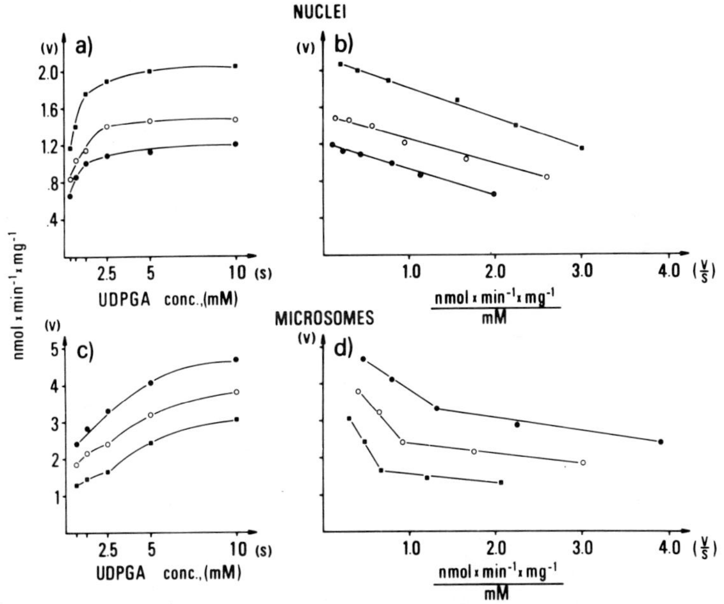

Figure 37.1 Effect of the concentration of UDPGA on GT activity. UDPGA concentration ranged between 0.32 and 10 mmol/l. The concentration of 1-naphthol was kept constant at 0.5 mmol/l. (**a**) and (**c**) saturation curves, (**b**) and (**d**) transformation of the activities into Eadie–Hofstee plots. ●—● = patient 5; ○—○ = patient 8; ■—■ = patient 12

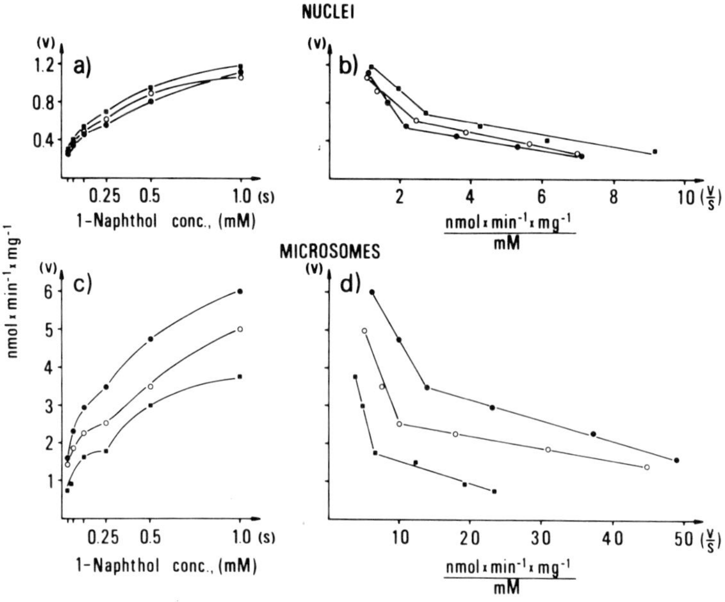

Figure 37.2 Effect of the concentration of 1-naphthol on the GT activity. The concentration of 1-naphthol ranged between 0.032 and 1 mmol/l, whereas that of UDPGA was 5 mmol/l. (**a**) and (**c**), saturation curves, (**b**) and (**d**) transformation of the activities into Eadie–Hofstee plots. ●—● = patient 5, ○—○ = patient 8; ■—■ = patient 12

Table 37.1 UDP-Glucuronyltransferase activity (nmol min^{-1} mg^{-1}) in the nuclear and microsomal fractions of human liver

Patient	*Sex*	*Age* (years)	*Nuclei*	*Microsomes*	*Nuclei/microsomes*
1	F	34	0.93	5.02	0.18
2	M	39	1.49	6.41	0.23
3	F	39	0.76	3.77	0.20
4	F	40	1.01	2.54	0.40
5	F	41	1.13	3.87	0.29
6	F	43	0.90	5.03	0.18
7	F	50	1.23	6.87	0.18
8	F	51	1.13	3.39	0.33
9	F	55	1.00	3.30	0.30
10	F	56	1.69	5.05	0.33
11	M	60	0.80	3.27	0.24
12	F	61	1.03	2.42	0.42
13	F	65	1.70	4.60	0.37
14	F	69	0.72	2.93	0.24
Mean		50.2	1.11	4.17	0.28
± SEM		3.0	0.08	0.37	0.02

Table 37.2 Kinetic parameters of UDP-glucuronyltransferase in the nuclear fraction of the human liver. The concentration of 1-naphthol was kept constant at 0.5 mmol/l. The concentrations of UDPGA ranged between 0.32 and 10 mmol/l

Patient	*Sex*	*Age* (years)	V_{max} (nmol min^{-1} mg^{-1})	K_m (mmol/l)
5	F	41	1.20	0.24
8	F	51	1.54	0.32
12	F	61	2.14	0.31
Mean			1.63	0.29
± SEM			0.27	0.02

Table 37.3 Kinetic parameters of UDP-glucuronyltransferase in the microsomal fraction of human liver. The concentration of UDPGA ranged between 0.32 and 10 mmol/l. The concentration of 1-naphthol was kept constant at 0.5 mmol/l. The subscripts 1 and 2 refer to the first and second phase of the curve, respectively. The first phase was obtained at concentrations of UDPGA ranging between 0.32 and 2.5 mmol/l; and the second one at concentrations ranging between 2.5 and 10 mmol/l

Patient	*Sex*	*Age* (years)	V_{max_1} (nmol min^{-1} mg^{-1})	V_{max_2}	K_{m_1} (mmol/l)	K_{m_2}
5	F	41	3.65	5.42	0.32	1.63
8	F	51	2.54	4.84	0.24	2.65
12	F	61	1.81	4.20	0.26	3.83
Mean			2.67	4.83	0.27	2.70
± SEM			0.53	0.35	0.02	0.64

Table 37.4 Kinetic parameters of UDP-glucuronyltransferase in the nuclear fraction of human liver. The concentration of UDPGA was kept constant at 5 mmol/l. The concentration of 1-naphthol ranged between 0.032 and 1 mmol/l. The subscripts 1 and 2 refer to the first and second phase of the curve, respectively. The first phase was obtained at concentrations of 1-naphthol ranging between 0.032 and 0.25 mmol/l; and the second one at concentrations ranging between 0.25 and 1 mmol/l

Patient	*Sex*	*Age* (years)	V_{max_1} (nmol min^{-1} mg^{-1})	V_{max_2}	K_{m_1} (mmol/l)	K_{m_2}
5	F	41	0.69	1.64	0.07	0.50
8	F	51	0.81	1.45	0.08	0.33
12	F	61	0.82	1.56	0.06	0.31
Mean			0.77	1.56	0.07	0.38
± SEM			0.04	0.05	0.01	0.06

Table 37.5 Kinetic parameters of UDP-glucuronyltransferase in the microsomal fraction of human liver. The concentration of UDPGA was kept constant at 5 mmol/l. The concentration of 1-naphthol ranged between 0.032 and 1 mmol/l. The subscripts 1 and 2 refer to the first and second phase of the curve, respectively. The first phase was obtained at concentrations of 1-naphthol ranging between 0.032 and 0.25 mmol/l; and the second one at concentrations ranging between 0.25 and 1 mmol/l

Patient	*Sex*	*Age* (years)	V_{max_1} (nmol min^{-1} mg^{-1})	V_{max_2}	K_{m_2} (mmol/l)	K_{m_1}
5	F	41	3.96	7.88	0.05	0.32
8	F	51	2.84	7.25	0.03	0.48
12	F	61	2.14	6.22	0.06	0.62
Mean			2.98	7.12	0.05	0.47
± SEM			0.53	0.48	0.01	0.09

The activity of the epoxide hydrolase was measured towards styrene oxide in the nuclear and microsomal fractions from six liver biopsies (patients 1,2,7,10,13,14). The hydrolase activity ($\bar{x} \pm$ SEM) was 1.44 ± 0.33 (nuclei) and 13.28 ± 1.18 (microsomes) nmol min^{-1} mg^{-1}. The nuclear to microsomal epoxide hydrolase activity ratio ($\bar{x} \pm$ SEM) was 0.12 ± 0.03. The nuclear to microsomal ratio ($\bar{x} \pm$ SEM) of GT, assayed in the same fractions, was (0.25 ± 0.03) significantly different from those found for styrene oxide hydrolase. When the nuclear to microsomal ratios for GT were plotted against those for the epoxide hydrolase no correlation was found (Figure 37.3).

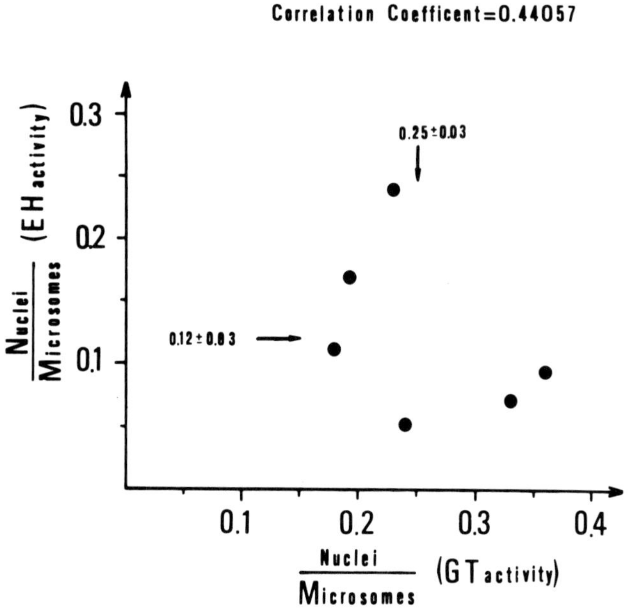

Figure 37.3 Correlation between the nuclear/microsomal ratios of epoxide hydrolase (EH) and those of glucuronyltransferase (GT). Each point is the mean of two determinations. The liver biopsies were from the patients 1,2,7,10,13,14

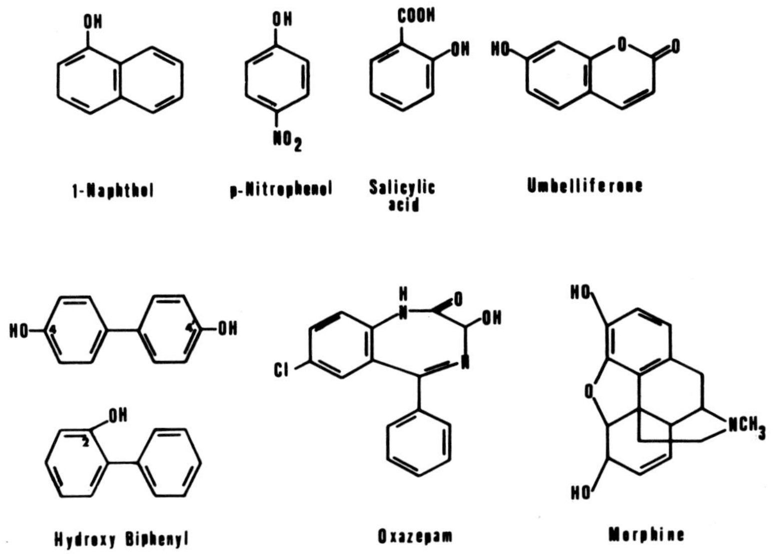

Figure 37.4 Chemical structure of eight substrates for glucuronyltransferase

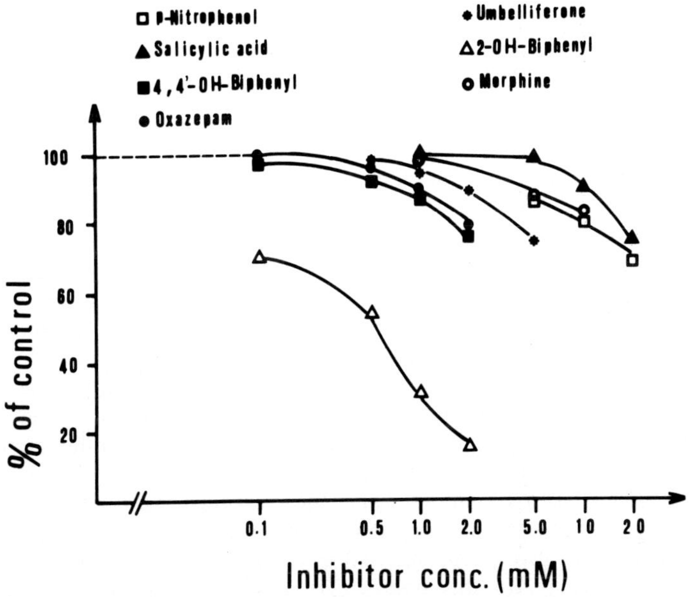

Figure 37.5 Effects of seven substrates for glucuronyltransferase on the rate of 1-naphthol glucuronidation in human liver microsomes

Table 37.6 Effects of various compounds on the rate of 1-naphthol glucuronidation[1]. Data ($\bar{x} \pm$ SEM) are expressed as percentage of control

	Nuclei	*Microsomes*	*Level of significance*[3] *between nuclei and microsomes*
Control[2]	100	100	n.s.
20 mmol/l Salicylic acid	65±2	70±1	n.s.
20 mmol/l *p*-Nitrophenol	64±2	66±3	n.s.
2 mmol/l Umbelliferone	94±4	93±1	n.s.
2 mmol/l 4-4′-Hydroxy biphenyl	71±3	79±3	n.s.
2 mmol/l 2-Hydroxy biphenyl	14±2	13±2	n.s.
1 mmol/l Oxazepam	60±2	80±5	$p<0.02$
10 mmol/l Morphine	93±3	84±1	n.s.

[1] Each figure is the mean of six livers.
[2] Controls contained the same volume of dimethylsulphoxide as the samples.
[3] Student's *t*-test for paired data
n.s. = not significant

The effects of different concentrations of *p*-nitrophenol, salicylic acid, umbelliferone, 4,4′-hydroxy biphenyl, 2-hydroxy biphenyl, oxazepam and morphine (for chemical structures *see* Figure 37.4) on the rate of 1-naphthol glucuronidation were first studied on the microsomal preparation from one human liver biopsy (Figure 37.5). The study was then repeated on the nuclear and microsomal fractions from six biopsies (patients 1,2,7,10,13,14) using only one concentration of each compound. The results are shown in Table 37.6. The compound 2-hydroxy biphenyl (2 mmol/l) exerted the maximum inhibitory effect. Whilst the lowest effect was obtained with umbelliferone (2 mmol/l) and morphine (10 mmol/l).

DISCUSSION

The present paper provides the first information on GT activity in the nuclear fraction from human liver. Our data show that 1-naphthol is glucuronidated in nuclei at a rate about one fourth that in microsomes.

After the first study on nuclear GT in rat liver[3], several investigators confirmed the original finding using different substrates such as *o*-aminophenol[10,11], 4-methyl-umbelliferone[12], bilirubin[11], 5-hydroxytryptamine[11], *p*-nitrophenol[12,13], 1-naphthol[12], testosterone[12] and phenolphthalein[12]. Bansal *et al.*[14] reported that various oxygenated derivatives of benzo(a)pyrene (B(a)P) were glucuronidated in the rat liver membranes. In particular, the nuclear activity, expressed on the basis of mg protein, was higher than the microsomal one towards 2-OH-B(a)P; 3-OH-B(a)P; 4-OH-B(a)P; 7-OH-B(a)P; 8-OH-B(a)P and 10-OH-B(a)P. Antoine *et al.*[15] studied GT towards eight aglycones, including morphine and chloramphenicol, in rat liver nuclear membranes. *o*-Aminophenol was also glucuronidated in the nuclear fraction obtained from embryo-chick liver[16]. In this tissue, GT activity was detectable only after induction[16]. Finally, the rate of 1-naphthol glucuronidation was measured in the nuclear fraction of liver, lungs and kidneys from baboons[6].

The interpretation of the nuclear activities of those enzymes, which were believed to reside in the microsomal fraction only, may be difficult because of the suspicion that endoplasmic contaminants obscure the true nuclear metabolic capacity. However, the nuclear to microsomal ratios of the activities of different drugs metabolizing enzymes could be expected to be similar if the nuclear activities are due to microsomal contaminants only. In our material, the nuclear/microsomal ratios for GT and epoxide hydrolase were significantly different, and no correlation existed between the activities of the two enzymes. Wishart and Fry[11] have demonstrated that Triton X-100, Lubrol, deoxycholate, digitonin and UDP-*N*-acetyl glucosamine have different effects on rat liver nuclear compared to microsomal GT.

With UDPGA as the variable substrate, nuclear GT followed Michaelis–Menten kinetics, whereas the microsomal enzyme obeyed biphasic kinetics. Such different kinetic patterns could be a proof of different properties of GT in the two subcellular fractions. Alternatively, the microenvironment influences the enzyme. Our previous studies on morphine glucuronidation in human fetal[17,18] and adult[19] human liver microsomes have shown that morphine GT obeyed Michaelis–Menten kinetics. It may, thus, be concluded that different forms of GT have different affinities for the endogenous substrate. Bock and associates[8] have reported a K_m for GT of 0.4 mmol/l when 1-naphthol (0.5 mmol/l) was the second substrate and human liver homogenate was the enzyme source. This figure is close to that we report here (0.27 mmol/l) with microsomes, when UDPGA concentrations ranged between 0.32 and 2.5 mmol/l.

The kinetics of GT, studied at varying concentrations of 1-naphthol, were characterized by two phases both in the nuclear and microsomal fractions. This finding is not surprising since such a type of kinetics was earlier reported with 1-naphthol in human liver homogenate[8,20]. Nuclear and microsomal GT differ in their V_{max}, since their K_m for the first and the second phases are similar.

In order to determine if differences were detectable in the catalytic site of the nuclear and microsomal enzymes, we studied the effects of seven substrates for GT on the rate of 1-naphthol glucuronidation. Oxazepam was the only tested compound which exerted different inhibitory effects on the nuclear and microsomal GT, since it preferentially inhibited the nuclear enzyme. A recent commentary reports that oxazepam is neither a typical substrate for GT_1, nor[21] for GT_2. Nevertheless, it is more powerful as an inhibitor on morphine glucuronidation[17,19,22]. The rate of 1-naphthol glucuronidation was notably reduced by 2-hydroxy biphenyl. This compound too does not belong to the group of typical substrates[21] for GT_1 or GT_2. A stronger inhibitory effect on the rate of naphthol glucuronidation was seen with *p*-nitrophenol, salicylic acid and umbelliferone, which together with 1-naphthol, belong to GT_1 substrates[21].

ACKNOWLEDGEMENTS

The authors are indebted to Dr M. Saviozzi for help in the morphologic study, Mrs F. Cosci for the secretarial work, and Mr C. Puccini for technical assistance. This work was supported by the CILAG Foundation and the Italian Association for Cancer Research.

References

1. Franke, W. W., Deumling, B., Ermen, B., Jarasch, E. D. and Kleining, H. (1970). Nuclear membranes from mammalian liver. *J. Cell Biol.*, **46,** 379–95
2. Kasper, C. B. (1971). Biochemical distinctions between the nuclear and microsomal membranes from rat hepatocytes. *J. Biol. Chem.*, **246,** 577–81
3. Amar-Costesec, A., Beaufay, H., Wibo, M., Thinés-Sempoux, D., Feytmans, E., Robbi, M. and Berthet, J. (1974). Analytical study of microsomes and isolated subcellular membranes from rat liver. *J. Cell. Biol.*, **61,** 201–12
4. Romano, M., Facchinetti, T. and Salmona, M. (1983). Is there a role for nuclei in the metabolism of xenobiotica? A Review. *Drug Metab. Rev.*, **14,** 803–29
5. Pacifici, G. M., Colizzi, C., Giuliani, L. and Rane, A. (1984). Nuclear epoxide hydrolase in the human fetal and adult liver. *Pharmacology*, **28,** 321–8
6. Pacifici, G. M. and Rane, A. (1983). Profile of drug metabolizing enzymes in the nuclei and microsomes of hepatic and extrahepatic tissues from monkeys. In Rydström, J., Mantelius, J. and Bengtsson, M. (eds.). *Extrahepatic Drug Metabolism and Chemical Carcinogenesis*, pp. 33–7 (Elsevier Science Publishers B.V.)
7. Pacifici, G. M., Lindberg, B., Glaumann, H. and Rane, A. (1983). Styrene oxide metabolism in Rhesus monkey liver: Enzyme activities in subcellular fractions and in isolated hepatocytes. *J. Pharmacol. Exp. Ther.*, **226,** 869–75
8. Bock, K. W., Brunner, G., Hoensch, H., Huber, E. and Josting, D. (1978). Determination of microsomal UDP-glucuronyltransferase in needle-biopsy specimens of human liver. *Eur. J. Clin. Pharmacol.*, **14,** 367–73
9. Lowry, O. H., Rosebrough, N. J., Farr, A. L. and Randall, R. J. (1951). Protein measurement with the Folin phenol reagent. *J. Biol. Chem.*, **193**, 265–75
10. Wishat, G. J. and Fry, D. J. (1977). Uridine diphosphate glucuronyltransferase activity in nuclei and nuclear envelopes of rat liver and its apparent induction by phenobarbital. *Biochem. Soc. Trans.*, **5,** 705–6
11. Wishat, G. J. and Fry, J. (1980). Evidence from rat liver nuclear preparations that latency of microsomal UDP-glucuronyltransferase is associated with vesiculation. *Biochem. J.*, **186,** 687–91
12. Zalescki, J., Bansal, S. K. and Gessner, T. (1982). Nuclear membrane-bound UDP-glucuronyltransferase of rat liver. *Can. J. Biochem.*, **60,** 972–9
13. Elmamlouk, T. H., Mukhtar, H. and Bend, J. R. (1981). The nuclear envelope as a site of glucuronyltransferase in rat liver, properties of and effect of inducers on enzyme activity. *Pharmacol. Exp. Ther.*, **219,** 27–34
14. Bansal, S. K., Zaleski, J. and Gessner, T. (1981). Glucuronidation of oxygenated benzo(a)pyrene derivatives by UDP-glucuronyltransferase of nuclear envelope. *Biochem. Biophys. Res. Commun.*, **98,** 131–9
15. Antoine, B., Magdalon, J. and Siest, G. (1983). Functional heterogeneity of UDP-glucuronyltransferases in different membranes of rat liver. *Bioch. Pharmacol.*, **32,** 2629–32
16. Wishart, G. J. and Fry, D. J. (1976). Apparent induction by phenobarbital of uridine diphosphate glucuronyltransferase activity in nuclear envelopes of embryo-chick liver. *Biochem. Soc. Trans.*, **4,** 265–6
17. Pacifici, G. M. and Rane, A. (1981). Inhibition of morphine glucuronidation by oxazepam in human fetal liver microsomes. *Drug Metab. Disp.*, **9,** 569–72
18. Pacifici, G. M., Säwe, J., Kager, L. and Rane, A. (1982). Morphine glucuronidation in human fetal and adult liver. *Eur. J. Clin. Pharmacol.*, **22,** 553–8
19. Säwe, J., Pacifici, G. M., Kager, L., von Bahr, C. and Rane, A. (1982). Glucuronidation of morphine in human liver and interaction with oxazepam. *Acta Anaesth. Scand.*, **74,** 47–51
20. Bock, K. W., Lilenblum, W. and von Bahr, C. (1984). Studies on UDP-glucuronyltransferase in human liver microsomes. *Drug Metab. Disp.*, **12,** 93–7
21. Bock, K. W., Burchell, B., Dutton, G. J., Hänninen, O., Mulder, G. J., Owens, I. S., Siest, G. and Tephly, T. R. (1983). Commentary. UDP-glucuronyltransferase activities. Guidelines for consistent interim terminology and assay conditions. *Biochem. Pharmacol.*, **32,** 953–5
22. Pacifici, G. M. and Rane, A. (1982). Renal glucuronidation of morphine in the human fetus. *Acta Pharmacol. Toxicol.*, **50,** 155–60

38
Increased activity of certain iso-enzymes of cytochrome P-450 and UDP-glucuronyltransferases in the liver of cigarette smokers

R. FLEISCHMANN, U. STÄRZ AND H. REMMER

SUMMARY

10–20 mg Human liver from biopsy samples removed for diagnostic purpose have been used to prepare microsomes, and to determine the activity of certain cytochrome P-450 and UDP-glucuronyltransferase isoenzymes, as well as some other enzymes involved in drug metabolism, by using different substrates as indicators.

Smokers oxidize benzpyrene and ethoxycoumarin and also conjugate 1-naphthol with significantly increased rates if compared with non-smokers.

A quantitative calculation of the particular matter inhaled by the smoker indicates that very powerful unknown inducing compounds could be present in tobacco smoke.

These findings may explain certain observations of reduced action, as well as increased elimination rate, of certain drugs used in therapy.

INTRODUCTION

The Boston Collaborative Drug Surveillance Program revealed that smokers responded to certain drugs much less than non-smokers[1]. The investigators tested theophylline[2], chlorpromazine[3] and a number of widely used sedatives[1]. They assumed an increased drug metabolism, but they were unable to explain why they observed a diminished action of benzodiazepines but not of barbiturates if they prescribed these drugs for smokers. Several other reports described a decreased effectiveness of propoxyphene, a drug related to methadone[4], and pentazocine[5]. Surprisingly, the action of anticoagulants, which is diminished during treatment with phenobarbital and some other drugs, was not changed[6].

Pharmacokinetic studies concerning the fate of these and several other drugs confirmed that the elimination rate of most of the mentioned compounds is increased in smoking individuals[7], but they are of limited value for detecting the cause of an increased drug metabolism. Animal studies for elucidating the impact of tobacco smoke on drug oxidation and conjugation using *in vitro* tests might explain an increased metabolism[8], but their relevance to drug actions in man is questionable.

Having experience with the isolation of microsomes from liver biopsy samples removed from patients for diagnostic purposes[9,10], we used small amounts not needed by the pathologist, of just 10–20 mg wet weight, for determining the oxidation- and conjugation-rate of different substrates preferentially metabolized by certain isoenzymes of cytochrome P-450 mono-oxygenase and UDP-glucuronyltransferase.

METHODS

The methods are described in detail elsewhere[11]. The microsomal protein isolated in each biopsy sample amounted to 200–500 μg, just sufficient for two to five tests. Having at our disposal only a small quantity of microsomes, we abandoned cytochrome P-450 determinations, preferring to measure the conversion rate of certain substrates under conditions of enzyme saturation, in order to obtain information about qualitative changes in the isoenzyme pattern of cytochrome P-450 and UDP-glucuronyltransferase in the liver of smoking individuals.

In the first series of experiments we tested a number of oxidation reactions and NADPH-dependent cytochrome c-reductase. If the amount of microsomal enzymes permitted it, epoxide hydrase and glutathione-S-transferase activities were included in the test. We used [^{3}H]benzo(a)pyrene-4,5-oxide and 1-chloro-2,4-dinitrobenzol, respectively, as substrates. The latter test was carried out by Dr Oesch and his group in Mainz. The activity of the glutathione-S-transferase was determined in the 100 000 *g* supernatant of liver biopsy samples. The activity of the glucuronyltransferase was measured with highly sensitive methods by using [^{14}C]naphthol, morphine and bilirubin[11] as substrates.

Only data from those individuals with apparently normal livers were included in the investigation. They were obtained from patients selected for liver biopsy because of cholelithiasis, Morbus Hodgkin and uncertain liver diseases which had to be verified by histological examinations. Since the results in normal, and fatty liver, without any other histological alterations, did not reveal any significant changes, these data were also included in the control group. No difference was found when we evaluated the results according to age and sex of the patients. After carefully interviewing all patients, we included in the group of smokers those patients who admitted to smoking more than 10 cigarettes daily. We excluded those individuals drinking alcohol or using drugs before or during the diagnostic examination, in order to avoid a possible influence of ethanol on the activity of drug metabolizing enzymes which might last for 1 week or even more after abstaining from alcohol. Alcohol drinkers were patients consuming 1 l beer (40–50 ml ethanol) or an equivalent amount of alcoholic beverages per day. The determination of γ-glutamyltranspeptidase (γ-GT) in the serum of all patients served as control for a non-admitted alcohol consumption.

RESULTS

The results (Table 38.1) demonstrate that the overall oxidation rate of benzpyrene and the hydroxylation of ethoxyresorufin is significantly increased (50–70%), but no enhanced oxidation of ethoxycoumarin could be detected if smokers were compared with non-smokers. The other microsomal enzymes did not reveal changes in activity.

Table 38.1 Activity of several drug metabolizing enzymes in the liver of smokers and non-smokers

		Smokers			Non-smokers		
	Substrate	*n*	$\bar{x}$	*SD*	*n*	$\bar{x}$	*SD*
Cyt. P-450 mono-oxygenase	benzo(a)pyrene (pmol)	17	109	49*	35	66	18
	7-ethoxyresorufin (pmol)	13	123	65*	35	70	30
	7-ethoxycourmarin (pmol)	17	357	136	27	307	104
Cyt. P-450 reductase	cyt. c (nmol)	17	189	37	32	193	45
Epoxide hydrase	[^{3}H]benzo(a)pyrene-epoxide (nmol)	5	10.6	2.5	7	7.0	1.6
Glutathione-S-transferase	1-chloro-2,4-dinitrobenzol (μmol)	3	2.0	1.0	5	1.8	0.5
γ-Glutamyltranspeptidase(U/l) in serum		17	32	29	35	25	24

Values are based on mg microsomal protein per min
* $p<0.05$, using the Dunnet-test
SD = standard deviation
n = number of liver microsomal samples assayed

It is well known from experiments with animals that phenobarbital and polyaromatic hydrocarbons specifically induce certain isoenzymes of cytochrome P-450 and certain well characterized UDP-glucuronyltransferases[12,13]. Phenobarbital increases the activity of a transferase which glucuronidates morphine and bilirubin, whereas benzpyrene enhances the glucuronidation of naphthol. Therefore, in a second collection of liver biopsy samples we tested whether a similar correlation can be found in smokers and non-smokers (Table 38.2).

Hepatic microsomes isolated from smokers glucuronidate 1-naphthol with a highly significant increased rate, 50% greater than hepatic microsomes from non-smokers; whereas UDP-glucuronyltransferase activities towards morphine or bilirubin were not enhanced in hepatic microsomes from smokers when compared to non-smokers.

Table 38.2 Microsomal glucuronidation rate of three different compounds with liver microsomes from smokers and non-smokers

Substrate	*UDP-Glucuronyltransferase activity* (nmol min^{-1} mg of protein^{-1}) *Smokers*			*Non-smokers*		
	n	$\bar{x}$	*SD*	*n*	$\bar{x}$	*SD*
1-Naphthol	30	20.9	8.9	49	14.6	6.9*
Morphine	11	1.1	0.6	26	0.9	0.6
Bilirubin	11	0.5	0.6	24	0.4	0.4

* $p<0.001$
SD = standard deviation
n = number of samples assayed

The results are comparable to animal studies. Rats pretreated with benzpyrene or methylcholanthrene also demonstrate an increase in 1-naphthol conjugation[12] and an enhanced oxidation of benzpyrene and ethoxyresorufin[14].

However, our own experiments with rats revealed certain differences (Fleischmann, R., Stärz, U. and Remmer, H., unpublished work). We have determined that benzpyrene treatment of rats not only enhanced the 1-naphthol glucuronidation and the oxidation of benzpyrene and ethoxyresorufin, but also the oxidative dealkylation of 7-ethoxycoumarin. These results suggest that differences exist between the inducing action of tobacco smoke in man, which did not increase the 7-ethoxycoumarin oxidation, and the inducing action of benzpyrene treatment of rats.

DISCUSSION

Quantitative reasons also speak against benzpyrene as an inducing agent in tobacco smoke. Its amount in the main stream of tobacco smoke is well known. A smoker of 20 cigarettes daily inhales not more than 20–30 μg of benzpyrene, i.e. 0.3–0.4 μg/kg body weight[15], but at least 5 mg/kg are needed for induction of similar enzymes in the rat liver. Even if we take into account the total amount of all combustion products (several hundreds) in the particular matter[15], the smoker does not inhale more than 10-15 mg condensed material when smoking a cigarette without a filter, and about 1–1.5 mg with a filter. Smoking 20 cigarettes daily, he is exposed to 20–200 mg (0.3–3 mg/kg) of non-volatile combustion products. These considerations point to unknown inducing compounds in tobacco smoke which are much more effective than benzpyrene.

It might be possible that such highly active substances are also responsible for the carcinogenic action of tobacco smoke, which is 10 000 times more mutagenic in the Ames-test than the amount of benzpyrene which it contains[15].

The presence of highly active inducing compounds in the particular phase of tobacco smoke was also revealed by pharmacokinetic studies in smokers and non-smokers receiving oral phenacetin[16]. The results indicated that the highly enhanced oxidative dealkylation of phenacetin to paracetamol predominantly occurred in the intestinal mucosa. Most of the condensed matter of tobacco smoke does not reach the small bronchi but is removed with the sputum and swallowed. The oral ingestion explains its inducing action on mucosa as well as liver cells.

Circumstantial evidence indicates the presence of unknown chemical substances, with an extraordinary inducing power on certain drug metabolizing enzymes, in tobacco smoke which might be identical with the compounds having similar inducing activities on the mucosa of the intestine and being present in barbecued meat[17].

The postulated highly inducing chemicals in our environment exceed the inducing activity of well-known drugs, as quantitative considerations indicate: drugs act as inducers if prescribed in a dose about several hundred mg per day or at least 5 mg/kg[18]. Chemicals in tobacco smoke seem to be effective in doses which are several orders of magnitude less. Drugs and the unknown chemical compounds also differ qualitatively in their inducing properties.

The best evidence for the existence of unknown most active inducers is the agreement of our *in vitro* data, using model substrates, with the pharmacokinetic and therapeutic results published in the literature[1,7]. Most remarkable in this respect is oxazepam[19], which predominantly loses its effect by conjugation. Its diminished therapeutic efficacy, if prescribed to smoking individuals, is now explainable. Oxazepam is, as far as we know, the first example of a drug the conjugation of which is increased.

ACKNOWLEDGEMENTS

We are grateful to Dr Oesch, Mainz, for supplying us with [^{3}H]benzo(a)pyrene-4,5-oxide. These studies were suported by Deutsche Forschungsgemeinschaft (Grant F1 78/5).

References

1. Boston Collaborative Drug Surveillance Program. (1973). Clinical depression of the central nervous system due to diazepam and chlordiazepoxide in relation to cigarette smoking and age. *N. Engl. J. Med.*, **288,** 277–80
2. Pfeifer, H. J. and Greenblatt, D. J. (1978). Clinical toxicity of theophylline in relation to cigarette smoking. A report from the Boston Collaborative Drug Surveillance Program; Boston University Medical Center. *Chest*, **73,** 455–9
3. Swett, C. (1974). Drowsiness due to chlorpromazine in relation to cigarette smoking. *Arch. Gen. Psychiat.*, **31,** 211–3
4. Boston Collaborative Surveillance Program. (1973). Decreased clinical efficacy of propoxyphene in cigarette smokers. *Clin. Pharmacol. Ther.*, **14,** 259–63
5. Keeri-Szanto, M. and Pomeroy, J. R. (1971). Atmospheric pollution and pentazocine metabolism. *Lancet*, **1,** 947–9
6. Mitchell, A. A. (1972). Smoking and warfarin dosage. *N. Engl. J. Med.*, **287,** 1153–4
7. Jusko, W. J. (1978). Role of tobacco smoking in pharmacokinetics. *J. Pharmacokinet. Biopharm.*, **6,** 7–39
8. Welch, R. M., Cavallito, J. and Loh, A. (1972). Effect of exposure to cigarette smoke on the metabolism of benzo(a)pyrene and acetophenetidin by lung and intestine of rats. *Toxicol. Appl. Pharmacol.*, **23,** 749–58
9. Schoene, R., Fleischmann, R. A., Remmer, H. and von Oldershausen, H. F. (1972). Determination of drug metabolizing enzymes in needle biopsies of human liver. *Eur. J. Clin. Pharmacol.*, **4,** 65–73

10. Fleischmann, R., Mattenheimer, H., Holmes, A. W. and Remmer, H. (1975). Micromethod for the preparation of a microsomal fraction from rat and human liver by differential sedimentation. *Biochem. Biophys. Res. Commun.*, **62,** 289–95
11. Fleischmann, R., Stärz, U. and Remmer, H. (1984). UDP-glucuronyltransferase activities in human liver microsomes: Substrate specificities, influence of different diseases, alcohol and cigarette smoke. *Eur. J. Clin. Pharmacol.* (submitted for publication)
12. Bock, K. W., Fröhling, W., Remmer, H. and Rexer, B. (1973). Effects of phenobarbital and 3-methylcholanthrene on substrate specificity of rat liver microsomal UDP-glucuronyltransferase. *Biochim. Biophys. Acta*, **327,** 46–56
13. Remmer, H., Bock, K. W. and Rexer, B. (1975). Relationship between microsomal hydroxylase and glucuronyltransferase. In Cooper, D., Rosenthal, O., Snyder, R. and Witmer, C. (eds.). *Cytochromes P-450 and b-5: Structure, Function and Interaction.* pp. 335–41. (New York, London: Plenum Press)
14. Burke, M. D., Prough, R. A. and Mayer, R. T. (1977). Characteristics of a microsomal cytochrome P-448 mediated reaction. Ethoxyresorufin *O*-de-ethylation. *Drug Metab. Dispos.*, **5,** 1–8
15. Weisburger, J. H., Cohen, L. A. and Wynder, E. L. (1977). On the etiology and metabolic epidemiology of the main human cancers. In Hiatt, H. H., Watson, J. D. and Winsten, J. A. (eds.). *Origins of Human Cancer.* Vol. 4, pp. 567–602. (Cold Spring Harbor Lab.)
16. Pantuck, E. J., Hsiao, K.-C., Maggio, A., Nakamura, K., Kuntzman, R. and Conney, A. H. (1973). Effect of cigarette smoking on phenacetin metabolism. *Clin. Pharmacol. Ther.*, **15,** 9–17
17. Conney, A. H., Pantuck, E. J., Hsiao, K.-C., Garland, W. A., Anderson, K. E., Alvares, A. P. and Kappas, A. (1976). Enhanced phenacetin metabolism in human subjects fed charcoal-broiled beef. *Clin. Pharmacol. Ther.*, **20,** 633–42
18. Remmer, H. (1972). Induction of drug metabolizing enzyme system in the liver. *Eur. J. Clin. Pharmacol.*, **5,** 116–36
19. Ochs, H. R., and Otten, H. (1981). Einfluß von Alter, Geschlecht und Rauchgewohnheiten auf die Kinetik von Oxazepam. *Verh. Dtsch. Ges. Inn. Med.*, **87,** 1205–8

39
Continuous enzymatic formation of glucuronides with the lipophilic hollow fibre technique *in vitro* and *in vivo*

G. BRUNNER, F. TEGTMEIER AND D. VELASQUEZ

ABSTRACT

Glucuronidation of a large number of endogenous and exogenous toxins was carried out over extended periods of up to 48 hours by the use of the lipophilic hollow fibre membrane technique. Substrate containing media (blood, buffer, waste fluids) were circulated through lipophilic hollow fibres. Solubilized crude UDP-glucuronyltransferase and cofactor UDPGA were circulated on the outside of the hollow fibres.

Lipophilic substrates accumulate in and penetrate the lipophilic membranes, and are rendered hydrophilic by glucuronic acid conjugation on the enzyme side. The newly formed glucuronides cannot rediffuse through the lipophilic membranes, and thus can be removed continuously from the enzyme side by coupled dialysis. Up to now the following components have been conjugated *in vitro* by this method: phenol, *p*-cresol, paracetamol, *p*-nitrophenol, 1-naphthol, 2-naphthol, lithocholic acid, enterolactone, enterodiol and secoisolariciresinol. *In vivo* extracorporeal glucuronidation of phenol was carried out with this technique in the rabbit. This technique allows the application of highly active soluble enzyme preparations, without immunological hazards *in vivo*, for extracorporeal glucuronidation and a continuous production of glucuronides as reference substances for basic research.

INTRODUCTION

Controlled glucuronide formation of exogenous and endogenous compounds is of interest for four reasons:

(1) It could be used *in vivo* for the glucuronidation of exogenous and endogenous toxins in severe liver disease (phenols, amines, bile acids, bilirubin, catechols, etc.).

(2) It could be used *in vivo* for exogenous intoxications of hydroxylated aromatic drugs and toxins (paracetamol, morphine, naphthol, etc.).

(3) It could be used for the production of reference substrates for research purposes (lignans, bile acids, phenols, etc.).

(4) It could be applied *in vitro* for the detoxification of waste fluids.

For *in vivo* application and for the commercial production of glucuronides it is essential to 'immobilize' the enzyme, to assure the absence of immunological hazards in *in vivo* application, and to avoid loss of enzyme after *in vitro* application. The classic immobilization technique through covalent binding of enzyme to carrier materials results in severe loss of enzyme activity[1]. The new liquid lipid membrane technique allows the use of enzymes in biological fluids without immobilization[2], and thus without loss of enzyme activity. It also offers optimal cofactor supply because no cofactor is lost, except for enzymatic reactions[3]. The aim of our experiments was to investigate the possibilities of the use of hollow fibre lipid membranes for the continuous glucuronidation of endogenous and exogenous toxins.

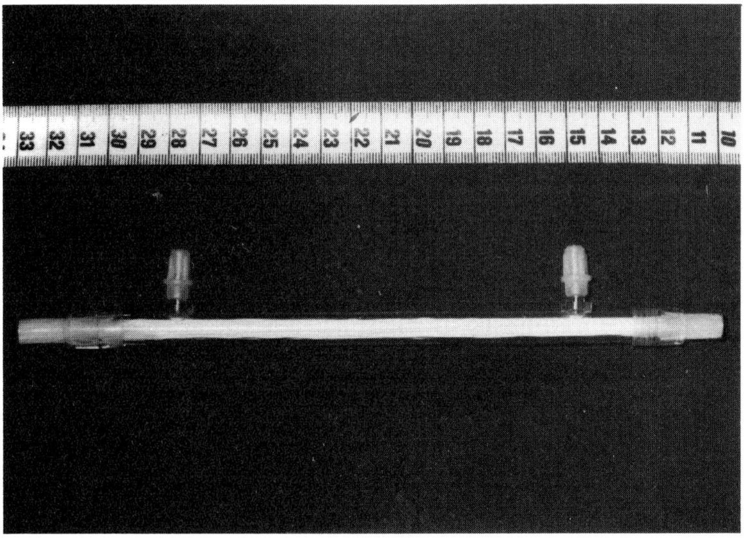

Figure 39.1 Lipid hollow fibre module used for continuous transmembranous glucuronidation

MATERIALS AND METHODS

Experimental set up

Polypropylene hollow fibres, the pores of which were filled with liquid phase, as previously described[2], were incorporated into a flow module (Figure 39.1).

This module with a membrane surface of 76 cm² was used in the experimental set up shown in Figure 39.2 (module A). Substrate-containing media (vessel

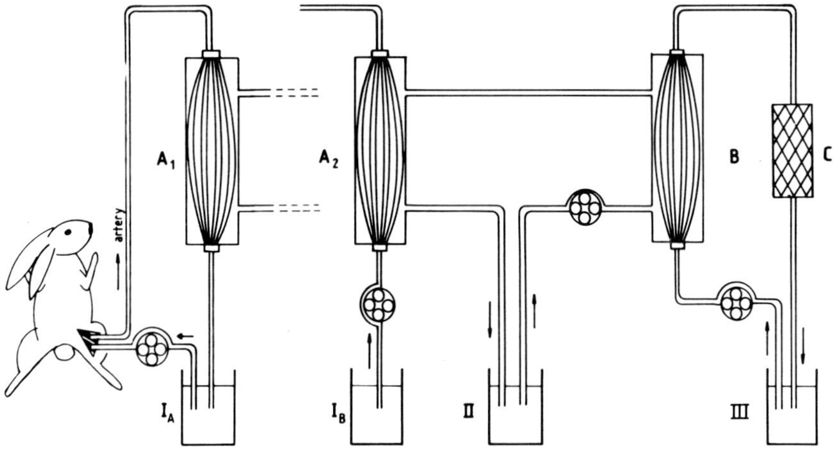

Figure 39.2 Experimental set up used for *in vitro* and *in vivo* glucuronidation experiments. A_1 and A_2 = lipid hollow fibre module, B = dialysing module, C = glucuronide extraction module, I_A = blood reservoir, I_B = toxin reservoir, II = enzyme-cofactor reservoir, III = reservoir for dialysing medium

I_A and I_B) were pumped through the interior of this module, while the enzyme UDP-glucuronyltransferase was circulated through the fibre-surrounding chamber together with the cofactor UDPGA (vessel II). For the removal of water soluble glucuronidation products a hydrophilic dialysing module was connected to the enzyme side of the system (module B).

The glucuronides passing the dialysing membrane were selectively retained on a reversed phase silica gel filled column (LiChroprep® RP-18 Merck Darmstadt) (module C). Modules A and B were purchased from Fesenius AG., Bad Homburg, Germany. Module C was a standard separation column. For kinetic *in vitro* experiments substrate was passed through module A_2 in an open circuit to maintain constant substrate concentrations. For *in vivo* experiments a closed circuit was used (A_1).

Enzyme preparation

Soluble UDP-glucuronyltransferase was prepared in crude form from pig liver microsomes by the same method as previously described for rabbit liver microsomes[4]. Protein content of the enzyme mixture in vessel II was adjusted to 2 mg/ml in all experiments with enzyme activities for *p*-nitrophenol ranging from 20 nmol mg^{-1} min^{-1} to 25 nmol mg^{-1} min^{-1}.

Experimental parameters

In vitro flow rates of substrates solution through module A_2 was 2.5 ml/min. For optimal glucuronide yield expensive substrates were pumped at rates of only 0.05 ml/min. *In vivo* the blood flow through module A_1 varied between 3.0 and 4.5 ml/min depending on the driving force of the artery of the animals.

The natural arterial flow in the rabbits was approximately 18 ml/min. When connected to the module the flow was reduced to 3.0–4.5 ml/min. The flow rate of the enzyme mixture through modules A and B was adjusted to 2.5 ml/min for all experiments. The flow on the stripping side through column C was also adjusted to 2.5 ml/min.

Toxin concentrations used in the system *in vitro* were 2 mmol/l for 1-naphthol and 2-naphthol, 1 mmol/l for phenol and *p*-cresol, 50 μmol/l for lithocholic acid, 2 mmol/l for all lactones and 0.1 mmol/l for paracetamol. The enzyme mixture used consisted of:

Enzyme protein	2.0 mg/ml
UDPGA	5.0 mmol/l
$MgCl_2$	5.0 mmol/l
Tris–HCl, pH 7.4	100 mmol/l
D-Saccharic acid-1,4-lactone	5.0 mmol/l

Cholate concentrations in vessels II and III were 0.06 mg/100 ml. *In vivo* serum concentrations of phenol in rabbits varied between 0.1 and 0.4 mmol/l. The experimental conditions applied to the *in vivo* detoxification were identical in respect to the enzyme reaction mixture and its flow rate. The continuous *in vivo* intoxication of the rabbit was carried out as described in detail elsewhere[5].

Analytical methods

UDPGA and the glucuronides were determined by isotachophoresis on a LKB Tachophor 2127 as previously described[6]. The analyses were carried out with a polytetrafluorethylene (PTFE) capillary (40 cm×0.5 mm ID) at 20°C. The zones were detected by UV-signal (254 nm) and thermosignal. The leading electrolyte system was 10 mmol/l HCl corrected to pH 3.3 by the addition of β-alanine. This system also contained 0.25% hydroxypropylmethylcellulose (HPMC) to reduce electroendosmosis. The terminating electrolyte was 10 mmol/l hexanoic acid. The total analysis time was approximately 30 minutes. For bile acid glucuronidation a modified buffer system had to be applied[7].

Phenol determination in the *in vivo* experiment was performed by gas chromatography after extraction from serum as separately described[5].

RESULTS

In vitro experiments

Four different groups of endogenous and exogenous substrates were submitted to enzymatic ether linking glucuronidation in direct batch – and transmembranous lipid hollow fibre experiments (Table 39.1). All phenolic compounds could be glucuronidated in both systems. Of the three lignanes tested two could be conjugated with both systems, while enterodiol, due to its more hydrophilic character, was conjugated only in the batch system at a low turnover rate[8].

Table 39.1 Glucuronidation of four different groups of substrates observed in batch and in lipid hollow fibre experiments. ● Glucuronidation in batch detectable. ■ Glucuronidation with lipid hollow fibre technique detectable. □ Glucuronidation with lipid hollow fibre technique not detectable

Phenols			*Lignanes*			*Bile acids*			*Alkaloids*		
Paracetamol	●	■	enterolactone	●	■	lithocholic acid	●	■	morphine	●	■
1-Naphthol	●	■	enterodiol	●	□	chenodeoxycholic acid	●	□			
2-Naphthol	●	■	secoisolariciresinol	●	■	cholic acid	●	□			
p-Cresol	●	■									
Phenol	●	■									
Catechol	●	■									
5-OH-Indol	●	■									

Of the bile acids only lithocholic acid could be glucuronidated in both systems, while chenodeoxycholic acid and cholic acid were not conjugated with the present lipid membrane system. Morphine was conjugated in both batch and lipid hollow fibres.

A typical *in vitro* closed circuit glucuronidation experiment is shown in Figures 39.3 and 4.

The transmembranous transfer rates and the K_m values of a typical representative substrate of each group are shown in Table 39.2. The rate of glucuronidation observed is dependent on the membrane transfer rate and on the individual K_m values of the substrates. The ratio of glucuronide formed to cofactor UDPGA consumed was 55% for batch and lipid membrane devices. When the cofactor was supplied from vessel III via module B the maximal ratio was 75%[9]. The latter device is of special interest for the commercial production of glucuronides.

In vivo experiments

The liquid lipid hollow fibre membrane device could be connected to healthy and intoxicated rabbits without any side-effects. No significant haemolysis or thrombocyte loss could be detected. The reaction rate on the enzyme side was

Table 39.2 K_m-values and membrane transfer values of some selected phenols, lignanes, bile acids and alkaloids. Membrane transfer measured in a polypropylene hollow fibre module without liquid lipid 'coating'. Substrate concentration 1.0 mmol/l, substrate flow 5.4 ml/min, flow of 'stripping medium' 3.0 ml/min

Substrate	*K_m-value* (mmol/l)	*Membrane-transfer* (nmole h^{-1} m^{-2})
Phenol	0.75	217
p-Cresol	0.45	409
Morphine	0.30	147
Lithocholic acid	0.04	26 (0.5 mmol/l in the presence of 0.03 ml/100 ml Zwittergent®)
Enterodiol	0.23	6
Secoisolariciresinol	0.22	137
Enterolactone	0.30	147

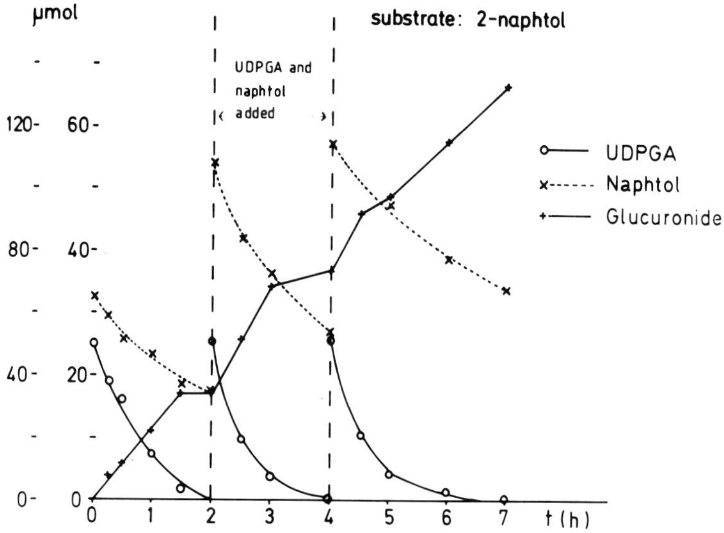

Figure 39.3 Transmembranous glucuronidation of 2-naphthol in a closed circuit experiment. Addition of cofactor and substrate restores decreasing glucuronidation rate

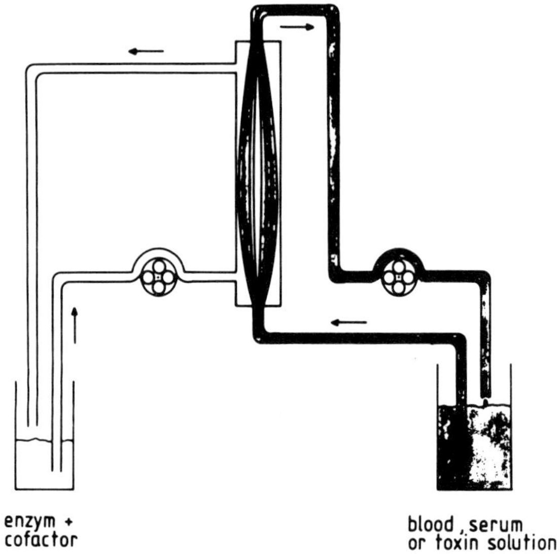

Figure 39.4 Closed circuit for transmembranous glucuronidation

several times higher than the diffusion rate of the phenol through the lipid coated membrane. All phenol penetrating the membrane from the animal was rapidly converted to its glucuronide (Figure 39.5). By increasing the membrane surface area an increase in glucuronide production could be observed (Figure 39.5). A similar effect could be observed when the thickness of the lipid membrane was decreased (Figure 39.6).

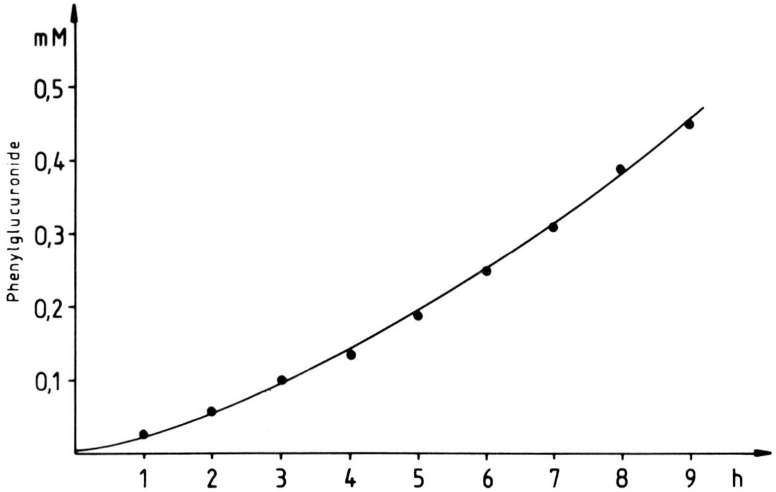

Figure 39.5 Increase in phenylglucuronide concentration on the enzyme side during transmembranous *in vivo* glucuronidation in a rabbit with phenol intoxication. Serum phenol concentration 0.32 mmol/l, blood flow 4.5 ml/min, 25 ml cofactor-enzyme solution (*see* materials and methods) circulated at 2.5 ml/min

DISCUSSION

The experiments demonstrate that with the lipid hollow fibre technique, glucuronidation reactions can be carried out over extended periods under easily controlled and standardized conditions for a large number of substrates. The system is also effective *in vivo*, and is aimed at a partial artificial support of liver detoxification. The lipid hollow fibre enzyme device is applicable only for highly lipophilic substrates as can be seen in Table 39.1. The higher the affinity of the substrate to the enzyme, the better is the permeability of the lipid membrane towards this substrate. The aim of our work is to improve the liquid lipid phase within the pores of the lipophilic hollow fibres nearer to the quality of physiological membranes. While at present the basic experiments were carried out with lipids on a paraffin basis, future work is directed to the use of the components of the fluid mosaic model[10].

From the present results observed in the rabbit experiments it can be deduced that enzymatic glucuronidation could extracorporally also be applied in man. With an observed transmembranous glucuronidation activity in the lipid hollow fibre system of 53.6 nmol cm^{-2} h^{-1} related to a 0.3 mmol/l phenol concentration in the blood, it is possible to remove 0.536 mmol toxin per hour with a hollow fibre surface of 1.0 m, and 250 ml crude rabbit UDP-glucuronyltransferase with a protein content of 3 mg/ml and a specific activity towards phenol of 15 nmol min^{-1} mg^{-1} protein. 1.0 m^2 membrane surface is the size frequently used in the commercially available hollow fibre devices of dialysis and plasma separation. The amount of 0.536 mmol phenol is within the magnitude of phenols observed in the circulating blood of patients in liver failure.

This technique is applicable not only for glucuronidation reactions. It has

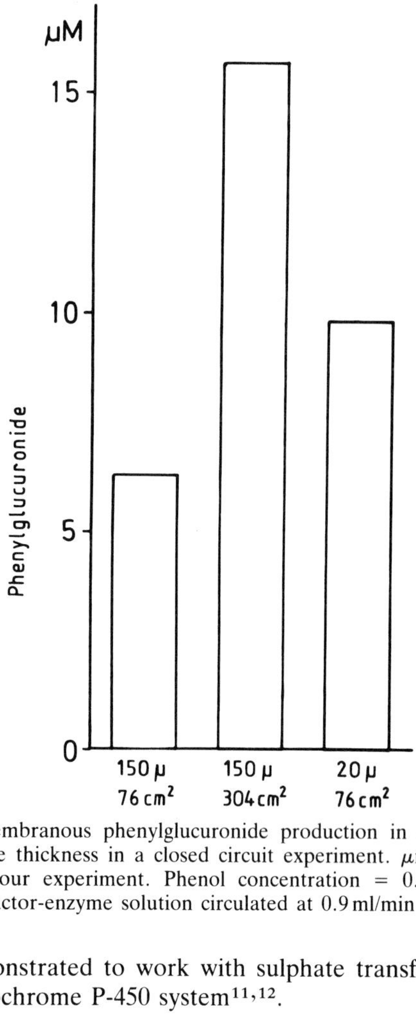

Figure 39.6 Transmembranous phenylglucuronide production in relation to membrane surface and membrane thickness in a closed circuit experiment. µmol Phenylglucuronide formed during a 5 hour experiment. Phenol concentration = 0.3 mmol/l circulated at 3.5 ml/min. 25 ml Cofactor-enzyme solution circulated at 0.9 ml/min

already been demonstrated to work with sulphate transferase, methyltransferase and the cytochrome P-450 system[11,12].

ACKNOWLEDGEMENT

The lignanes were a kind gift from Dr K. Setchell, Harrow, England.

References

1. Brunner, G., Holloway, C. J. and Lösgen, H. (1979). Large agarose beads for extracorporeal detoxification systems. 2. Preparation and enzymatic properties of agarose-bound UDP-glucuronyltransferase. *Int. J. Artif. Organs*, **2,** 163
2. Brunner, G. and Tegtmeier, F. (1984). Enzymatic detoxification using lipophilic hollow fibre membranes. I. Glucuronidation reactions. *Art. Organs*, **8,** 125
3. Brunner, G. and Tegtmeier, F. (1984). New technologies for extracorporeal enzymatic

detoxification. In: Paul, J. P. (ed.). *Biomaterials in Artificial Organs*. (London: MacMillan Press)

4. Holloway, C. J., Husmann-Holloway, S. and Brunner, G. (1981). Assay of UDP-glucuronyltransferase with mixtures of acceptors using analytical capillary isotachophoresis. *Electrophoresis*, **2,** 25
5. Velasquez, D., Tegtmeier, F. and Brunner, G. *In vivo* enzymatic detoxification in the rabbit using lipophilic hollow fibre membranes. I. Glucuronidation of phenol. *Int. J. Artif. Organs* (submitted)
6. Holloway, C. J., Husmann-Holloway, S. and Brunner, G. (1980). New method for the quantitative assay of the enzymatic hydrolysis of UDP-glucuronic acid using analytical capillary isotachophoresis. *J. Chromatog.*, **188,** 235
7. Tegtmeier, F. and Brunner, G. Rapid determination of bile acid glucuronides and bile acid sulphates using analytical capillary isotachophoresis. *Electrophoresis* (submitted)
8. Tegtmeier, F., Brunner, G. and Setchell, K. *FEBS Lett.*, Enzymatic synthesis and purification of lignane glucuronides (submitted)
9. Tegtmeier, F., Belsner, K. and Brunner, G. Enzymatic synthesis of glucuronides using lipophilic hollow fibre membranes. In preparation
10. Singer, S. J. and Nicolson, G. L. (1972). The fluid mosaic model of the structure of cell membranes. *Science*, **175,** 720
11. Tegtmeier, F. and Brunner, G. Enzymatic detoxification using lipophilic hollow fibre membranes. II. Sulfation reactions. *Artif. Organs* (in press)
12. Belsner, K., Tegtmeier, F. and Brunner, G. Enzymatic detoxification using lipophilic hollow fibre membranes. III. Hydroxylation reactions. In preparation for *Artif. Organs*

40
Effect of hepatic dysfunction on the kinetics of some drugs that are glucuronidated

R. A. BRANCH AND E. JACQZ

Numerous studies have evaluated the influence of both acute and chronic liver disease on the pharmacokinetic disposition of drugs that are eliminated following metabolism by the mixed function oxidase enzymes[1-3]. With few exceptions, the efficiency of the elimination process, or drug clearance, is impaired in both acute and chronic liver disease, and in many cases the extent of impairment in drug clearance is related to the extent of hepatic dysfunction. In contrast, there is less information available about drugs whose primary route of elimination is via glucuronidation.

Interest in the pharmacokinetics of drugs eliminated by glucuronidation was stimulated within our group, at Vanderbilt University, by a series of studies in which the disposition of four benzodiazepines was investigated in patients with cirrhosis. The benzodiazepines included two that are initially metabolized by oxidative metabolism, diazepam[4] and chlordiazepoxide[5], and two that are mainly metabolized by glucuronidation, oxazepam[6] and lorazepam[7]. The dispositions of these four drugs were studied in a group of normal subjects and a group of patients with cirrhosis. The pharmacokinetic parameters of each drug are listed in Table 40.1. The plasma clearance of both diazepam and chlordiazepoxide was decreased by approximately 50% in cirrhotic patients compared to controls, and resulted in a prolongation of the elimination halflife. With chlordiazepoxide, the change in the elimination halflife was greater than the change in clearance, because of an associated increase of the volume of distribution due to changes in protein binding. Such qualitative or quantitative changes are well established in liver disease[8]. In contrast, the plasma clearance of both oxazepam and lorazepam was not altered by hepatic dysfunction. The doubling of the mean elimination halflife of lorazepam in cirrhosis was also due to an increase in the volume of distribution caused by a reduction of this drug's plasma binding which was not observed wih oxazepam. In a subgroup of subjects, both lorazepam and antipyrine clearance were measured on separate

Table 40.1 Comparison of pharmacokinetics of four benzodiazines in normal subjects and patients with cirrhosis

	Clearance (ml min^{-1} kg^{-1})			*Halflife* (min)		
	Control	*Cirrhosis*	*% Change*	*Control*	*Cirrhosis*	*% Change*
Diazepam	26.6±41	13.8±2.4*	−48	7±14	106±15	+126
Chlordiazepoxide	15.3±4.4	7.7±2.1*	−50	24±12	63±27*	+163
Oxazepam	136±17.5	155.5±31.5	+14	3.6±0.3	3.8±0.5	+3.5
Lorazepam	0.75±0.23	0.81±0.48	+8	22±5	32±10*	+44

* $p < 0.05$ in comparison to control

occasions. In patients with impaired antipyrine clearance due to cirrhosis, the lorazepam clearance was the same as in normal subjects (Figure 40.1) This observation indicates that glucuronidation of lorazepam is preserved in patients with hepatic disease even when oxidative metabolism is impaired.

The preservation of glucuronidation in liver disease could be partially explained by a relative resistance of the glucuronidation pathway to hepatic damage, due to a deep localization of the enzymes within the microsomes[9]. In addition, glucuronyltransferases are a heterogenous group of enzymes, highly concentrated in the liver[10], but also widely distributed in the gut, lung and kidney[11]. In man, the eliminations of both oxazepam and lorazepam are by low clearance processes. Thus, preservation of their rates of glucuronidation

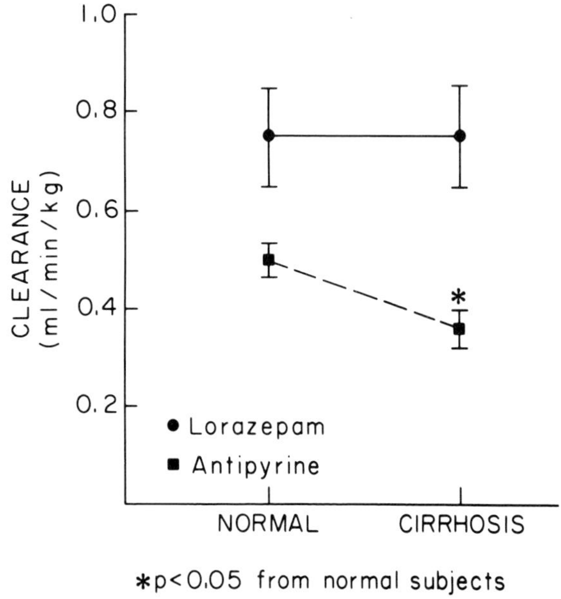

Figure 40.1 The clearance of lorazepam and antipyrine. Each drug was measured in each subject in a group of normal subjects and a group of patients with cirrhosis. (Adapted from Kraus *et al.*, Ref. 7)

could be due to conserved extrahepatic metabolism. However, hepatic glucuronyltransferases should be responsible for at least part of the metabolism of drugs that are glucuronidated with a high hepatic clearance. Consequently, we studied the pharmacokinetics of morphine, which is extensively and rapidly glucuronidated, in both normal subjects and patients with liver disease[12]. In normal subjects, the plasma concentration–time curve following intravenous administration declined biexponentially with a β-phase halflife of approximately 2.5 hours and a plasma clearance of 1200 ml/min, which is in excess of anticipated liver plasma flow, implying some extrahepatic metabolism (Figure 40.2). The morphine glucuronide plasma concentration–time profile was charac-

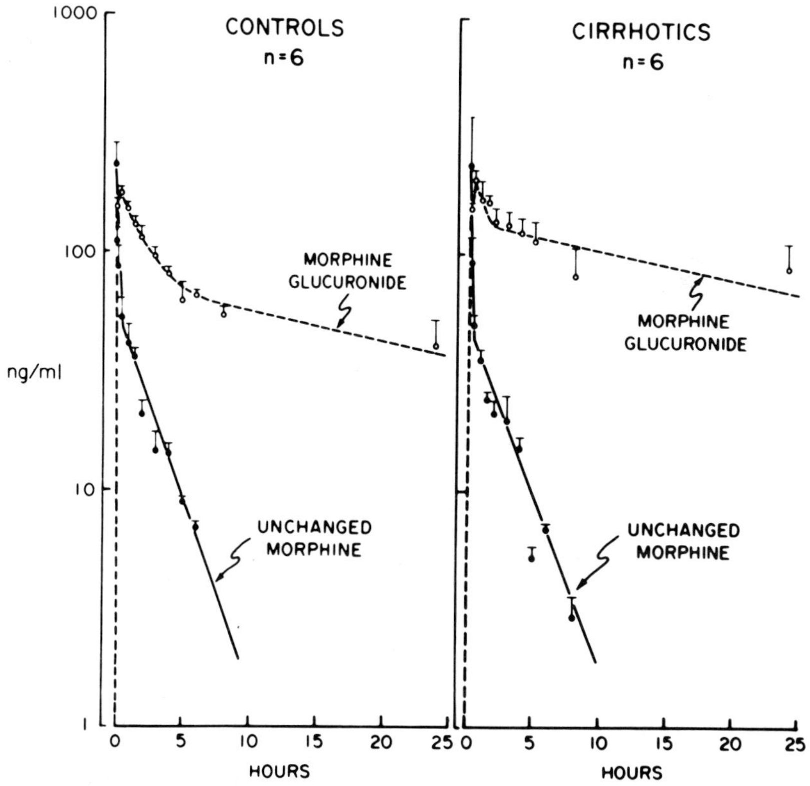

Figure 40.2 Pharmacokinetics of morphine in normal subjects and patients with cirrhosis. (From Patwardhan *et al.*, Ref. 12)

terized by an early rapid rise to almost ten-fold greater levels than the aglycone, and then declined biexponentially with a late phase halflife considerably longer than the unchanged morphine (Figure 40.2). In six cirrhotics who had evidence of impaired hepatic function as judged by a 40% reduction in indocyanine green plasma clearance, the plasma concentration–time profiles of both morphine and morphine glucuronide were the same as in normal subjects. These observations suggest that even though an unknown proportion of morphine is glucuronidated in extrahepatic sites, it is likely that there is conserved intrahepatic glucuronidation. Similar evidence to this has been obtained with labetolol[13], which is also glucuronidated with a high clearance. Following intravenous administration, total clearance of labetolol is unaffected by liver disease, yet when it is given orally, the normal low systemic availability is increased, presumably due to the development of portasystemic shunts, allowing absorbed drug to bypass the liver. This indicates that the liver is contributing to presystemic elimination in normal subjects.

In experiments in man, it is difficult to distinguish between intrahepatic and extrahepatic contributions to total clearance. We have, therefore, undertaken two further lines of enquiry in experimental animals. In the first, we have investigated extrahepatic glucuronidation in studies in the dog. In the second we have investigated hepatic glucuronidation in the isolated perfused rat liver and hepatic microsomes from control rats and carbon tetrachloride pre-treated rats.

In the dog, the pharmacokinetics disposition of both lorazepam and morphine were studied in sham-operated dogs and dogs with hepatectomy. Hepatectomy was performed by hepatic devascularization in conjugation with a porto–caval shunt, but leaving the liver *in situ* to minimize trauma[14]. Sham-operated dogs had a porto–portal shunt inserted, maintaining a normal portal blood flow, and the hepatic arterial blood flow was left intact. In hepatectomized dogs, the clearance of both lorazepam and morphine were significantly reduced compared to control (Table 40.2), indicating relative extrahepatic contributions of 11% and 44%, respectively. Despite the loss of the major site of glucuronidation, the appearance of lorazepam glucuronide and morphine glucuronide in plasma was prompt, and there were similar concentration–time profiles in hepatectomized dogs to control dogs. These results confirm that the liver is the major organ responsible for the glucuronidation for two drugs which are rapidly eliminated by glucuronidation in this species. Despite the important role of the liver, extrahepatic drug metabolizing enzymes contribute to their metabolism, and the initial appearance of the glycone in plasma is as rapid in hepatectomized dogs as in control dogs, raising the possibility that factors other than glucuronyltransferase activity might be important determinants of the elimination of the glycone once it is formed.

Table 40.2 Effect of hepatectomy on the pharmacokinetics of lorazepam and morphine in the dog

	Clearance ($ml\ min^{-1}\ kg^{-1}$)			*Halflife* (min)		
	Control dogs	*Hepatectomized dogs*	*% Change*	*Control dogs*	*Heptectomized dogs*	*% Change*
Lorazepam	29.7±4.2	3.3±3.0	−89	74±12	338±34	+365
Morphine	62.3±15.3	27.3±4.1	−66	79±21	200±76	+153

In further experiments focusing on glucuronidation in the liver, we have investigated the effect of acute liver injury in the rat, using carbon tetrachloride as a hepatotoxin, and lorazepam as a model drug which is metabolized by both oxidative metabolism and glucuronidation in this species[15]. In initial studies, we confirmed that total systemic clearance in the intact rat was quantitatively similar to hepatic clearance in the isolated perfused rat liver, and that glucuronidation accounted for approximately 25% of hepatic clearance in isolated perfused livers from normal rats. Following carbon tetrachloride pretreatment, total lorazepam clearance was significantly reduced by 63% (Table 40.3).

Table 40.3 The effect of carbon tetrachloride on lorazepam disposition in the isolated perfused rat liver

	Control	*CCl_4*	*% Change*
Lorezepam clearance (ml/min)	9.7±4.9	3.6±1.9*	−63
Recovery glucuronide (% of dose)	79±15	130±26*	+64
Lorazepam glucuronide clearance (ml/min)	2.6	1.56	−40
Lorazepam non-glucuronide clearance (ml/min)	7.4	2.04	−72

* $p<0.05$ in comparison to control

However, the recovery of lorazepam glucuronide in bile, perfusate and liver was increased by 64% in the hepatotoxic rats, suggesting that hepatic production of the glucuronide is spared in this form of hepatic damage. The efficiency of glucuronidation can be quantitated in control and hepatotoxic rats by calculating glucuronide clearance from the total recovery of glucuronide in bile, perfusate and liver tissue divided by the area under the plasma concentration–time curve of lorazepam in the perfusate. Using mean data from this experiment, there was a 40% reduction in glucuronide clearance, but a greater 72% reduction in non-glucuronide or oxidative clearance (Table 40.3). Thus, it appears that the intrahepatic glucuronidation of lorazepam is affected to a lesser extent than the oxidation of lorazepam following acute carbon-tetrachloride toxicity.

In subsequent studies, we have used the same hepatotoxin to induce acute hepatic damage. We obtained hepatic microsomal preparations from control and carbon tetrachloride pretreated rats, and measured cytochrome P-450 and NADPH cytochrome c reductase concentrations, the activity of *p*-nitroanisole demethylation and aniline hydroxylation as indices of oxidative metabolism, and *p*-nitrophenol glucuronidation and *o*-aminophenol glucuronidation as indices of glucuronidation (Figure 40.3)[12]. All four indices of hepatic oxidative metabolism were reduced to an approximately equal extent by carbon tetrachloride pretreatment. In contrast, the two measures of glucuronidation obtained from freshly prepared microsomes were either increased or unchanged. These results indicate that in contrast to mixed function oxidase enzymes, there appears to be a relative preservation of glucuronyltransferase activity in the same microsomal membranes. It has previously been suggested that there is an incomplete expression of glucuronyltransferase activity in freshly prepared microsomes. In the present study, microsomes solubilized with Triton X-100 had a tenfold enhancement of glucuronyltransferase activity in control rats, but only a sixfold increase in carbon tetrachloride treated rats (Figure 40.4).

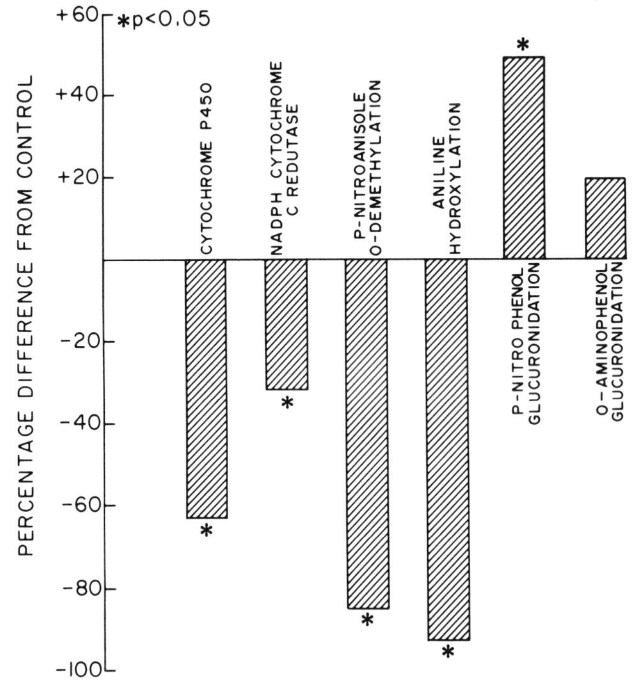

Figure 40.3 The effect of carbon tetrachloride pretreatment on indices of oxidative metabolism and glucuronidation in hepatic microsomal enzymes. (Adapted from Desmond *et al.*, Ref. 15)

Thus, it is possible that there is membrane activation of glucuronyltransferase in the presence of acute liver injury.

In conclusion, the glucuronidation of some drugs is maintained in the presence of hepatic dysfunction in patients with liver disease. The reason for this preservation is probably multifactorial, and includes the contribution of extrahepatic glucuronyltransferase, the possibility that glucuronyltransferase is not rate-limiting for the elimination of drugs which are glucuronidated, and that glucuronyltransferases in microsomal enzymes may be activated by hepatic disease processes. Irrespective of the mechanism, normal pharmacokinetic disposition of drugs that are glucuronidated in the presence of liver disease permits the clinician to use these drugs without having to anticipate dosage modification, on the basis of impaired drug elimination, when such drugs are indicated in patients with liver disease.

ACKNOWLEDGEMENT

This work was supported in part by USPHS Grant No. 31304.

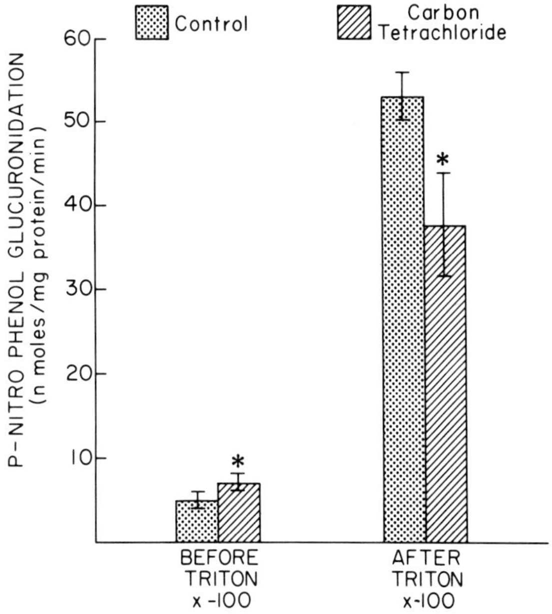

Figure 40.4 The effect of carbon tetrachloride pretreatment on *p*-nitrophenol glucuronidation in freshly prepared and Triton X100 solubilized microsomes. (Adapted from Desmond *et al.*, Ref. 15)

References

1. Wedlund, P. and Branch, R. A. (1983). Principles of drug dosage modification in liver disease. In Chernow, B. (ed.). *Pharmacological Approach to Critically Ill Patient*, pp. 84–114. (Baltimore: Williams and Wilkins)
2. Larry, D. and Branch, R. A. (1983). Clearance by the liver: current topics in understanding the hepatic disposition of drugs. *Semin. Liver Dis.*, **3,** 285–97
3. George, C. F. (1979). Drug kinetics and hepatic blood flow. *Clin. Pharmacokin.*, **4,** 433–48
4. Klotz, U., Avant, G. R., Hoyumpa, A., Schenker, S. and Wilkinson, G. R. (1975). The effects of age and liver disease on the disposition and elimination of diazepam in adult man. *J. Clin. Invest.*, **55,** 347–59
5. Roberts, R. K., Wilkinson, G. R., Branch, R. A. and Schenker, S. (1978). Effect of age and parenchymal liver disease on the disposition and elimination of chlordiazepoxide (Librium). *Gastroenterology*, **75,** 479–85
6. Shull, H. J., Wilkinson, G. R., Johnson, R. and Schenker, S. (1976). Normal disposition of oxazepam in acute viral hepatitis and cirrhosis. *Ann. Int. Med.*, **84,** 420–5
7. Kraus, J. W., Desmond, P. V., Marshall, J. P., Johnson, R. F., Schenker, S. and Wilkinson, G. R. (1978). Effects of aging and liver disease on the disposition of lorazepam. *Clin. Pharm. Ther.*, **24,** 411–9
8. Blaschke, T. P. (1977). Protein binding and kinetics of drugs in liver disease. *Clin. Pharmacokinet.*, **2,** 32–44
9. Popper, H. (1973). Structural aspects of hepatic biotransformation. In Goerk, W. and Sickinger, K. (eds.). *Drugs and the Liver*, pp. 39–50. (Stuttgart: K Schauttauer Verlag)
10. Dutton, G. J. (1980). Location of UDP-glucuronyltransferase in the cell. In *Glucuronidation of Drugs and Other Compounds*, pp. 23–8. (Boca Raton: CRC Press)

with sulphation, which has in general a lower capacity. A further important difference between glutathione and glucuronide conjugation is the relatively lesser importance of a deficiency of the conjugating agent or its cofactors for glucuronidation, at least under clinical circumstances. By contrast, glutathione depletion is common in liver disease and in intoxications, and therapeutic replacement is, therefore, contemplated.

The described versatility is also reflected in the presence of glucuronide conjugation activity in virtually all higher animals, only the insects use glucose; in fish, glucuronidation undergoes characteristic variations with climatic temperatures and is related to spawning. The activity is lower in neonatal mammals; on maturation, increases develop in two clusters of substrates with different corticosteroid sensitivity. Ontogenetic variations of the microsomal phospholipid membrane modify enzyme activity in a substrate specific fashion[7]. There are relatively few inhibitors of glucuronidation, e.g. furosemide and salicylamide[8], but many agents induce glucuronidation; almost all act non-specifically on other drug metabolizing systems and particularly almost always induce cytochrome P-450. However, they show, as will be discussed later, significant substrate specificity, as do the various glucuronyltransferases themselves. While these transferase isoenzymes need not vary in immunologic reactivity, they show different conjugating ability to various compounds.

Acquired reduction of glucuronidation is only rarely a clinical problem. It occurs mainly in intoxications, but may play a, so far poorly appreciated, role in the regulation of hepatic phenotypic expression. However, mutants of defective specific isoenzymes are known in animals and have clinical counterparts. The former include, besides the wellknown Gunn rat, defective in conjugation of bilirubin and related substances and with only partial reduction for some, but not for most other substrates; one strain of Wistar rat, defective in androsterone glucuronidation, and the Bolivian, but not the Brazilian, squirrel monkey[9], in which the bilirubin glucuronidation defect may result from abnormalities in membrane lipids. The classical clinical example is the bilirubin conjugation defect, partial in Gilbert's and complete in the Crigler–Najar syndrome.

Nevertheless, there is clinical, physiologic, biochemical, and pharmaco–toxicologic evidence for rate limitation of the steps in glucuronidation. Clinical observations include the increased bilirubinaemia from fasting in Gilbert's syndrome, presumably because of reduced availability of carbohydrate precursors, and the role of caloric deprivation in neonatal jaundice. It is not established whether the phenomenon also occurs in diabetes. Exhaustion of glucuronide conjugation, and its replacement by sulphation, may influence human intoxications like that by acetaminophen.

Physiologic evidence for rate limitation is the indication that glucuronidation follows Michaelis–Menten kinetics, at least if the latency of part of the enzyme reaction is eliminated. However, low water solubility interferes with kinetic analysis, even if binding proteins are added. Probably because the hydrophilic UDP-glucuronic acid does not readily pass through phospholipid membranes, for complete enzyme activity, either UDP-*N*-acetylglucosamine (or Mg^{2+}) is required to facilitate transport allosterically[10], or the membrane must be disturbed, for instance by detergents. Moreover, the enterohepatic circulation determines the action of glucuronides, which in turn depends on uptake by hepatocytes which for steroid glucuronates is sex dependent and saturable[11].

Biochemically, the availability of hexoses is rarely restricted, while lack of cofactors may reduce the precursor UDP-glucose, or with inhibited UDP-glucose dehydrogenase the conjugating agent UDP-glucuronic acid, as experimentally induced by administration of D-galactosamine or D-galactosone. Diethyl ether anaesthesia has a similar effect, which also includes other class II reactions[12], and thus reduces biliary excretion of a series of compounds. Acetaminophen also decreases UDP-glucuronic acid, presumably by binding, while butylated hydroxyanisol raises it. Similarly, increased available UDP-glucuronic acid enhances glucuronidation of bilirubin and particularly formation of diglucuronide in primate liver. This effect is, however, only significant with very high blood bilirubin concentrations.

From a pharmaco–toxicological standpoint, modified conjugation may alter the therapeutic effect of drugs, for instance tobacco smoke contains a, so far, unidentified inducing agent which reduces action and increases elimination of some medications.

The effect of liver cell injury on glucuronic acid conjugation is problematic. There are few indications of a reduction, if at all, more of ester than of ether conjugation. Impaired glucuronidation, possibly as a result of saturation from overdose and associated with a compensatory increase in sulphation, was reported in severe human and cat poisoning[13]; bile acid glucuronidation is reduced in cirrhosis. By contrast, most studies show either no effect of liver disease (except for chronic congestion) or even an increase, for instance in alcoholic liver injury or after experimental exposure to dimethylnitrosamine. Bile alcohol formation, a relatively small component of bile acid metabolism, is increased in primary biliary cirrhosis, in which other functional parameters show impairment. In an old hepatic test[14] the preference of glucuronidation of benzoic acid over hippuric acid formation was taken as a sign of liver injury.

Similarly, in cholestasis, hepatic glucuronidation of bilirubin appears increased, as is that of bile acids. The urinary excretion of bile acid glucuronates is enhanced in man, though less than that of sulphates, and other urinary glucuronates also increase after experimental bile duct ligation[15]. Bilirubin competes in bile acid conjugation. The conjugates are not detergent, but lithocholate glucuronide is cholestatic[16], though not cytotoxic. It has been wellknown for a long time that in cholestasis the urinary excretion represents a major pathway for the bile acids. Parenthetically, synthetic nor-bile acids are poorly conjugated with amino or glucuronic acids and, therefore, as weak acids are effectively reabsorbed in the bile ductules, and their 'chole-hepatic' circulation enhances choleresis.

Glucuronidation may respond to both liver cell injury and cholestasis biphasically with an increase followed sometimes by a final reduction, as seen in the perfused liver damaged by carbon tetrachloride. This biphasic reaction contrasts with the uniform inhibition of cytochrome P-450 dependent oxidation under various hepatotoxic regimens.

The most impressive example of preserved glucuronic acid conjugation in even severe liver cell injury, even if associated with cholestasis, comes from the Hyman van den Bergh-reaction, reported in 1917. Direct reacting, that means glucuronidated, serum bilirubin is indeed not reduced but markedly increased in all types of liver diseases associated with hepatocellular injury. Even in massive necrosis of the liver, excess conjugated bilirubin is found in serum, and thus at least bilirubin conjugation appears well preserved. It is an ironic contribution to the history of science that one of the most intelligent and knowledgeable clinical scientists, Isadore Snapper, was concerned for several decades with the van den Bergh's reaction, to the development of which he had contributed, as well as with glucuronic acid conjugation without ever relating the two processes to each other, a subsequent accomplishment of three other groups in the 1950s.

The explanation of the increase of glucuronidation in liver cell injury is probably the specific location of the system in the endoplasmic reticulum membrane. It has been known for years that the cytochrome P-450 monooxygenase system is closer to the cytoplasmic, and the glucuronide conjugation system closer to the luminal surface of the endoplasmic reticulum membrane. According to an old, simplistic concept[17], a disturbance of its cytoplasmic layer in liver injury reduces cytochrome P-450 activity, but increases activity of the now exposed conjugating system. Hepatocellular degeneration, often associated with increased activity of lipase C, an endogenous detergent, and with lipid peroxidation, may disturb the cytoplasmic layers of the phospholipid bilayer and thus facilitate the access of the hydrophilic UDP-glucuronic acid from the cytoplasm. This is in keeping with the activation of the latent conjugation by detergent agents and by the demonstration of exposed and buried transferases, the latter exhibiting a high K_m. The phospholipid membrane provides not only a barrier, but also positive and negative conformational constraints and thus impart a specificity which may, for instance, be altered in choline deficiency.

The role of glucuronidation in hepatic carcinogenesis is reflected in its increased activity in precancerous hepatocytic nodules, in which cytochrome P-450 activity is reduced. Both factors contribute to the decreased *in vitro* binding of carcinogens or other toxic chemicals and their inhibited uptake by the transformed hepatocytes and to the cells' known resistance to them. This resistance favours the preferential hepatocytic proliferation in the established models of chemical carcinogenesis, in part because of additional promoting influences. The promoter phenobarbital further enhances the glucuronidation. Some promoting agents induce specific molecular forms of UDP-glycosyltransferases[18]. In human carcinoma tissue, glucuronic acid conjugation, particularly of 1-naphthol, may exceed its sulphation, and this may assist in the selection of chemotherapeutic agents.

In general, glucuronic acid conjugation is not as much influenced as the other class II and particularly the class I reactions, by the multifactorial disturbances in a regulatory network which are characteristic of the various abnormal phenomena in liver diseases. Therefore, the pathological syndromes associated with glucuronidation are rather simple (one cause–one disease) effects, rare in human pathology and almost all experiments of nature. One is bilirubin gallstones from biliary supersaturation of unconjugated bilirubin or from bacterial deconjugation, bilirubin thus being lithogenic. The other is the mentioned genetic mutants such as Gilbert's disease and the rare Crigler–Najar syndrome.

From all these considerations, the glucuronic acid conjugation emerges as a high-capacity system involved in the clearance of many different substances, based on families of closely related transferase isoenzymes, and barely limited in clinical conditions by availability of the conjugating agent and/or its cofactors. Its function may be described as 'sanitary engineering', a term used at a previous Falk meeting[19]. However, the glucuronidation of so many different substances accounts for its implications in various aspects of biology and particularly pharmacology, and this symposium thus presented a panorama of observations dealing with divergent topics, including bile acids, bilirubin, sex hormones and drugs.

Another key problem is that of the various aspects of specificity. Species specificities of glucuronidation were emphasized, with some enzyme activities characteristic of man and chimpanzee only. The process is not restricted to hepatocytes and has been demonstrated, including variegated pharmacological effects, in many epithelia, such as in intestines, where bile acid glucuronidation declines from duodenum to colon, or in kidney and in bronchus, where it is preserved in short-term cultures of tumours, at least as far as 1-naphthol is concerned. Extrahepatic glucuronidation may account for its preservation in hepatectomized dogs. Pharmacokinetics have been studied in isolated cells from various organs of animal and man.

Specificity of location may concern the location in the hepatic acinus or lobule. Although immunocytochemically the hepatocytes (endoplasmic reticulum and nuclear envelope), but not non-parenchymal cells, have been stained throughout the lobule, and subpopulations of isolated cells showed no differences[20], most studies indicate a preferential localization in the centrolobular zone 3, with sulphation localized anteriorally, that means, in zone 2. Organelle localization shows distinct substrate variations, with the endoplasmic reticulum exhibiting highest activity, followed by nuclear envelope, Golgi zone, and finally, plasma membrane. While localized activity differed but little for some substrates and also for some inducers, others exhibited higher velocity in endoplasmic reticulum and nuclear envelope; the localization in the latter may serve to inhibit carcinogenesis. The potential for bilirubin glucuronidation may be equal in all the lipid membranes, but lack of latency in rough endoplasmic reticulum and nuclear envelope renders the former the major active site. The localization of the enzyme in the phospholipid membrane accounts for its latency, and the influence of this membrane on the enzyme's configuration may be specific.

Great specificity, including regio- and stereospecificity, implying positional characteristics, is expressed by the various substrates. In monkeys monoglucuronide formation of bilirubin has greater capacity than that of diglucuronides, probably because of two independent binding sites for UDP-glucuronic acid. However, with physiologic bilirubin levels, more di- than monoglucuronides are formed. Also the glucuronidation of bile acids varies, with highest activity for litho- and ursodeoxycholic acid. Similar structure–activity variations exist for steroids and drugs; substrates so far not considered include, besides clofibric acid[21], lignans, previously known in plants but now also recognized in man and animals; they have potential as anticancer agents because of the lower rate of some cancers in vegetarians who excrete them in higher amounts.

Inducing agents which prolong the lifespan of the transferases above their halflife of 24 hours, also have great substrate specificity, including regiospecificity of binding. Their effect may be dose related, for instance in the action of phenobarbital on bilirubin UDP-glucuronyltransferase, equal in rat and man. The mechanism of the inducers is not established. They may stabilize the enzyme, but may also alter Michaelis–Menten kinetics, suggesting changes in the phospholipid membrane depending latency of the enzyme. The corticosteroids may either increase all protein synthesis or raise activity of specific enzymes. Inhibitors, competitive or not, may also be specific.

The characteristics of the enzyme itself were demonstrated by peptide maps, amino acid composition, isoelectric point, antibody absorption, and particularly by estimation of the molecular weight, including analysis by radiation inactivation. Although the reliability of the molecular weight methods is not established, polypeptides between 41 000 and 57 000 were identified, which varied with both substrate and inducers. Transferases differ also by some being processed by proteolytic cleavage of extensions or by glycosylation. The approximately 50 000 peptides appear to be monomers, for instance transforming bilirubin to monoglucuronides with high V_{max}, other are tetramers, for instance for low V_{max} transformation of bilirubin monoglucuronide to diglucuronide. Dimers or tetramers seem to act on steroids and other chemicals. Their size may be related to the configuration of the binding sites.

Let us finally look into the future and point out approaches suggested by studies here presented. The reported cloning of the glucurosyltransferase with the assistance of β-galactosidase inducers, in progress with the subsequent sequencing, will provide specific data as to molecular size and configuration and the specificity of the various isoenzymes, as well as definite information on the binding sites and on affinity, replacing kinetic data which can be far less easily interpreted. Of great interest is the UDPGA independent conjugation with lipophilic sugars, so far only demonstrated for bile acid conjugation. The alterations of bile alcohol conjugation in genetic or disease acquired alterations of the bile acid metabolism offer interesting vistas, as does the possibility of using solubilized enzyme preparations combined with cofactors in extracorporeal systems to treat hepatic coma. Finally, the reported relation between bilirubin conjugation and sex hormones, which themselves undergo glucuronidation and which accounts for the higher unconjugated serum bilirubin levels in males after puberty, raises the interesting possibility that glucuronic acid conjugation of sex hormones may play an important regulatory role in development. Since conjugation of the hormones presumably reduces their biologic activity, the prenatal imprinting by sex hormones, particularly androsterone, which is held responsible for the development of secondary sex characteristics, may be regulated by glucuronide conjugation of the hormones.

Such speculations are the result of the stimulation obtained at this symposium, which clarified many problems in a complicated field. Therefore, not only the organizers and authors of this volume, but also the Falk Foundation deserve our appreciation.

References

1. Popper, H. (1984). The future of hepatology. *Hepatology*, **4,** 152–5
2. Keppler, D., Popper, H., Reutter, W. and Bianchi, L. (eds). (1984). *Mechanism of Hepatocytic Injury and Death*. (Lancaster: MTP Press)
3. Sugimoto, Y., Whitman, M., Cantley, L. C. and Erikson, R. L. (1984). Evidence that the Rous sarcoma virus transforming gene product phosphorylates phosphatidylinositol and diacylglycerol. *Proc. Natl. Acad. Sci. USA*, **81,** 2117–21
4. Arias, I. M. and Jakoby, W. B. (eds.). (1976). *Glutathione: Metabolism and Function.* (New York: Raven Press)
5. Belinsky, S. A., Kauffman, F. C., Sokolove, P. M., Tsukuda, T. and Thurman, R. G. (1984). Calcium-mediated inhibition of glucuronide production of epinephrine in the perfused rat liver. *J. Biol. Chem.*, **259,** 7705–11
6. Dutton, G. J. (1980). *Glucuronidation of Drugs and Other Compounds.* (New York: CRC Press)
7. Delpech, I., Kiffel, L., Magdalou, J., Siest, G., Martin, P., Bouchy, M. and André, J-C. (1984). Structural changes of liver microsomes in rat during neonatal life: influence on the glucuronidation rates of various substrates. *Biochem. Biophys. Res. Commun.*, **119,** 29–34
8. Boutin, J. A., Thomassin, J., Siest, G. and Batt, A-M. (1984). Inhibition studies of microsomal UDP-glucuronosyltransferase activities by furosemide and salicylamide. *Pharmacol. Res. Commun.*, **16,** 227–41
9. Portman, O. W., Alexander, M., Cornelius, C. E., Chowdhury, J. R., Chowdhury, N. R. and Arias, I. M. (1984). The effects of nutrition on unconjugated plasma bilirubin concentrations in squirrel monkeys. *Hepatology*, **4,** 454–60
10. Cummings, J., Graham, A. B. and Wood, G. C. (1984). Kinetic studies of latent microsomal UDP-glucuronyltransferases. Kinetics of glucuronidation in intact and perturbant-treated membranes. *Biochim. Biophys. Acta*(M), **771,** 127–41
11. Brock, W. J. and Vore, M. (1984). Characterization of uptake of steroid glucuronides into isolated male and female rat hepatocytes. *J. Pharmacol. Exp. Ther.*, **229,** 175–81
12. Aune, H., Hals, P-A., Hansen, B. I. and Aarbakke, J. (1984). Effect of diethylether on the formation of paracetamol sulphate and glucuronide in isolated rat hepatocytes. *Pharmacology*, **28,** 67–73
13. Savides, M. C., Oehme, F. W., Nash, S. L. and Leipold, H. W. (1984). The toxicity and biotransformation of single doses of acetaminophen in dogs and cats. *Toxicol. Appl. Pharmacol.*, **74,** 26–34
14. Snappper, I. and Saltzman, A. (1947). Excretion of benzoyl glucuronate as a test of liver function. *Am. J. Med.*, **2,** 334–41
15. Siegers, C-P. and Klaassen, C. D. (1984). Biliary excretion of acetaminophen in ureter-ligated rats. *Pharmacology*, **28,** 177–80
16. Oelberg, D. G., Chari, M. V., Little, J. M., Adcock, E. W. and Lester, R. (1984). Lithocholate glucuronide is a cholestatic agent. *J. Clin. Invest.*, **73,** 1507–14
17. Popper, H. (1975). Structural aspects of hepatic biotransformation. In Gerok, W. and Sickinger, K. (eds.). *Drugs and the Liver*, pp. 39–50. (Stuttgart: F. K. Schattauer Verlag GmbH)
18. Sato, K., Kitahara, A., Yin, Z., Waragai, F., Nishimura, K., Hatayama, I., Ebina, T., Yamazaki, T., Tsuda, H. and Ito, N. (1984). Induction by butylated hydroxyanisole of specific molecular forms of glutathione S-transferase and UDP-glucuronyltransferase and inhibition of development of γ-glutamyl transpeptidase-positive foci in rat liver. *Carcinogenesis*, **5,** 473–7
19. Popper, H. (1980). Summary. In Popper, H., Bianchi, L., Gudat, F. and Reutter, W. (eds.). *Communication of Liver Cells*, pp. 311–9. (Lancaster: MTP Press)
20. Tonda, K. and Hirata, M. (1983). Glucuronidation and sulfation of *p*-nitrophenol in isolated rat hepatocyte subpopulations. Effects of phenobarbital and 3-methylcholanthrene pretreatment. *Chem. Biol. Interact.*, **47,** 277–87
21. Odum, J. and Orton, T. C. (1983). Hepatic microsomal glucuronidation of clofibric acid in thc adult and neonate albino rat. *Biochem. Pharmacol.*, **32,** 3565–9

Section 10
Abstracts of Posters

Abstracts of Posters

ABSTRACT

1
Partial purification of UDP-glucuronyltranferase messenger RNA

M. R. JACKSON AND B. BURCHELL

A major step forward in the understanding of many of the interesting biological problems associated with UDP-glucuronyltransferase (GT) will no doubt be achieved by using cDNA probes from clones to GTmRNA[1].

A prerequisite to obtaining a cDNA clone for any low abundance message is to enrich the message of interest in the population to be cloned. This has previously been achieved in a number of ways, for example: (1) induction, (2) sucrose gradient fractionation, (3) denaturing agarose gels, (4) polysome immunoprecipitation and fractionation[2]. We have used all of these methods to partially purify GTmRNAs, assaying for biologically active message by *in vitro* translation in a rabbit reticulocyte lysate system[3], followed by immunoprecipitation[4] with sheep and rabbit anti GT sera.

We extracted poly $(A)^+$RNA from drug treated chick embryos or Wistar rats using the guanidine thiocyanate procedure[5] and oligo d(T) cellulose[6]. Fractionation of this poly $(A)^+$RNA on a low salt 5–20 g/100 ml sucrose gradient allowed partial purification and good recovery. This method has enabled us to purify rat GTmRNA to approximately 3% of the messages and to estimate the size of the assayed message. Rat GTmRNA sedimented at approximately 17S whilst chick embryo GTmRNA at approximately 21S on the sucrose gradient.

cDNA libraries have been constructed from this enriched RNA and we are now screening the clones to identify those of interest by differential hybridization[7] to [^{32}P]cDNA synthesized from crude poly $(A)^+$RNA or poly $(A)^+$RNA enriched for GTmRNA. Preliminary studies with polysome immunoadsorption[8] indicate this method will be valuable for preparation of poly $(A)^+$RNA very highly enriched in GTmRNA, which will improve the present screen.

References

1. Burchell, B., Kennedy, S., Jackson, M. and McCarthy, L. (1984). The biosynthesis and induction of microsomal UDP-glucuronyltransferase in avian liver. *Biochem. Soc. Trans.*, **12**, 50–3

2. Maniatis, T., Fritsch, E. F. and Sambrook, J. (1982). *Molecular cloning*. (Cold Spring Harbor Laboratory Publications)
3. Pelham, H. R. B. and Jackson, R. J. (1976). An efficient mRNA dependent translation system from reticulocyte lysates. *Eur. J. Biochem.*, **67,** 247–56
4. Fagan, J., Pastewka, J., Guengerich, F. and Gelboin, H. (1983). Multiple cytochrome P-450 are translated from multiple messenger ribonucleic acids. *Biochem. J.*, **22,** 1927–34
5. Chirgwin, J. M. *et al.* (1972). Isolation of biologically active ribonucleic acids from sources enriched in ribonucleases. *Biochemistry*, **18,** 5294–99
6. Aviv, H. and Leder, P. (1972). Purification of biologically active globin messenger RNA by affinity chromatography on oligothymidylic acid cellulose. *Proc. Natl. Acad. Sci. USA*, **69,** 1408–12
7. Grunstein, M. and Hogness, D. S. (1975). Colony hybridization: a method for the isolation of cloned DNAs that contain a specific gene. *Proc. Natl. Acad. Sci. USA*, **72,** 3961–5
8. Kraus, J. P. and Rosenberg, L. E. (1982). Purification of low abundance messenger RNAs from rat liver by polysome immunoadsorption. *Proc. Natl. Acad. Sci. USA*, **79,** 4015–9

ABSTRACT

2
Microsomal membrane integrity and expression of UDP-glucuronyl-tranferase activity in response to UDP-*N*-acetylglucosamine

I. SCRAGG, W. J. ARION AND B. BURCHELL

UDP-glucuronyltransferase (GT) activity is 'latent' in microsomes and can be specifically activated up to 5-fold by UDP-*N*-acetylglucosamine (UDP-GlcNAc)[1,2] or non-specifically activated up to 20–fold by membrane perturbation[3]. UDP-GlcNAc has been classified as a physiological regulator of GT since the presence of physiological concentrations of UDP-GlcNAc are required during the assay of microsomal GT activity to raise the reaction rate up to 60% of the level observed in isolated hepatocytes[4]. Stimulation of GT by UDP-GlcNAc has been observed only in untreated, intact microsomal fractions; GT is rendered insensitive to UDP–GlcNAc if the membrane integrity is destroyed with detergent[2,5].

We have used microsomal mannose-6-phosphatase activity as a measure of microsomal membrane integrity[6], to study effects of detergent and UDP-GlcNAc on 1-naphthol GT activity.

Washed rat liver microsomes were prepared in 0.25 mol/l sucrose/ 5 mmol/l HEPES (pH 7.4) and stored at 20 mg/ml at −70°C; storage resulted in no increase in mannose-6-phosphatase activity.

Microsomes, pretreated with a range of concentrations of Lubrol 12A9, a non-ionic detergent, caused an increase in mannose-6-phosphatase activity, and maximum expression of mannose-6-phosphatase was achieved at a detergent concentration of 0.25 mg detergent/mg protein. A very similar pattern of increase of 1-naphthol GT activity was determined in parallel assays of the same samples. Thus the expression of mannose-6-phosphatase directly correlates ($r = 0.998$) with the expression of 1-naphthol GT in microsomes and the expression of the activity was related to the intactness of the membrane.

Microsomes were also pretreated with increasing concentrations of UDP-GlcNAc; low 'physiological' concentrations of UDP-GlcNAc had no effect on mannose-6-phosphatase activity but activated 1-naphthol GT 2-fold. Higher concentrations of UDP–GlcNAc 0.8–8 mmol/l (final assay concentrations) activated mannose–6–phosphatase and produced a further activation of 1-naphthol GT.

We conclude from this work that:

(1) Microsomes which are 100% intact might (theoretically) not display 1-naphthol GT activity.
(2) Physiological concentrations of UDP-GlcNAc give maximal stimulation of GT *in vitro*.
(3) It appears that UDP–GlcNAc or some other factor is essential to allow physiological expression of transferase activity, unless the endoplasmic reticulum *in vivo* has a different structure to isolated microsomes.

References

1. Pogell, B. M. and Leloir, L. F. (1961). Nucleotide activation of liver microsomal glucuronidation. *J. Biol. Chem.*, **236,** 279–91
2. Winsnes, A. (1969). Studies on the activation *in vitro* of glucuronyltranferase. *Biochim. Biophys. Acta*, **191,** 279–91
3. Dutton, G. J. and Burchell, B. (1977). Newer aspects of glucuronidation. *Prog. Drug. Metab.*, **2,** 1–70
4. Otani, G., Abou-El-Malkarem, M. M. and Bock, K. W. (1976). UDP-glucuronyltransferase in perfused rat liver and in microsomes. III Effects of galactosamine and carbon tetrachloride on the glucuronidation of 1-naphthol and bilirubin. *Biochem. Pharmacol.*, **25,** 1293–7
5. Winsnes, A. (1971). The effects of sulfhydryl reacting agents on hepatic UDP-glucuronyltransferase *in vitro*. *Biochim. Biophys. Acta*, **242,** 549–59
6. Arion, W. J., Ballas, L. M., Lange, A. J. and Wallin, B. K. (1976). Microsomal membrane permeability and the hepatic glucose-6-phosphatase system. *J. Biol. Chem.*, **251,** 4901–7

ABSTRACT

3
On the conjugation of digitoxigenin-digitoxosides by a specific form of UDP-glucuronosyltransferase of dogs

A. SCHMOLDT, B. HERZFELDT AND L. VON MEYERINCK

In contrast to all other species, including man, digitoxin (dt-3) is rapidly eliminated in dogs, especially as hydrophilic compounds.

In the present study we investigated the *in vitro* conversion of dt-3 into hydrophilic metabolites. With liver microsomes of Beagle dogs dt-3 and its cleavage products digitoxigenin-*bis* digitoxoside (dt-2), digitoxigenin-mono-digitoxoside (dt-1), and digitoxigenin (dt-0) were tested as substrates for microsomal UDP-glucuronosyltransferase(s).

The highest conjugation rates were found for dt-1 and dt-3. The dt-3 conjugation rate exceeded that of all other species (rat, guinea-pig, cat, rabbit, human) tested so far.

Table

Substrate	*app.* V_{max} (pmoles mg micr. prot^{-1} min^{-1})	*app.* K_m (μmol/l)
dt-3	400	117
dt-2	157	7
dt-1	850	8
dt-0	200	145

The app. K_m-values for dt-1 and dt-2 are comparably low as found for dt-1 in rats

Competitive inhibitors for glucuronidation of dt-3 are dt-2 and dt-1, whereas dt-0, testosterone, and pregnanediol exhibited non-competitive inhibition. 4-hydroxy-biphenyl and *p*-nitrophenol inhibited uncompetitively.

In conclusion, the high elimination rate of dt-3 in the dog is mainly due to the high UDP-glucuronosyltransferase activity for dt-3. There is further evidence for a specific form of the conjugating enzyme in the dog responsible for the glucuronidation of digitoxigenin-digitoxosides.

ABSTRACT

4 UDP-Glucuronosyltransferase activity toward digitoxigenin-mono-digitoxoside in neonatal rats

J. B. WATKINS AND C. D. KLAASSEN

Glucuronidation is low or undetectable in embryonic and early fetal tissues and changes to adult levels at rates depending on the acceptor, tissue and species. Because other data indicate there may be a specific UDP-glucuronosyltransferase (GT) in the liver of adult rats that glucuronidates digitoxigenin-monodigitoxoside (DIG), the development of GT activity in neonatal rats toward DIG was compared with that of other acceptors. Conjugation of *p*-nitrophenol and 1-naphthol was higher at birth and decreased to adult levels by 20 days of age. Glucuronidation of chloramphenicol, morphine, valproic acid and bilirubin increased from birth to adult activity by 20 days of age. Conjugation of phenolphthalein, oestrone and diethylstilboestrol was low in 1-day-old rats and higher than adult in 20-day-old animals. In contrast, glucuronidation of DIG was barely detectable (9% of adult) in 20-day-old rats. Administration of 3-methylcholanthrene on days 6–9 significantly stimulated GT activity toward naphthol, *p*-nitrophenol and morphine, whereas phenobarbital precociously increased conjugation of chloramphenicol, morphine, valproic acid and diethylstilboestrol. Pregnenolone-16α-carbonitrile enhanced the development of GT activity toward morphine, chloramphenicol, valproic acid, bilirubin, diethylstilboestrol and oestrone. Glucuronidation of DIG was not increased after 3-methylcholanthrene or phenobarbital, but can be induced somewhat after pregnenolone-16α-carbonitrile to 7% of adult values in 10-day-old rats. Thus, development and inducibility of GT activity toward DIG are different than those for the other acceptors, suggesting there may be another GT in rat liver which is responsible for the conjugation of DIG.

ACKNOWLEDGEMENT

This work is supported by USPHS grants ES07079 and ES03192.

ABSTRACT

5
Immunochemical studies on the properties and biosynthesis of UDP-glucuronosyltransferase of Reuber hepatoma cells

B. S. BOCK-HENNIG, G. SCHMID-OTT AND K. W. BOCK

The H-4-II-E cell line of a Reuber hepatoma combines rapid growth with stable expression of microsomal cytochrome P-450 dependent mono-oxygenase and UDP-glucuronosyltransferase (UDPGT). Ouchterlony double-diffusion analysis revealed partial identity between the hepatoma enzyme and the 3-methylcholanthrene-inducible rat liver enzyme. Immunochemical staining of hepatoma microsomal proteins separated by SDS-PAGE ('Western blot' analysis) showed major immunoreactive protein bands at about MW 61 000, whereas in liver microsomes the band at 61 000 as well as three bands in the 54 000 region (at 52, 54 and 56 000) were stained. Recently the 61 000 and 54 000 bands could be partially separated during enzyme purification of the liver enzyme (G. Schirmer, unpublished).

The enzyme was labelled by growing cells in the presence of [^{3}H]L-leucine for 8 h. After a 16 h chase period, cells were harvested, lysed with 1% sodium cholate and the enzyme was immunoprecipitated using rabbit IgG against rat liver UDPGT. SDS-PAGE of the immunoprecipitate showed a single radioactive peak. UDPGT activity towards 1-naphthol was increased 1.6-fold 24 h after the addition of benz(a)anthracene and dexamethasone, although the increase was much less than that found with mono-oxygenase activities towards benzo(a)pyrene (80-fold) or ethoxyresorufin (100-fold). Under these conditions [^{3}H]L-leucine incorporation into immunoprecipitated UDPGT was significantly enhanced (1.9-fold) indicating increased enzyme synthesis *de novo*. Based on the decay of radioactivity in the immunoprecipitated UDPGT a turnover of about 32 h was estimated.

The results indicate the suitability and limitations of H-4-II-E cells for investigating the biosynthesis of UDPGT. More work is needed to elucidate whether the UDPGT proteins at 61 and 54 000 are different gene products or post-translational modifications of a common gene product.

ABSTRACT

6 Prevention of toxic oxidation–reduction cycles between quinones and quinols by glucuronide formation

K. W. BOCK, W. LILIENBLUM AND B. S. BOCK-HENNIG

Aromatic compounds are often oxidized to phenols and quinones which undergo toxic oxidation–reduction cycles with the continuous and overstoichiometric production of reactive oxygen species. Furthermore, reactive electrophilic phenoxy radicals are formed in these redox cycles, which may also contribute to the cytotoxicity of phenols. It was investigated to what extent conjugation with glucuronic acid or sulphate may prevent toxic redox cycles. (1) Addition of benzo(a)pyrene-3,6-quinone (BP-3,6-quinone) or menadione to hepatocytes or Reuber H-4-II-E hepatoma cells significantly increased oxygen consumption. For example, addition of 25 nmoles BP-3,6-quinone to 10^6 hepatocytes stimulated oxygen consumption by 2-3 nmoles/min. (2) When glucuronidation was inhibited by salicylamide, oxygen consumption after 1 h was higher than in controls without the inhibitor due to the higher quinone concentration. In addition, inhibition of conjugation by salicylamide increased the cytotoxicity of BP-3,6-quinone, as indicated by the dose-dependent decrease of [^{3}H]thymidine incorporation into DNA of hepatoma cells. (3) The conversion of BP-3,6-quinone to the corresponding quinol glucuronides was more than 10-fold higher in hepatocytes from 3-methylcholanthrene-treated rats than in hepatocytes from phenobarbital-treated rats or untreated controls. These observations indicate that a 3-methylcholanthrene-inducible enzyme form of UDP-glucuronosyltransferase is mainly responsible for the inactivation of the quinol, in line with previous studies in subcellular systems (*FEBS Lett.*, **121,** 269 (1980)).

The results suggest that glucuronidation together with sulphation effectively prevent toxic redox cycles between quinones and quinols in the intact cell.

ABSTRACT

7
Induction of bilirubin UDP-glucuronosyltransferase by carboxylic acids: structure–activity relationships

S. FOURNEL, J. MAGDALOU, J. THOMASSIN, G. SIEST AND J. CALDWELL

Clofibrate and other chemically related compounds increase bilirubin UDP-glucuronosyltransferase. As their carboxylic acid-containing structure may play a role in the extent of enzyme induction, the effect of treatment by ten arylcarboxylic acids was investigated on bilirubin conjugation by rat liver microsomes. A daily injection for 5 days ($100\,mg\,day^{-1}\,kg^{-1}$ body weight) differentially affected the enzyme activity. For example, while benzoic acid or diphenylacetic acid had no effect in this respect, hydratropic acid, triphenylacetic acid or 4-chlorophenoxypropionic acid significantly enhanced bilirubin conjugation. Determination of structure–activity relationships showed that the number of phenyl or methyl groups, as well as their position on the molecule, influenced, to a great extent, the enzyme induction. Among the physicochemical parameters tested by multiple linear regression, the lipophilicity of the carboxylic acid molecule, its overall reactivity expressed as the difference between Homo and Lomo energy*, and the net charge of the carboxyl group oxygen were related (r = 0.935) to the induction level of bilirubin UDP-glucuronosyltransferase.

Work is in progress to elucidate the induction mechanism by carboxylic acids.

* Homo, highest occupied molecular orbital
Lomo, lowest occupied molecular orbital

ABSTRACT

8
Glucuronosyltransferase heterogeneity: modification of activity after xenobiotic administration

A. MYARA AND F. TRIVIN

UDP-glucuronosyltransferases (UDPGT) are enzymes involved in the metabolism of detoxification assumed by the liver. Multiple forms of these enzymes remain unknown. The aim of this present work was to study the behaviour of glucuronosyltransferases after treatment of Wistar and Gunn rats by two xenobiotics: phenobarbital and hydrocortisone (respectively, 0.40 mmol/kg and 25 μmol/kg body weight, daily for 4 days). The UDPGT activities were evaluated towards four substrates: bilirubin, *p*-nitrophenol, harmol and 4-methylumbelliferone, on liver microsomal preparations, after dialysis for 1 h against EDTA (10 mmol/l) containing β-mercaptoethanol (0.2 mmol/l). Between the Gunn and the Wistar group, net differences were noted. After phenobarbital administration, no bilirubin UDPGT activity remained detectable in Gunn liver microsomes, whereas it was increased (+197%) with the Wistar group; similar observations have been noted with harmol UDPGT: in the Wistar group, the activity for this aglycone was increased (+103%), while it was not modified in Gunn rats. With *p*-nitrophenol UDPGT, response to induction was weak and quite the same in Wistar and Gunn rats. Yet, the molecular form which conjugates 4-methylumbelliferone seemed to be different between the two groups: induction was weak with Wistar rats (+12.3%) and important with Gunn rats (+62.6%). Effects of hydrocortisone were different. In the Wistar group, glucuronide conjugation of bilirubin and harmol decreased (respectively, −51.3% and −39%), whereas no significant modifications were observed with the two other aglycones. In the Gunn group, only the activity towards 4-methylumbelliferone was modified (−54.7%). These results show the heterogeneity of UDPGT, tested towards various substrates, various xenobiotics and various strains of rats.

ABSTRACT

9
Latency of UDP-glucuronyltransferase in intact endoplasmic reticulum and cryosensitization of the ER-membrane permeability barrier

T. HALLINAN, D. BROWN, A. E. RONHILD DE BRITO AND K. PENDLEBURY

Evidence has been advanced that latency of UDP-glucuronyltransferase in microsomes is artefactual, being absent in sheets of endoplasmic reticulum (ER) surrounding isolated nuclei. We approached this question by permeabilizing rat hepatocytes with filipin, which selectively lyses plasma membranes by complexing their abundant cholesterol while the cholesterol-poor ER-membranes remain electronmicroscopically intact.

Adding 50–300 μmol/l filipin increased, about 2-fold, hepatocyte glucuronidation of 0.5 mmol/l 1-naphthol using 1 mmol/l UDP-glucuronic acid, but more filipin caused no further marked increase. However, 500 μmol/l filipin had no effect on naphthol glucuronidation by isolated microsomes ± 0.5 mmol/l UDP-*N*-acetylglucosamine (UDPNAG), although glucuronidation was stimulated about 2.7-fold by UDPNAG in filipinized hepatocytes.

Adding 4–5 mg/ml digitonin to filipin-permeabilized hepatocytes fragmented their previously intact ER into very small (strained?) vesicles and greatly stimulated naphthol glucuronidation 6.5–10.5 fold, comparable to stimulation of microsomal glucuronidation by digitonin. It thus appears that naphthol glucuronidation is latent in permeabilized hepatocytes in which the ER is intact.

Freezing suspensions of guinea-pig liver microsomes in a −20°C deep-freeze, in 0.154 mol/l KCl, 0.25 mol/l mannitol or 0.15 mol/l Tris-HCL pH 7.2 largely or completely removed the latencies of three microsomal enzyme systems, 1-naphthol glucuronyltransferase, nucleoside diphosphatase and mannose 6-phosphatase. Freezing in KCl with liquid N_2 and then at −70°C conserved glucuronyltransferase-latency and freezing in water was not very membrane-olytic. Rabbit, but not mouse or rat liver microsomes are also readily cryosensitized at −20°C but glycerol or sucrose cryoprotected enzyme latencies.

ABSTRACT

10
Activity of the UDP-glucuronyl-transferase enzyme in rat liver with increased bile acid synthesis

V. LAPOSTOLLE

Changes in the bile salt pool interfere with cholesterol, phospholipid and bile acid metabolism which might interfere with the functional dynamics of microsomal membranes.

The aim of this study was to investigate the activity of the *p*-nitrophenol UDP-glucuronyltransferase enzyme deeply encased in the microsomal membrane, in rats with increased biliary salt synthesis which occurs at least in part in microsomes.

Male Wistar rats had either a chronic bile fistula (CBF) implanted for 4 days or were fed 4% cholestyramine (Ch) for 5 days. Appropriate control groups were used. Liver weight/body weight percentage (LW/BW), microsomal proteins (MP) and cytochrome P-450 (cyt. P-450) contents, and *in vitro* *p*-nitrophenol UDP-glucuronyltransferase activity (UDPGT) were measured. Results are given below as % of control groups.

Table

	LW/BW	*MP*	*Cyt. P-450*	*UDPGT*
CBF	NS	NS	NS	−30
Ch	NS	NS	+33	+37

NS = non-significant difference

The difference in *p*-nitrophenol UDP-glucuronyltransferase activity between the two models indicate that factors other than the direct stimulation of bile acid synthesis could play a role whatever its exact mechanisms. It is likely that the loss of lipids (cholesterol and phospholipids) and electrolytes in bile during biliary drainage, interfere directly or indirectly with either the availability of glucuronic acid or the activity of the enzyme.

ABSTRACT

11
Regulation of hepatic UDP-glucuronyltransferase activity in the rat by gastrointestinal polypeptide hormones

G. L. RICCI, V. BALDASSARRE, G. LONGO, J. FEVERY,
G. ZANNINELLI, K. P. M. HEIRWEGH AND J. DE GROOTE

Injection of glucagon[1] and secretin[2] at pharmacological rates were reported to increase bilirubin (BR) UDP-glucuronyltransferase in the rat and the action to reach a maximal effect at 90 min. The aim of present work was to investigate whether: (1) vasoactive intestinal polypeptide (VIP), structurally sharing many similarities in the amino acid sequence with the other two polypeptides, has a similar effect, and (2) glucuronidation of a different substrate (*p*-nitrophenol; *p*-NP) is changed.

Male Wistar rats 220–280 g were equipped with a catheter into the right jugular vein and fasted overnight. They were treated with glucagon 100 μg/- (n = 11), secretin 0.4–0.5 c.u./- (n = 10), V.I.P. 300 ng/-h^{-1} 100 g b.wt.$^{-1}$ (n = 11) or NaCl 0.16 mol/l (n = 13) for 120 min. The homogenates (1 g wet liver wt./10 ml sucrose 0.25 mol/l–EDTA 1 mmol/l) were activated with an equal volume of digitonin at different concentrations (1, 2, 3, 5 or 10 mg/ml, final concentration) for 60 min on ice; glucuronidation rate of BR and *p*-NP was assayed with 0.25 mmol/l of acceptor substrate and 5 mmol/l UDP-glucuronic acid. Subcellular fractionation was carried out by differential centrifugation according to De Duve *et al.*[3].

RESULTS

Maximal activation of enzyme rate was reached at a digitonin concentration of 5 mg/ml (final). UDP-glucuronyltransferase specific activity is summarized in the following table.

With secretin a conjugation rate comparable to maximal activation (93±4%) was reached with half the optimal concentration of digitonin.

In order to better understand the apparent selectivity of actions on the two

Table

	n	p-*NP* (nmol min^{-1} mg prot^{-1})	*BR* (nmol 10 min^{-1} mg prot^{-1})
NaCl 0.16 mol/l	13	7.14±1.35	2.70±0.25
Glucagon	11	10.18±1.10*	3.22±0.35*
Secretin	10	6.72±1.21	3.16±0.15*
VIP	11	11.41±1.78**	2.54±0.26

Mean±1 SD; * $p<0.05$; ** $p<0.01$

transferases, the specific activities have been plotted as one function of the other. In the plot of the enzyme activities after NaCl 0.16 mol/l, secretin and VIP three clusters of points with a fair overlapping were obtained. The glucuronidation activity for *p*-NP inversely correlated with that for BR ($r = -0.874$; $p<0.01$). No relationship was present in the plot of the two enzyme activities after pretreatment with glucagon. Subcellular distribution of glucuronidation was rather similar in all groups: both BR and *p*-NP UDP-glucuronyltransferase were mostly located in the microsomal fraction (P) with changes similar to those observed in the homogenate. Recovery of BR-UDP-glucuronyltransferase in N_3 (mainly nuclear envelopes) and in ML (large particles) fraction after pretreatment with secretin was increased ($p<0.05$). No differences were present between groups in protein concentration and cholesterol and phospholipd composition of microsomes.

CONCLUSIONS

Glucagon, secretin and VIP are able to modify the activity of hepatic UDP-glucuronyltransferase; the effect appears to be both polypeptide and substrate specific, in agreement with the concept of functional heterogeneity of the enzyme. The relationship between the activities of BR and *p*-NP suggests that the mode of action of secretin and VIP is different from that of glucagon. It is speculated that this action consists of discrete physical changes, interplaying with the different polarity of the two substrates. The result would be a modification in the overall rate of conjugation.

References

1. Constantinopoulos, A. and Matsaniotis, N. (1978). *Gastroenterology*, **75,** 468
2. Ricci, G. L. and Fevery, J. (1979). *Biochem. J.*, **182,** 881
3. De Duve, C., Pressman, B. C., Giannetto, R., Wattiaux, R. and Appelmans, F. (1955). *Biochem. J.*, **60,** 604

ABSTRACT

12
The formation of bilirubin diglucuronide from bilirubin monoglucuronide

E. R. GORDON

Two pathways localized at different subcellular sites have been proposed for the hepatic conversion of bilirubin monoglucuronide (BMG) to bilirubin diglucuronide (BDG): (1) a microsomal glucuronyltransferase system[1,2] requiring UDPGA and (2) a UDPGA independent transglucuronidation reaction catalysed by an enzyme in the canalicular liver plasma membrane (cLPM)[3]. The existence of this latter system has been questioned and considered by some to be accounted for by dipyrrole exchange[4]. To examine this problem, we compared the capacity of hepatic microsomes and highly purified cLPM to form BD from BMG either enzymatically and/or by dipyrrole exchange. In this latter reaction BMG is cleaved non-enzymatically, and random recombination of the dipyrroles occurs. The products are bilirubin, BMG and BD in a ratio of 1:2:1, and the isomeric composition of the products are IIIα, IXα, and XIIIα in the ratio of 1:2:1.

The microsomes, in the presence of UDPGA, quantitatively converted BMG to BG without a change in isomeric configuration or the formation of bilirubin. In contrast, cLPM did not convert BMG to BD either enzymatically or by dipyrrole exchange. Dipyrrole exchange was detected if the preparations of BMG were not pure or if the reaction media was made acidic (pH 4.6 or 1.8). Ascorbic acid (1 mmol/l) inhibited this reaction.

These studies definitely demonstrate that the endoplasmic reticulum, and not the cLPM, is the hepatocellular site of bilirubin diglucuronide formation.

References

1. Gordon, E. R. and Goresky, C. A. (1980). *Can. J. Biochem.*, **58,** 1302–10
2. Blanckaert, N., Gollan, J. L. and Schmid, R. (1979). *Proc. Natl. Acad. Sci. USA*, **76,** 2037–41
3. Jansen, P. L. M., Chowdhury, J. R., Fischberg, E. B. and Arias, I. M. (1977). *J. Biol. Chem.*, **252,** 2710–16
4. Sieg, A., Van Hess, G. P. and Heirwegh, K. P. M. (1982). *J. Clin. Invest.*, **69,** 347–57

ABSTRACT

13
Evidence against enzymatic formation of bilirubin diglucuronide in rat liver plasma membranes

A. SIEG AND K. P. M. HEIRWEGH

An enzyme with high specific activity in plasma membrane enriched fractions (PMEF) from rat liver has been reported to transform 2 moles of bilirubin monoglucuronide (BMG) into 1 mole each of bilirubin (B) and bilirubin diglucuronide (BDG) *in vitro*[1] and *in vivo*[2]. The mechanism of the reaction has not yet been established, but could involve transglucuronidation or dipyrrole exchange occurring between BMG molecules. We repeated the incubations of BMG with PMEF from Wistar and Gunn rat liver and compared it to incubations of BMG with human erythrocyte ghosts (HEG).

RESULTS

The reaction mechanism is dipyrrole exchange, not transglucuronidation, as the formation of BDG and B out of 2 moles of BMG was paralleled by an increase of the IIIα and XIIIα isomers of the β-aglycone. The dipyrrole exchange proceeded with comparable rates in the presence of PMEF and HEG and independently of protein concentration (0–613 μg/ml). Heat denaturation of the proteins (10 min at 100°C) did not result in decreased reaction rates. Thus BMG incubated with PMEF from rat liver or HEG is converted into B and BDG by spontaneous, non-enzymatic dipyrrole exchange.

ACKNOWLEDGEMENT

Supported in part by the Deutsche Forschungsgemeinschaft.

References

1. Jansen, P. L. M., Chowdhury, J. R., Fischberg, E. B., Daniller, A. and Arias, I. M. (1977). *J. Biol. Chem.*, **252,** 2710
2. Chowdhury, J. R., Jansen, P. L. M., Fischberg, E. B., Daniller, A. and Arias, I. M. (1978). *J. Clin. Invest.*, **21,** 191

ABSTRACT

14
UDP-glucuronyltransferase-catalysed deconjugation of bilirubin and other glucuronides

P. L. M. JANSEN, H. T. M. CUYPERS AND W. H. M. PETERS

Bilirubin monoglucuronide (BMG) and the glucuronides of *p*-nitrophenol (PNPgluc), 4-methylumbelliferone (4MUBgluc) and phenolphthalein (Phgluc) are rapidly deconjugated when incubated with UDP and rat liver microsomes. These reactions are catalysed by UDPGT and not by β-glucuronidase because: (1) all reactions were done in the presence of 7 mmol/l saccharo-1,4-lactone, a potent β-glucuronidase-inhibitor; (2) with B-[^{14}C]monoglucuronide as substrate, UDP-[^{14}C]glucuronic acid was identified as the reaction product, (3) Gunn rat microsomes, lacking bilirubin UDGPT, do not catalyse BMG deconjugation.

The conditions and kinetic parameters for these reactions are indicated in the table.

Table

Substrate	$K_m^{x\text{-gluc}}$*	K_m^{UDP}*	K_i^{ATP}*	V_{max}**	optimum pH
BMG	n.d.	12.3×10^{-3}	↑	360×10^{-3}	5.1
PNPgluc	1.4	0.62	0.27	29.8	5.1
4MUBgluc	0.5	0.27	0.43	14.0	5.4
Phgluc	0.2	0.53	0.22	1.2	6.5

* mmol/l;
** nmoles mg protein^{-1} min^{-1}
n.d. not determined

ATP and detergents stimulate BMG deconjugation in a mutually independent and additive way; the other deconjugation reactions are competitively inhibited by ATP (K_i^{ATP}, *see* Table) and detergents have no effect.

CONCLUSIONS

Bilirubin UDPGT appears to have very special properties which sets it apart from the other UDPGT-isoenzymes: (1) Bilirubin UDPGT is lacking in the

Gunn rat, whereas many other glucuronidation reactions are present albeit in a defective way; (2) as for the reverse reaction, bilirubin UDPGT is partly latent and is stimulated by ATP in a probably allosteric way; the other deconjugation reactions are non-latent and competitively inhibited by ATP; (3) BMG formation is catalysed by a monomeric enzyme of MW 41 500, whereas most other glucuronidation reactions are catalysed by di- or tetrameric enzymes[1] of MW varying from 73 500–175 000.

Reference

1. Peters, W. H. M., ter Haar, E. M., Nauta, H. and Jansen, P. L. M. (1983). *Hepatology*, **3**, 811

ABSTRACT

15 Effects of ioglycamide on bilirubin conjugation and transport in the rat

V. MESA, J. FEVERY, J. DE GROOTE AND K. P. M. HEIRWEGH

Iodinated contrast agents seem to share the secretory pathway with bilirubin conjugates but not with bile acids. We studied the effects of ioglycamide on bilirubin (B) metabolism in Wistar rats. This compound does not undergo conjugation. A maximal biliary secretion rate of ioglycamide (T_m: 4.3±0.3 μmoles^{-1} min^{-1} kg b.wt.$^{-1}$) was obtained at infusion rates of 5.5 μmoles min^{-1} kg^{-1} (n = 12). Ioglycamide induced a dose-dependent choleresis as 22 ml of bile was excreted per mmol of ioglycamide. Bile acid output was not affected. Despite a 340% increase of bile flow during ioglycamide-T_m the biliary output of UCB and of B monoglucuronide (BMG) decreased to 13% of control values and the excretion of BDG to 52%. UCB and BMG changed in parallel suggesting that UCB might be formed by deconjugation of BMG. During ioglycamide treatment, BDG became by far the predominant pigment in bile (87%±6 of total pigment vs 61%±4 in basal conditions, n = 12) and in serum: BDG rose from traces to 1.15±0.17 μmol/l, BMG from 0.04 to 0.71±0.10 μmol/l, whereas UCB dropped from 0.82±0.12 to 0.32±0.04 μmol/l. Conjugates in serum thus increased from 5% to 85% of total bilirubin. It was calculated that 1 μmol of bile pigment was retained per 1000 μmol ioglycamide secreted. All effects were fully reversible. To investigate why BDG became the predominant bile pigment, bilirubin UDP-glucuronyltransferase was measured. At low bilirubin concentrations (25 μmol/l) BDG amounted to 60% of total conjugates formed, at 164 μmol/l it was only 2–10%. Ioglycamide did not alter transferase activity nor the ratio of BDG : BMG formed. We suggest that ioglycamide mainly inhibits the excretion of BMG (and less that of BDG). The BMG retained in the hepatocyte *in vivo* would undergo more efficient transformation to BDG, and UCB might also become more efficiently conjugated. An additional inhibition of deconjugation of BDG by ioglycamide cannot be excluded.

ABSTRACT

16 Direct demonstration of BDG formation by chemical isomerization of BMG

S. ADACHI, Y. ADACHI, T. UESUGI AND K. KAMISAKA

The mechanism of BDG formation is still controversial. In the present report, we investigated BDG formation from BMG using the direct HPLC method[1].

Conversion of BMG into BDG by chemical isomerization was maximum at pH 6.5 during incubation for 5 min at 37°C. This conversion of BMG was significantly reduced by sodium ascorbate, GSH, cysteine, dithiothreitol, NADH or NADPH. Moreover, serum albumins and the 105 000 *g* supernatant fraction of rat liver also strongly stabilized BMG. The reaction of BMG (18.5 nmol) with 0.25 mg of rat liver plasma membrane for 5 min at 37°C produced about 8.5 nmol of BDG which was rich in the IXα and XIIIα isomers, and an equimolar of BR was also formed which abounded in the IIIα and IXα isomers. In contrast, BMG was strongly stabilized in the incubation with 10 mg of the rat plasma membrane. Moreover, the existence of 10 mmol/l of sodium ascorbate in the reaction mixture completely inhibited the BDG formation. Therefore, it has been revealed that the formation of BDG observed in the former reaction is due to the chemical isomerization of BMG.

Homozygous Gunn rats receiving i.v. injection of BMG (100 nmol) excreted about 75–90% of the BMG dose into the bile within 1 h, but no BDG formation was observed during the experimental period.

From these results, we have concluded that the transglucuronidation is not proved as the mechanism of BDG biosynthesis.

Reference

1. *J. Chromatog.*, **277**, 308, 1983

ABSTRACT

17 Bucolome *N*-glucuronide

K. MOHRI, T. UESUGI AND K. KAMISAKA

Bucolome (BC, 5-butyl-1-cyclohexylbarbituric acid), which was developed as an anti-inflammatory drug, is a potent choleretic in the rat. We have reported here on the isolation and characterization of a novel bucolome *N*-glucuronide (BC-NG), and on its biosynthesis. BC-NG may be the first *N*-glucuronide identified as a major metabolite of barbiturates.

BC-NG was isolated from the bile of rat, after i.p. injection of BC, by means of silica gel column chromatography (eluent: $CHCl_3$–MeOH). The binding of the glucuronyl group on the 3-N position of BC in β-configuration was proved by measuring [^{13}C]NMR, PMR, GC-Mass, IR and UV spectra in addition to some chemical and enzymatical methods.

The excretion of BC-NG into the bile and urine in rat was measured by HPLC method using ODS columns (eluent; pH 5.7, 0.05 mol/l phosphate buffer–MeOH, 35/50, v/v). After injection of 50 mg BC i.p., about 50–60% of the dose was excreted into the bile as BC-NG within 5 h, but the urinary excretion of BC-NG was less than 1% of dose.

Rat liver microsomes showed the activity of UDP-glucuronate-dependent BC-NG formation. The activity was maximal at around pH 7.4 (0.1 mol/l Tris–HCl). Mg^{2+} (10 mmol/l) and glucaro-1,4-lactone (5 mmol/l) increased BC-NG formation. Treatment of the microsomes with digitonin or lubrol WX stimulated the conjugating activity. BC-NG formation was also catalysed by both liver microsomes of guinea-pig and rabbit.

ABSTRACT

18
Biosynthesis of dulcin *N*-glucuronide

T. UESUGI, K. KAMURA, T. UEMATSU AND K. KAMISAKA

Dulcin *N*-glucuronide (D-NG) was first isolated from the urine of a rabbit given dulcin[1]. In the present report, the biosynthesis of D-NG was studied in several animals using the HPLC method. Dulcin metabolites were separated with ODS columns (10 μm). A 5 : 2 mixture by volume of water and *n*-propanol was used as eluent with the addition of 0.1 mg/100 ml of cetyltrimethyl ammonium bromide. All separations were carried out at the flow-rate of 1.0 ml/min.

The excretion of dulcin metabolites was studied in rat, guinea-pig, rabbit and human. After oral dosage of dulcin (50–100 mg), D-NG excretion was observed only in rabbit. In other species, the major metabolites were the *o*-glucuronide and/or the *o*-sulphate of *p*-hydroxyphenylurea originated in the de-ethylation of dulcin.

The rabbit liver microsomes catalysed UDP-glucuronate-dependent *N*-glucuronidation of dulcin, but the conjugation was not observed with the liver microsomes of mice, rat and guinea-pig. The conjugating activity of rabbit microsomes was maximal at pH 8.2 and around 20 mmol/l of Mg^{2+}. Lubrol WX, digitonin and sodium cholate stimulated the activity, but Triton X-100 and Emulgen 911 diminished it. All of them stimulated the conjugating activity towards *p*-nitrophenol.

The results suggest that the rabbit liver possesses at least an unique UDP-glucuronyltransferase which is quite distinct from the enzyme(s) in other animals.

Reference

1. Akagi, M., Aoki, I. and Vematsu, T. (1966). *Chem. Pharm. Bull.*, **14,** 1

ABSTRACT

19 The identification of non-steroidal oestrogen glucuronides in human urine

M. AXELSON, J. SJÖVALL AND K. D. R. SETCHELL

Two oestrogens of plant origin, equol (7-hydroxy-3-(4′-hydroxyphenyl)-chroman and daidzein (4′, 7-dihydroxy-isoflavone) have been identified for the first time in human urine. Both compounds were characterized as monoglucuronide conjugates using selective liquid-chromatographic isolation methods and gas chromatography-mass spectrometry. Equol is a weak oestrogen with antioestrogenic properties, possessing 10^{-3}–10^{-5} times the activity of oestradiol, to which it bears some structural similarity. It has previously been found in the urine of animals grazing certain species of clover. High blood concentrations of this compound lead to an infertility syndrome in sheep referred to as clover disease.

The dietary origin of equol in humans was therefore investigated, and experiments with different diets showed that soya food has a remarkably high content of an equol precursor, which was isolated and identified as the glucoside of daidzein. This phyto-oestrogen is converted into equol by intestinal bacterial degradation, conjugated with glucuronic acid and is then excreted in urine. The excretion of equol in human urine, which is normally in the range of the classical oestrogens, increased 100–1000-fold to about 4–6 mg per 24 h after ingestion of a single meal containing 40 g soya meal. The widespread use of soya beans as a protein food source makes it important to determine possible biological effects of equol upon the menstrual cycle of women and the development and/or treatment of hormone-dependent tumours.

ABSTRACT

20
Glucuronidation and urinary excretion of hyodeoxycholic acid in man

M. PARQUET, A. RAIZMAN, N. BERTHAUX AND R. INFANTE

Urinary excretion of endogenous bile acids in man is extremely low, although in cholestatic patients, significant amounts of glucuronidated bile acids can be recovered in urine. Recent studies[1] have shown that when hyodeoxycholic acid (HDCA) (normally found in rat and pig bile) is administered to cholecystectomized (T-tube) gallstone patients, surprisingly high amounts of glucuronidated HDCA were excreted in urine, indicating an unusual metabolic pathway.

Intestinal absorption, biotransformation and urinary excretion of HDCA and HD-cholylglycine have been studied in normal subjects.

SUBJECTS

HDCA administration

Five healthy volunteers received 0.5 g or 1 g HDCA orally. One also received 20 μCi [^{14}C]HDCA. Urine was collected at 24 h intervals for 3 days.

HD-Cholylglycine administration

Two healthy volunteers received 1 g HD-cholylglycine orally. Urine was collected at 12 h intervals for 1 day.

METHODS

Aliquots of urine were lyophilized and bile acids extracted and purified on a XAD-2 column. Bile acids were determined and identified by GLC, TLC and spectrophotometry combined with hydrolysis by 3α-hydroxysteroid dehydrogenase, cholylglycine hydrolase and/or glucuronidase.

RESULTS

HDCA administration

A high proportion of the initial dose was excreted in urine as HDCA-glucuronide within 72 h : 19 and 23% in the two male subjects and 19, 20 and 50% in the three females. The highest urine concentration was observed in the first 24 h samples (males : 219 μmol/l, 106 μmol/l, females : 208 μmol/l, 287 μmol/l, 605 μmol/l).

HD-Cholylglycine administration

Significant amounts of HDCA were excreted in urine as HDCA glucuronide within the 12 h of ingestion. Its concentration was higher at 12–24 h than at 0–12 h (subject A: 75–213 μmol/l; B: 198–362 μmol/l).

CONCLUSION

In normal subjects, HDCA undergoes extensive glucuronidation and urinary excretion as in T-tube patients with partly interrupted enterohepatic circulation, showing that HDCA is a good substrate for UDP-glucuronosyltransferase. Excretion of this polar glucuronide is shared between biliary and renal pathways, the latter via the blood circulation. After HD-cholylglycine administration HDCA was isolated from urine as the glucuronide, suggesting glycine deconjugation prior to intestinal absorption and further biotransformation.

Reference

1. Sacquet, E., Parquet, M., Riottot, M. *et al.* (1983). *J. Lipid Res.*, **14,** 604–13

ABSTRACT

21 Indications for an endogenous thioglucuronide in serum, urine and bile

A. TANGERMAN

Thioglucuronides studied so far were all of xenobiotics. They have been identified as excretory products, suggesting that this class of compounds is an end product of metabolism. We describe a compound, most likely methyl-β-D-thioglucuronide, in serum, urine and bile of humans.

Addition of acid to serum, urine or bile results in a release of a finite amount of methanethiol. Filtration experiments have shown that this methanethiol arises from a compound (I) with a molecular weight of less than 500. Based on the following findings, it is suggested that this compound is methyl-β-D-thioglucuronide:

(1) Reaction of methanethiol with rat liver microsomes results in the formation of a compound which also gives methanethiol on acid hydrolysis. The synthesis was strongly dependent on the concentration of UDP-glucuronic acid, suggesting the formation of a thioglucuronide.
(2) Compound (I) is easily hydrolysed by acid to give the free thiol and is stable to alkali. The same was found in the literature for alkyl-thioglucuronides.
(3) Compound (I) is resistant against β-glucuronidase. The same was observed in the literature for alkyl-thioglucuronides.
(4) The concentration of (I) in the urine of normal humans amounts to 15–40 μmol/l, while that in bile amounts to about 0.20 μmol/l. It may, therefore, be concluded that (I) is exclusively excreted in the urine. This is in accordance with the rule that glucuronides of small molecular weight (*c.* 300) appear mainly in the urine, whereas those of high molecular weight (*c.* 700) appear mainly in the bile.

The concentration of (I) in the serum of normals amounts to about 0.20 μmol/l.

Compound (I), if methyl-β-D-thioglucuronide, is the first endogenous thioglucuronide described in literature. A definite proof can be given by comparing (I) with the synthetic methyl-β-D-thioglucuronide.

ABSTRACT

22
The α-glucuronide of *N*-nitrosomethyl-tert-butylamine and its identification in urine of rats by ion pair HPLC

G. ROßNAGEL AND M. WIESSLER

Conjugates of α-hydroxylated nitrosamines have not been found up to now *in vivo* or *in vitro*. We developed chemical methods to synthesize such conjugates and began our studies with the non-carcinogenic *N*-nitrosomethyl-tert-butylamine. The synthetic glucuronide enabled us to develop an analytical procedure based on ion pair HPLC, to detect the compound in the urine of rats. Recovery experiments showed that the conjugate could be isolated quantitatively.

^{14}C-labelled nitrosamine was synthesized. After administration to male Sprague Dawley rats a radioactive metabolite which appeared to be the glucuronide was detected in urine (HPLC retention time corresponded to that of the synthetic standard). The metabolite has been identified indirectly on the basis of hydrolysis by β-glucuronidase. Inhibition of β-glucuronidase by saccharic acid 1,4-lactone yielded the intact metabolite.

ABSTRACT

23
Glucuronidation and sulphation reactions in rabbit kidney proximal tubule cells

J. J. HJELLE, G. A. HAZELTON, C. D. KLAASSEN AND J. T. HJELLE

Although the kidney has been shown to glucuronidate and sulphate a number of substrates, the intrarenal localization of enzymes and co-substrates, and particularly their enrichment in proximal tubules, remains to be adequately investigated. Thus, kidneys from female rabbits were dissected and homogenates of cortex, outer-stripe of the medulla, whole kidney and proximal tubules[1] were prepared. UDP-glucuronosyltransferase (UDPGT) and sulphotransferase (ST) activities toward 1-naphthol (1-NAP) were highest in tubules (2.86±0.36 and 0.247±0.034 nmoles product min^{-1} mg $protein^{-1}$) compared to outer stripe (45 and 38% of tubule activity, respectively), cortex (61 and 18%) and whole kidney (62 and 15%). Similarly, UDP-glucose dehydrogenase activity was highest in tubules (1.5 fold greater than the other regions). Moreover, UDP-glucuronic acid concentration was greater in cortex than medulla (120±8 and 64±6 nmoles/g tissue). Substrate specificity studies of UDPGT in tubules showed higher activities (nmoles product min^{-1} mg $protein^{-1}$) toward 1-NAP (2.3±0.05), 4-nitrophenol (1.7±0.1), 4-hydroxybiphenyl (6.3±0.7) and diethylstilboestrol (1.3±0.1) than oestrone, acetaminophen, chloramphenicol and digitoxigenin-monodigitoxoside. Analytical subcellular fractionation of tubules in sucrose gradients revealed that UDPGT activity, and a minor portion of the ST activity, distributed with the microsomal markers while the majority of ST activity overlapped the cytosolic marker. In conclusion, proximal tubule cells are major contributors to phase II biotransformations in the kidney.

ACKNOWLEDGEMENT

This work is supported by USPHS grants ES 07079, ES 03192 and AM 28644.

Reference

1. Hjelle, J. J. *et al.* (1981). *Kid. Int.*, **20,** 71

ABSTRACT

24
Effect of chronic ethanol administration on glucuronidation of *p*-nitrophenol (PNP) in microsomes and the isolated perfused liver in the rat

M. MITCHELL, S. HALL AND R. A. BRANCH

Chronic ethanol ingestion can influence the oxidative metabolism of many drugs. However, it is unknown whether drug elimination following glucuronidation is altered. We have investigated the glucuronidation of PNP in male Wistar rats, pair-fed either a high ethanol diet (36%) or an isocaloric diet for 6 weeks. Following addition of PNP (50 mmol/l) to a 100 ml reservoir of a recirculating isolated perfused liver, perfusate concentrations declined initially as an apparent zero process, changing to an exponential rate of elimination. Maximal rates of PNP elimination were 6.2 ± 0.5 and $5.1 \pm 0.6\,\mu$mol/min in control and ethanol treated rats, respectively. The terminal halflife in ethanol treated group (173 ± 42 min) was significantly ($p < 0.05$) longer than controls (94 ± 12 min). Accumulation of PNP glucuronide in perfusate was similar. However, PNP glucuronide excretion in bile was reduced by approximately 30% in both the first and second hour of perfusion in ethanol pretreated rats ($p < 0.05$). PNP sulphate in perfusate and bile was not different between groups. Hepatic UDPGA concentrations in liver were similar in both groups of rats (421 ± 24 vs. 433 ± 44 nmol/gm liver, respectively). K_m and V_{max} parameters, determined in both freshly prepared and Triton X100 solubilized microsomes using bisubstrate kinetics, were not significantly different between groups. The predicted maximal rate of glucuronide production from freshly prepared microsomes was slightly less than the observed maximal rate of glucuronide production in the intact liver, while the apparent K_m parameters *in vitro* were considerably less than in the isolated perfused liver. These results suggest that firstly, glucuronyltransferase activity is not the only rate-limiting step in PNP glucuronide elimination in the normal liver and secondly, chronic pretreatment with ethanol inhibits PNP glucuronide elimination by effecting a rate-limiting mechanism other than glucuronyltransferase activity. We postulate that altered elimination is due to inhibition of biliary secretion of PNP glucuronide.

ABSTRACT

25
Normal disposition of temazepam in cirrhosis and a significant enterohepatic circulation of this drug in man

P. DESMOND, H. GHABRIAL, K. WATSON, P. HARMAN, K. BREEN AND M. MASHFORD

Temazepam which is metabolized to an ether glucuronide, was given orally to 14 normals and 14 cirrhotics. There was no significant difference in $t_{\frac{1}{2}abs}$, $t_{\frac{1}{2}\beta}$ or apparent oral clearance. This phenomenon, also seen with other drugs subject to glucuronidation, may have multiple mechanisms. Effects of cirrhosis on biliary excretion and any enterohepatic circulation have not been considered. To examine this concept, disposition of temazepam was studied in five patients with T-tube biliary diversion. All bile drainage and urine were collected for 48 hours. $t_{\frac{1}{2}\beta}$ was lower (5.7±0.5 h vs 15.2±1.6 h) and apparent oral clearance higher (2.3±0.3 vs 1.4±0.1 ml min^{-1} kg^{-1}) compared to the control values. Recovery from urine of temazepam as the glucuronide was similar, and thus differences in absorption cannot explain the findings. Mean temazepam recovery in bile was 8% of dose, and thus interruption of an enterohepatic circulation could contribute to the striking findings.

ABSTRACT

26
Effect of liver diseases on the glucuronidation kinetics of 4-methylumbelliferone

H. D. KUNTZ, U. FEMFERT AND B. MAY

Clinical experience concerning hepatic dysfunction and its effect upon drug disposition is fragmentary. The important question whether selective specificity for certain sensitive processes may be present is still open. The absence of any useful indirect indicator of the liver's ability to transform a particular drug has given rise to the development of the concept of using appropriate marker drugs. The choleretic and biliary antispasmodic drug hymecromone (7-hydroxy-4-methyl-2H-1-benzopyrane-2-on; 4-methylumbelliferone; 4-MU) is metabolized in humans mainly (> 98%) via glucuronidation without any significant phase-I-transformation being involved.

After intravenous administration of 200 mg 4-MU the pharmacokinetics of the mother drug and the glucuronide were studied using a newly developed HPLC procedure[1].

The elimination process of 4-MU from plasma formally corresponds to an open three-compartment model. The clearance of the glucuronide is described by an open two-compartment system. The glucuronidation reaction is rapid: the maximum plasma glucuronide concentration measured is reached within 3 minutes after administration. The glucuronide – but not 4-MU itself – is excreted biliarily.

Patients with various liver diseases (acute hepatitis, chronic active liver disease, liver cirrhosis) did not show any retardation of the glucuronidation reaction: the halflife of 4-MU/4-MUG and the 'glucuronidation index' were normal. In patients with chronic congestion of the liver, a drastically retarded elimination of the formed glucuronide was observed, the clearance of 4-MU remained unaltered.

As judged from toxicological considerations and the general feasibility of the test in the clinical setting, 4-MU is highly recommended as a useful marker for the quantitative evaluation of the liver's glucuronidation capacity *and* the biliary excretion rate.

Reference

1. Femfert, U., Kuntz, H. D. and May, B. (1983). Rapid high performance liquid chromatographic method for the measurement of hymecromone and its conjugates in blood plasma or serum at concentrations attained during therapy. *J. Chromatogr.*, **278,** 452–7

ABSTRACT

27
Substrate activation in the clinical pharmacokinetics of 4-methylumbelliferone glucuronidation

U. FEMFERT, H. D. KUNTZ AND B. MAY

Pharmacokinetically, the glucuronidation of 4-methylumbelliferone is a triphasic process which can be described formally by an open three-compartment model with unidirectional elimination from a peripheral compartment. The rapidness of the time events, however, makes any compartmental distribution highly improbable.

From the parameterization of the kinetic data it can be demonstrated that the effect of 4-methylumbelliferone concentration (S) on the activity (v) of the glucuronidating enzyme does not comply with the Michaelis formulation of enzyme action. Since there is obviously no apparent interaction of a catalytic site with another site (catalytic or modifier) as judged from Klotz and Scatchard analyses, the observed phenomenon must be considered as a modification of the mechanism operative at the active site.

Our model assumes that the free enzyme may exist in two conformations, E and E^+. Both conformations are considered to be in equilibrium, with E being the thermodynamically more stable, dominating conformation. The interconversion process $E \rightarrow E^+$ is assumed to be slow, and it is further assumed that there is no greater affinity of the substrate for one of the conformational states, and that the binding of substrate will be *per se* without any effect on enzyme conformation. In the course of the reaction pathway there will be an obligatory rate-limiting conformational change at the active site of the enzyme-substrate complex, and at the end of the reaction cycle the enzyme will be regenerated in the thermodynamically unfavourable conformation E^+:

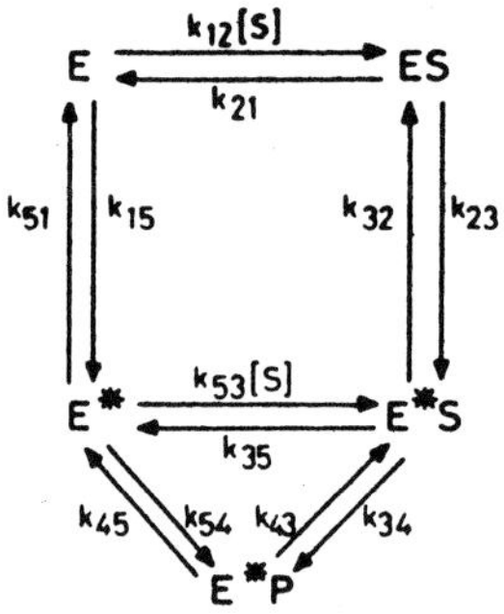

If the time required for the enzyme to relax to state E is smaller than the average time interval before another substrate molecule binds, $k_{51} > k_{53}$, the reaction path will be a function of the substrate concentration. As long as $k_{51} > k_{53}$ (S) the entire cycle will be valid, unless with higher substrate concentrations k_{53} (S) will become greater than k_{51}, and the reaction proceeds via the short cut $E^+ + S \rightarrow E^+S \rightarrow E^+ + P$

ABSTRACT

28
Diethyl ether anaesthesia depresses the biliary excretion of acetaminophen

J. B. WATKINS, C.-P. SIEGERS AND C. D. KLAASSEN

The biliary excretion of acetaminophen and its metabolites over 8 h was determined in rats exposed to diethyl ether by inhalation for 1 h. Additional rats were anaesthetized with urethane (1 g/kg i.p.) while control animals were conscious throughout the experiment (surgery was performed under hexobarbital narcosis: 150 mg/kg i.p.; 30 min duration). The concentration of UDP-glucuronic acid was decreased 80% in livers from ether-anaesthetized rats but was not reduced in urethane-treated animals when compared to that in control rats. The concentration of reduced glutathione was not affected by either urethane or diethyl ether. Basal bile flow was not altered by the anaesthetic agents. Bile flow rate after acetaminophen injection (100 mg/kg i.v.) was increased slightly over basal levels for 2 h in hexobarbital-treated control rats, was unaltered in urethane-anaesthetized animals, and was decreased throughout the 8 h experiment in rats exposed to diethyl ether for 1 h. In control and urethane-anaesthetized animals, approximately 30–35% of the total acetaminophen dose (100 mg/kg i.v.) was excreted into bile in 8 h, while only 16% was excreted in rats anaesthetized with diethyl ether. Urinary elimination (60–70% of the dose) was not altered by exposure to ether. Separation of metabolites by reverse phase high pressure liquid chromatography showed that ether decreased the biliary elimination of unchanged acetaminophen and its glucuronide, sulphate and glutathione conjugates by 47, 40, 49 and 73%, respectively, as compared to control rats. Excretion of unchanged acetaminophen and the glutathione conjugate into bile was depressed in urethane-anaesthetized animals by 45 and 66%, respectively, whereas elimination of the glucuronide and sulphate conjugates was increased by 27 and 50%, respectively. These results indicate that biliary excretion is influenced by the anaesthetic agent, and that diethyl ether depresses conjugation with sulphate and glutathione as well as glucuronic acid.

ACKNOWLEDGEMENT

This work is supported by USPHS grants ES07079 and ES03192.

ABSTRACT

29
Glucuronide conjugation and biliary excretion of paracetamol in diabetic and hyperthyroid rats

C.-P. SIEGERS, W. LOESER AND M. YOUNES

The biliary excretion of unchanged paracetamol (P) and its glucuronide-, sulphate- and glutathione-conjugates was studied in bile-fistula rats after an i.v. dose of 100 mg/kg P. Experimental diabetes was accomplished by four daily doses of 75 mg/kg streptozotocin, hyperthyroidism by four daily doses of T_3 (0.1 mg/kg i.p.). In diabetic rats bile flow was significantly reduced during the 8 h sampling period. Excretion of the P-sulphate and P-glucuronide into the bile were markedly diminished, whereas excretion of the P-GSH and unchanged P were not affected. In hyperthyroid rats no marked effects on bile flow and the excretion of P and conjugates were observed, except for a slight increase in the amounts of P-sulphate and P-glucuronide. In diabetic rats the impairment of glucuronide conjugation may be related to a decrease in the synthesis of UDPGA or glucuronyltransferase activity, the data reported in the literature are contradictory. The reduced biliary excretion of P-sulphate, however, seems to be due to an enhanced renal elimination of the sulphate during the diabetic state.

ABSTRACT

30
Comparison of hepatic and extrahepatic glucuronidation using *in vivo* and *in vitro* methodology

M. MISTRY AND J. B. HOUSTON

The glucuronidation of morphine (M), naloxone (N), etorphine (E) and buprenorphine (B) has been investigated in female Sprague-Dawley rats using a specific radiometric assay. Incubation of each compound individually with UDP-glucuronic acid and either hepatic or intestinal microsomes results in V_{max} and K_m of 0.65±0.07, 0.77±0.02, 1.00±0.03 and 0.79±0.05 nmole $min^{-1}mg$ $protein^{-1}$, and 0.212±0.026, 0.076±0.002, 0.01±0.001 and 0.036±0.01 mmol/l for liver, and 0.16±0.02, 0.54±0.09, 2.31±0.07 and 0.42±0.03 nmole $min^{-1}mg$ $protein^{-1}$ and 0.32±0.065, 0.53±0.13, 0.095±0.022 and 0.091±0.015 mmol/l for intestine for M, N, E and B, respectively. The rank order of the *in vitro* intrinsic glucuronidating activity (using the index V_{max}/K_m) is the same for each tissue: M<N<B<E with a 30-fold range of activities. *In vivo* disposition studies involving judicious choice of route of administration (intra-arterial, intravenous via jugular or hepatic portal, intraduodenal) have been used to assess the role of the intestine, liver and lung in the overall first-pass metabolism of each compound. Comparison of blood concentration–time data demonstrate that pulmonary extraction is not important for either compound and the intestinal extraction ratio for M(0.33), N(0.57), and B(0.48) is statistically significant, but less marked than the hepatic extraction ratios of 0.47, 0.80, 0.87 and 0.72 for M, N, E, and B, respectively. Calculation of intrinsic *in vivo* glucuronidating activity (intrinsic clearance) shows a rank order of M<B<N<E over a range of 70 to 630 ml $min^{-1} kg^{-1}$. Correction for the degree of binding to blood constituents (intrinsic clearance of unbound drug) changes the rank order to M<N<B<E (range 110–2000 ml $min^{-1} kg^{-1}$) which is in agreement with *in vitro* studies.

ABSTRACT

31
On the use of nor-antipyrine as a test substance for the assessment of glucuronidation vs. sulphation *in vivo*

J. BÖTTCHER, H. BÄSSMANN AND R. SCHÜPPEL

Nor-antipyrine (NORA), the *N*-demethylated phase I metabolite of antipyrine in man, rat and rabbit, turned out to represent a useful tool for the assessment of glucuronidation versus sulphation and their interrelationship *in vivo*.

A loading dose of NORA is completely conjugated in these species to form nor-antipyrine-5-enol-glucuronide and nor-antipyrine-5-enol-sulphate. Both conjugates have been isolated from urine and characterized directly by FD-mass spectrometry, ^{13}C-NMR, ^{1}H-NMR and UV spectroscopy. Quantitation of both conjugates is effected either by TLC, after selective hydrolysis[1] or directly by RP-HPLC-assay of intact conjugates[2]. NORA is conjugated in a species and dose dependent manner, which may be expressed as the ratio of urinary NORA-sulphate vs. NORA-glucuronide. At a dose level of 10 mg/kg p.o., NORA-sulphate/NORA-glucuronide ratios are as follows: man 0.1, rabbit 0.4, rat 2.6.

A dose dependent shift from sulphation to glucuronidation is observed in the rat. At increasing dose, 4–40 mg/kg (23–230 μmol l^{-1} kg^{-1}), the glucuronidation becomes the more important conjugation reaction in the rat. The ratio of NORA-sulphate/NORA-glucuronide shifts from 5.8 to 0.9.

Induction of UDP-glucuronyltransferases by phenobarbital in rats gives rise to a marked change in the conjugation pattern of NORA, in that the formation of NORA-glucuronide is greatly enhanced at the expense of NORA-sulphate.

The conjugation pattern of NORA may thus serve as a sensitive probe for detecting and analysing changes in phase II metabolism *in vivo*.

References

1. Böttcher, J. *et al.* (1984)
2. Bässmann, H. *et al.* (1984)

ABSTRACT

32
Glucuronidation of morphine and β-sympathomimetics in isolated rat intestinal epithelial cells

A. SJ. KOSTER, A. C. FRANKHUIJZEN-SIEREVOGEL AND
J. NOORDHOEK

The intestinal glucuronidation of morphine and several β-sympathomimetics (*see* Table) was investigated in isolated mucosal cells of the rat intestine. Most of these drugs are known to undergo (intestinal) first-pass metabolism *in vivo*. Glucuronidation of morphine was measured by HPLC analysis of the formed morphine 3-glucuronide. Glucuronides of the β-mimetics were measured by ion-pair HPLC analysis (with electrochemical detection) of the free drug, liberated by β-glucuronidase treatment of the cell incubate. The β-mimetics were extracted with ethylacetate containing 10 mmol/l bis(ethylhexyl) phosphoric acid.

Table

Substrate	*Cellular* V_{max} (pmole min^{-1} mg cell $protein^{-1}$)	*Cellular* K_m (mmol/l)	*Intrinsic clearance* (ml min^{-1} kg rat^{-1})
Morphine	102± 7	0.17±0.03	0.90
Orciprenaline	176± 34	1.33±0.34	0.20
Terbutaline	72± 23	0.70±0.49	0.15
Fenoterol	228± 25	0.62±0.17	0.55
Salbutamol	1081±215	1.11±0.36	1.46
Ritodrine	747± 46	0.08±0.03	14.01
Bamethan	530± 26	<0.01	>79.50

Glucuronidation of all drugs tested could be clearly measured. Comparison with literature data and *in vivo* experiments indicates, however, that a quantitatively reliable prediction of intestinal presystemic elimination of these drugs cannot be made with V_{max} and K_m values only; additional factors (e.g. uptake of the substrate and transport of unmetabolized substrate by the mucosal blood flow) have to be taken into consideration.

Glucuronidation of morphine in isolated cells could be completely inhibited by the addition of 1-naphthol (0.05 mmol/l), salicylamide (1 mmol/l) or fenoterol (5 mmol/l). Glucuronidation of fenoterol could be reduced by adding 1-naphthol (0.2 mmol/l: 50% inhibition), salicylamide (5 mmol/l: 40% inhibition) or morphine (5 mmol/l: 15% inhibition). It seems likely that these interactions are mainly caused by depletion of UDPGA. Data obtained with microsomes suggest that 1-naphthol and morphine are metabolized by different forms of UDP-glucuronosyltransferase; fenoterol is probably glucuronidated by the latter form.

The results indicate that intestinal cells can be used to predict intestinal first-pass metabolism (at least qualitatively), and that phenolic food constituents (e.g. 1-naphthol) and non-prescription drugs (e.g. salicylamide) may affect the intestinal first-pass metabolism of morphine and fenoterol.

ABSTRACT

33
UDP-Glucuronosyltransferase heterogeneity: contribution of the kinetic constants and the physicochemical properties of the aglycones

J. THOMASSIN, A. CARTIER, J. MAGDALOU, J. A. BOUTIN AND G. SIEST

In an attempt to elucidate the molecular basis of UDP-glucuronosyltransferase heterogeneity, the kinetic constants (K_m^{app}, V_{max}^{app}) of the rat liver microsomal enzyme were determined towards 34 hydroxylated aglycones. These data were related to the physicochemical properties of the substrates as determined by CNDO* calculation based on energetic and structural criteria. By multidimensional analysis, it was possible to classify the aglycones according to these parameters. The non-substituted phenols which are planar molecules presented a high V^{app} and were strictly transformed by a GT_1 form. The substituted phenols as well as the monoterpenoic alcohols were conjugated at a lower V_{max}^{app} by another form of UDP-glucuronosyltransferase (GT_2). On the other hand, the K_m^{app} values were not different between the two groups.

Interestingly, the coumarinic compounds which are planar molecules behave differently according to the position of the hydroxyl group. By comparison of the conjugation rate of the 7- and 4-hydroxycoumarin, which possess essentially the same physicochemical properties, we have shown with the microsomal enzyme that the 7-hydroxycoumarin was conjugated 20 times faster than the corresponding 4-hydroxy compound. The same results were obtained with enzyme purified from liver of rats treated with phenobarbital or 3-methylcholanthrene. Steric hindrance may play an important role on the conjugation reaction. In conclusion, we observed that the V_{max}^{app} and not the K_m^{app} were related to the physicochemical properties of the aglycones. For the non-coumarinic compounds V_{max}^{app} was essentially related to the electzonic parameters. It seems that the conjugation rate depends essentially on the reactivity of the hydroxyl group. Moreover, the planar or non-planar structure of the aglycone was not enough to explain its conjugation by one enzyme form.

* CNDO: complete neglect of differential overlap

ACKNOWLEDGEMENT

This work was supported by a grant from PIRMED (1982).

Index